The History and Influence
of the
American Psychiatric Association

The History and Influence
of the
American Psychiatric Association

Walter E. Barton, M.D.

Past President, Former Medical Director, and
50-Year Life Fellow of the American Psychiatric Association;
Professor of Psychiatry (Emeritus), Dartmouth Medical School

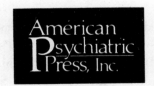

American Psychiatric Press, Inc.
1400 K St., N.W.
Washington, D.C. 20005

DEDICATION

To Carol Davis, Jean Jones, and Zing Jung

Cover design by Great, Inc.
Text design by Richard E. Farkas
Typeset by Mid-Atlantic Photo Composition
Printed by RR Donnelley & Sons Co.

Library of Congress Cataloging-in-Publication Data

Barton, Walter E., 1906—
  The history and influence of the American Psychiatric Association.

  Bibliography: p.
  Includes index.
  1. Psychiatry—United States—History. 2. American Psychiatric Association—History. I. American Psychiatric Association. II. Title. [DNLM: 1. Psychiatry—history—United States. 2. Societies, Medical—history—United States. WM 1 A512B]
RC443.B35   1986   616.89'006073   86-17250
ISBN 0-88048-231-1 (alk. paper)

Contents

List of Illustrations

1. Church and Hospital de San Hipolito (the dome-topped building behind) in Mexico City, the first mental hospital in the New World (1566–1986). Photo by José Antonio Martinez. Courtesy of Ramón Parres.

2. The old Pennsylvania Hospital, where the first hospital unit for care of the insane was provided in the colonies (1752). Courtesy of George S. Layne, M.D., of Bristol, Pennsylvania.

3. The first mental hospital in the United States, Williamsburg, Virginia, 1773 (from an original etching by John E. Costin).

4. Benjamin Rush (1746–1813), father of American psychiatry. A copy of the Peale portrait (in Independence Hall) with hands from a portrait by Sully.

5. Samuel B. Woodward (1787–1850), cofounder of the American Psychiatric Association and its first President. Courtesy of the National Library of Medicine.

6. Francis T. Stribling (1810–1874), cofounder of the American Psychiatric Association. Courtesy of the National Library of Medicine.

7. The home of Thomas Kirkbride and the Jones Hotel. Courtesy of the National Library of Medicine.

8. The Founding Fathers. Courtesy of the American Psychiatric Association Archives.

9. Amariah Brigham (1798–1849), founder and first Editor of the *American Journal of Insanity* (July 1844).

10. Dorothea Dix (1802–1887), social reformer, founder of 32 mental hospitals. Copy for the American Psychiatric Association of a portrait by Samuel Waugh (1865). Original in Dixmont Hospital.

11. Thomas B. Kirkbride (1809–1883), founding father, first Secretary, and officer of the Association for 26 years.

12. Isaac Ray (1807–1881), founding father and internationally renowned medico-legal expert.

13. Adolph Meyer (1866–1950), dominant psychiatrist in the U.S. for 50 years. Author of the concepts "psychobiologic whole" and "common sense psychiatry." President of the American Psychiatric Association in 1927.

14. Silas Wier Mitchell (1829–1914), founder and first President of the American Neurological Association (1875). Poet, novelist, and catalyst to change the American Psychiatric Association.

15. Clifford W. Beers (1876–1943), founder of the mental hygiene movement (1909) and of the national citizens organization (left). Clarence M. Hincks (1885–1964), founder of the Canadian Mental Health Association (1918) and its head for 30 years. For eight years (1930–1938) he served as Director for the U.S. and Canadian Associations (right).

16. Thomas W. Salmon (1876–1927), played a key role in the development of military psychiatry in World War I. Director of the National Mental Health Association. He became the first nonsuperintendent President of the American Psychiatric Association, 1923–1924.

17. Organization meeting, American Board of Psychiatry and Neurology, October 1934. Front row: C. Cheney, C. Macfie Campbell, Walter Freeman, H. Douglas Singer, Adolf Meyer, and George Hall. Back row: F. Ebaugh, L. Casamajor, J.A. Jackson, L. Ziegler, L.J. Pollack, and E.G. Zabriskie.

18. Left to right, Top: Harry Solomon, Robert Felix, Karl Bowman
    Middle: William Menninger, Francis Braceland
    Bottom: John Whitehorn, Zigmund Lebensohn, Karl Menninger.

19. The Medical Directors and Executive Secretary.
    Top: Austin Davies—Executive Secretary (1932–1964)
    Middle: Daniel Blain (1948–1958), Matthew Ross (1959–1963)
    Bottom: Walter E. Barton (1964–1974), Melvin Sabshin (1974–present)

20. The Parsons Mansion (1910). Note gas light, brick gate entrance to rear, absence of planting.

21. The Museum Building (1967) on R Street.

22. Parsons library at 1700 18th St. N.W., Washington, D.C.
    Bottom: The Modern Founders Room, American Psychiatric Association, 1959.

23. The American Psychiatric Association headquarters building, 1400 K St. N.W., Washington, D.C.

24. View of the present American Psychiatric Association lobby.

Preface

History is " . . . a tale of social and economic conflict over the emergence of new hierarchies of power and authority, new markets and new conditions of belief and experience. . . . In America, no one group has held so dominant a position in this new world of rationality and power as has the medical profession." *

Several excellent histories of psychiatry have been written, along with a few biographies of its great men and women. Four books have been written about the history of the American Psychiatric Association (1–4). Other books have been written about the history of concepts or movements, or about specific organizations. It is my intention to follow the development of psychiatry in America through the founding and growth of the American Psychiatric Association.

Early in the formative period of this nation an appeal went out to the heads of some 20 insane asylums then in existence, inviting them to join together to learn from each other. Thirteen superintendents of public and private insane asylums made the arduous journey to Philadelphia in 1844. The small group had a tremendous influence upon public opinion and upon action taken by the states.

---

* Reprinted from Starr P: The Social Transformation of American Medicine. New York, Basic Books, 1982. Copyright 1982 by Paul Starr. Reprinted by permission of the author and Basic Books.

It is my intention to focus on that group, to tell the story of its interests, actions, missed opportunities, and achievements, and to trace its survival into the present. That group, now called the American Psychiatric Association, has more than survived; it has had an enormous influence on the field of psychiatry. It is my intention to examine this influence, to elaborate on Gregory Zilboorg's statement, "The history of American psychiatry is the history of the American Psychiatric Association" (4).

There are three assumptions implicit in this book which affect our understanding of the recorded events. These assumptions relate to perspective, pace, and cycles. Perspective in historical terms means that ideas and events are viewed as products of the knowledge, skills, and values of their time. We do not evaluate them from today's vantage point, retrospectively. Pace in history is not an inexorable forward march. A few pioneers advance ideas that are years ahead of their time, while the main body eventually catches up. Others lag far behind, cling to the old and familiar, and are out of step with the forward pace. Change may be sudden or so slow as to be imperceptible. The cycle turns, old beliefs become new ones. The innovative idea, resisted as preposterous, gains adherents. Soon all jump on the wagon. The wheel is changed, redesigned, and modified until it scarcely resembles the original. Put back on the wagon it runs downhill and often out of sight, only to be forgotten. When the wheel is rediscovered it generates enthusiasm, is refurbished, and is presented as new. The cycle begins again.

Every resident in psychiatry and every psychiatrist and mental health professional should be familiar with the landmarks in the history of psychiatry. This book is for all of you.

Walter E. Barton, M.D.
Hartland, Vermont

References

1. Curwen J: History of the Association of Medical Superintendents of the American Institutions for the Insane from 1844 to 1874 Inclusive. Harrisburg, PA, Theodore F. Shaffer, 1875
2. Hurd H: The Institutional Care of the Insane in the U.S. and Canada (A Project of the History Committee). Baltimore, MD, Johns Hopkins University Press, 1916

3. Hall JK, Zilboorg G, Bunker HA (Eds): One Hundred Years of American Psychiatry, 1844–1944. A Project by the American Psychiatric Association in Celebration of its 100th Birthday. New York, Columbia University Press, 1944
4. McGovern CM: Masters of Madness: Social Origins of the American Psychiatric Profession. Burlington, VT, University of Vermont Press, 1985

Acknowledgments

I have been a history buff for most of my professional life. I read historical novels and history for enjoyment and relaxation. My obsessive nature has compelled me to put into bulging files, collected over the years, bits and pieces that "might come in handy sometime." Retirement has allowed me the time to write.

For more than 50 years I participated in the events set down here. Many of the most exciting and productive years of my life were spent working in the American Psychiatric Association. That experience introduced some personal bias which I have sought to overcome by checking facts remembered against the records, and against the perceptions of others.

Many persons have contributed to this project: staff and former employees of the American Psychiatric Association, past presidents, and many hospital administrators, librarians, and archivists around the country. It was my custom, when recorded history seemed vague on a point, or when I was unaware of a possible source, to write letters. I thank all those who filled in the gaps and directed me to the data I needed.

I am indebted in particular to the three persons to whom this book is dedicated. Carol Davis for 20 years sent me copies of articles on history and developed the files that formed the basis of the project. Her memory of significant APA events and her efficient filing system quickly produced needed documents. Jean Jones gathered historical tidbits. It was her enthusiasm for history that stimulated the intent to work on the project. Zing Jung carried the burden of searching for needed information once the project began.

Ramon Parres supplied essential historical data on Mexican history and Jack Griffin did the same for Canadian history. They also supplied the photographs of San Hipolito and Clarence Hincks.

Some of the illustrations are from Curwen's book *The Original 13*. Most are from the APA Archives, which William Baxter, archivist, supplied. The etching of Williamsburg is from an original by John E. Costin. He was commissioned by the American College of Mental Health Administration. The artist used an 1829 illustration from a sketch by Dickie Galt (descendant of Jahn Galt) and an architectural sketch by the Architectural Research Department of the Williamsburg Foundation.

I thank all the secretaries who typed early drafts and Peg Pearson who put the final manuscript on the word processor that made revisions easier.

Last, I thank all those who contributed material that made this book possible. In particular, I am indebted to George Mora, medical historian, for his critical review with major and minor suggestions that I hope have made this book more readable.

Roy Hoskins once said something that applies more to this book on history than to any other I have written: "If you find any of your flowers in my garden, I hope you will accept my thanks and know that I thought well of them."

WEB

1

The Beginning:
Development in the Care of
The Mentally Ill Before 1840

Socrates: Come lie down here.
Strepsiades: What for?
Socrates: Ponder awhile over matters that interest you.
Strepsiades: Oh, I pray, not there.
Socrates: Come, on the couch!
Strepsiades: What a cruel fate.
Socrates: Ponder and examine closely. Gather your thoughts
together, let your mind turn to every side of things. If
you meet with difficulty, spring quickly to some other
idea; keep away from sleep.
— Aristophanes, *The Clouds*, 423 B.C.

GOD AND MAN IN NATIVE AMERICA:
PRECURSORS OF MODERN MEDICINE

Early man worshipped the sun as the source of warmth, light,
and life. The moon and the stars above, the blowing winds,
crashing thunder, flashing lightning, and the changing seasons
were sources of mystery and stirred within man a recognition of
forces beyond his control. Evil spirits lurked in the dark, raged
against him in storms and volcanic eruptions, or seared the land in
drought. Supernatural forces caused misfortune, illness, and
death. Rituals were developed to win favor of the good and to
placate or drive out the evil. Selected priests, priestesses, and

1

shamans were invested with authority to deal with supernatural forces.

Mayan civilization emerged in 500 B.C. and flourished until A.D. 1519 in Oxaca, in Vera Cruz, and in the mountain valleys of the central plateau of Mexico. Mayan urban society encompassed social classes, professional groups, and a complex economy. During Europe's middle ages, Mayans developed precise prediction of solar and lunar eclipses and an accurate calendar. They had a writing system and a mathematical concept of zero.

An elite group in Mayan society, priests and chiefs were the guardians of knowledge and intervenors for the people in the worship of the gods. The moon goddess, Ixchel, was the patroness of fertility, weaving, and medicine (2–5).

In the early 15th century A.D., the Aztec prospered. Aztec physicians shared some of the priest's power and could intervene with the gods whose rage produced disease. These *ticiti* specialized in resolving the more severe anxieties, and were responsible for the health of the community. The prestige that physicians enjoyed was offset by the penalty of death should disease not be prevented. After a long apprenticeship, men and women equally shared the knowledge of herbs and "prognostic wisdoms." Dream interpreters used mushrooms and herbs (1). To achieve full status as a physician (which a woman could achieve only after menopause) one had to be judged fit to perform rites of segregation and other ceremonial acts. (To digress slightly, women were physicians in Egypt much earlier. A tablet dating from about 2730 B.C. describes a woman as Chief Physician. In the later Middle Kingdom in Egypt, women were prominent in the medical profession.) (6)

In the Aztec view, "Health was an integral part of the social progress, the image of the body was a continuation of nature; illness was an expression of social maladaption and a punishment of the gods" (2, p.4). With the exception of its use in ceremonies and religious rites, Aztec society forbade the use of alcohol and exacted the severest penalty for transgression. The vain god Tiolac produced illness (gout and paralysis) from cold and humidity, and punished those who abused alcohol with delirium. Tiazolteoti (another name for Venus) punished the sins of lust, filth, and obscenity. To allay the god's anger for wrongdoing when the patient was seriously ill, the physician searched and probed the mind until all sins were revealed. The spoken confession, a spiritual catharsis of the repressed guilt, produced the cure and the body was then purified by a steam bath (1). The elite group of physicians trained at the temple Calmecac, dedicated to the goddess Tiazolteoti, also used trephination, suggestion, and herbal potions (such as henbane, mushrooms, and those with peyote-like action) to gain insight into hidden thoughts and to regain the favor of the goddess (7).

The Spanish Conquest of 1511 fulfilled an ancient prophesy: white men with beards would arrive from the ocean and become new gods (2). Initially no resistance was offered, but destructive wars followed, led by Cortez in 1519. By 1521 an army of 400 Spaniards, assisted by 100,000 natives as allies, defeated the Aztecs. Consolidation and eventual change were gained by the missionaries who approached natives with humility, kindness, and compassion. But it was the military leaders who were determined to stamp out the pagan culture. Idols were smashed, books burned, and temples torn down to build churches (8, 9).

Forty-five years after the conquest of Cortez, the first mental hospital in the New World was established in Mexico City, modeled after those in Spain. The Hospital de San Hipolito was founded by Bernardino Alverez Herrara in 1566. He started a colony for the chronically ill, built six general hospitals, founded a religious order to care for the sick, and devoted his life to care of the ill. San Hipolito endured for 200 years (it was rebuilt in 1777) as a refuge for the exclusive care of the mentally ill and retarded (7). The hospital functioned until 1910, when patients were moved to newer facilities. The building still stands.

A second institution, Manicomio de la Canoa, was founded in 1687 when José Sayago (a carpenter) and his wife took mentally ill persons into their home (7). A priest helped to care for the patients, leading the church to build larger quarters. In the early 1800s it was a model institution, providing good care with occupational therapy and recreation. Mexico established two other mental hospitals before the 19th century: one in Guadalajara (1739) and one in Belem (1794) (1).

In 15th-century North America, hunters, trappers, fishermen, and farmers were mistakenly called Indians by explorers from Europe seeking a passage to India. The natives enjoyed a deep faith in supernatural forces which linked all living things. "To many Indians each animal, each tree and each manifestation of nature had its own spirit with which the individual could establish supernatural contact through his own spirit or that of an intermediary" (10). The Great Spirit was an all-powerful supreme being that could create other supernatural beings (as in our current religious belief in angels or demons). Ghosts of the dead (spirits) maintained an interest in the tribe and might be present on any occasion.

The medicine man was not set apart as a priest might be, but was part of the community (perhaps less skilled as a hunter or warrior) and was recognized as meditative and trustworthy. He learned his art from other shamans. The shaman saw illness as a disruption in the harmony among living things and his task was to restore balance. The medicine man could intercede for individuals and sometimes for whole groups. Good crops, a successful hunting expedition, or success in war might be secured by appeal to supernatural forces.

The ritual of communication with the spirit world varied with the tribe, as did the contents of the medicine bundle. The ritual might employ prayers, incantations, chanted songs, dreams, rattles, noises, or symbolic sand paintings. Some shamen wore carved and decorated masks to portray the spirit as revealed to the mask maker.

Shamen employed botanical substances such as alder bark for wounds, or moss boiled in spring water for stab wounds, or oil of soile for sores and burns. Cupping burns and drugs might also be used.

The Jesuit missionaries of the 17th century wrote, "Some have other diseases, which as it were inborn and concealed" (10). The other diseases that were concealed came from the depths of the soul and not through knowledge, in a primitive awareness of the unconscious and the conscious. Natural wishes were fulfilled in dreams. The dreams could mask the soul's true desires. It appears that the Indians were aware of the unconscious and the conscious, that thoughts were repressed, that desires of which an individual was unaware could cause illness. A form of psychotherapy uncovered the latent meaning of dreams by free association. Through this process, the shaman helped the individual to understand hidden wishes, resulting in improved functioning (10).

The concept of right of ownership of land of the red man was basically different from that of the white man. To the red man, land and its produce, like air and water, were free for the use of the group. No man might own land as personal property and bar others from it. A tribe might claim a territory for its use but it was held communally. Indians walked in soft soled shoes in the spring when the earth was pregnant so the Mother Earth's body would not be harmed. The shocking use by white men of a steel-bladed plow was seen as slicing open the breast of the Earth Mother (10).

The heritage of the Indian culture has enriched the world. The Indians introduced corn, potatoes, peanuts, squash, peppers, tomatoes, pumpkins, avocadoes, pineapples, cacao (chocolate), chickle (chewing gum), and tobacco; drugs such as cocaine, curare, chinchona bark (quinine), and cascara; and such things as canoes, snow shoes, moccasins, hammocks, kyacks, pipes, panchos, parkas, toboggans, and even rubber balls.

Native Americans in the northeastern region of the northern continent had developed a unique system of governance, probably before Columbus arrived. It would, in time, influence, in a strange way, both the evolution of democratic government and communist thinking.

In the year 1460, not far from the city we now know as Syracuse, the many clans (extended families) lived in the village of the Onondaga. The Long House People occupied bark-covered dwellings, some 10 fires long; each family resided in a section around its fire. In the sunlit open plowed field, the women planted and harvested maize, beans, squash, pumpkins, and sunflowers, while the older children, from a raised platform, guarded the crops from marauding animals and birds. The men, up at dawn, returned home with a goodly number of partridge and quail to eat at the next meal, with corn bread and boiled beans.

Everyone shared in the hard life. The men hunted, fished, and fought in the seemingly endless tribal conflicts. In between times, they made hooks, snares, traps, bark canoes, lodges, bows, arrows, stone knives, and axes. The women cured the deer and animal skins, made and adorned moccasins, leggings, shirts, and robes, plaited mats and baskets, gathered nuts, berries, and plants, tended the gardens, and raised the children (11).

Adodarhoh, the Chief of External Affairs (there was also a Chief of Internal Affairs), was a fearsome leader who believed that survival of the tribe depended on aggressive warfare. The councilors of the tribe, elected by the women (who also owned the clan's personal property), agreed with Adodarhoh. The Onondaga's Hiawatha, a wise and perceptive and much loved man, saw the loss of the young and the strong in skirmishes as decimating and weakening the tribe. His was a search for a way to end the strife and constant danger of attack from other tribes. When he was unable to reason with the tribal council and failed to influence them, he exiled himself and walked westward through the forest.

Wherever he camped, he was invited into the nearest village and there heard talk of a great one who also sought peace. After 23 days of travel, he found the man he sought, Dekanawida, in a Mohawk village (an exile from the Huron tribe). The two men were delighted to discover that they shared a common goal, which they set out to achieve. Together, they swayed the council of the mighty warrior Mohawk nation to lead the crusade for peace. Hiawatha, the disciple of Dekanawida, set out to win over the councils of four other tribes: Oneida, Cayuga, Seneca, and, finally, the Onondaga. The treaty was marked by the exchange of belts of wampum among the tribes as a reminder to preserve their words. Later the five-nation confederation was joined by the Tuscarora. The league of tribes brought peaceful relations from the Atlantic Ocean to the Great Lakes and unity in a democratic organization. The dream of the Great Peace became a reality (11).

> I am weary of your quarrels,
> Weary of your wars and bloodshed,
> Weary of your prayer for vengeance,
> Of your wranglings and dissensions;
> All your strength is in your union,
> All your danger is in discord;
> Therefore be at peace hence forward,
> And as brothers live together.
> —Henry W. Longfellow, *The Song of Hiawatha*, 1855 (12)

The search for peace would continue through the centuries. It would accelerate during the wars of the 20th century when psychiatrists would join others in efforts to reduce tensions among nations and to ban the use of nuclear weapons.

When the Jesuit priests discovered the federation of the Iroquois, they were amazed at the villages of long houses, surrounded by long palisades, and a vital agriculture with crops unknown to them. They noted the tribes' practice of virtue, their rigid code of honor and etiquette, and their deep religious beliefs.

Lewis Morgan, a lawyer and railroad lobbyist, published *League of the Ho-De-No-Sau-Nee* (Iroquois) in 1851. In this book he noted the pattern of government and structure: a council was selected by women; if performance was unsatisfactory, three warnings were given before the women removed him; voting was proportionate to numbers; a caucus was held in advance of a vote so that each tribe might speak with one voice; a unanimous decision was made after negotiation; and there was an oral constitution.

The confederation may have influenced colonists framing the federation of states, for Benjamin Franklin admired the organization of the League. It did influence the formation of the U.S.S.R. Morgan's book was the subject of notes left by an enthusiastic Karl Marx, who died while writing *Das Kapital*. Frederick Engel used the notes as a cornerstone of *The Origin of Family, Private Property and the State*. Land and waterways were not to be individually owned (as the Iroquois practiced). There were to be communal households and shared responsibilities (11).

The myth that native America, South and North, was inhabited by nomadic savages persists. A very different culture evolved at a slower pace than it did in Europe. However, the largest single dwelling in the world before 1066 (when the Battle of Hastings was fought) was in North America. In Chaco Canyon, New Mexico, was a four-story multiple dwelling known as Pueblo Bonita. It had 800 rooms, housed 1,200 people, and included 39 places of worship. When explorers came to the New World, it is estimated there were 20 million inhabitants in Mexico, 12 million in Peru, and 1 million in North America (13).

MEDICAL PSYCHOLOGY IN EUROPE: AMERICA'S ANTECEDENTS

The older civilizations in Europe and Asia recognized madness. There are references to madness and epilepsy in the Old Testament (14). The Egyptian and Hindu civilizations indicated a similar knowledge (15–18). The development of philosophic thought in Greece from 585 B.C. was followed by the clinical observations of Hippocrates, born on the island of Cos in 460 B.C. He left a heritage of writings in what probably constituted the library of the School at Cos (19). Plato (427–348 B.C.) suggested that the mad be kept off the streets and relatives fined if they were negligent in this duty.

Aristotle (384–322 B.C.) speculated on the location of psychological faculties and stressed observation and reason. It was Asclepiades of Bithynia (124 B.C.) and his followers, members of the priest–physician group, who were inheritors of the secrets of healing. They founded the organized healing centers—Aesculepian Temples—for the treatment of the sick (17). Asclepiades released the insane from dark cellars, used massage, wine tonics, exercise, and occupation. Healing in a religious retreat fostered diversion of the melancholy by means of sports, music, theatre, relaxation, use of odoriferous herbs, and sleep near the temple to win the favor of the gods and be cured (18). Not all the mentally ill were so fortunate, for the troublesome were chased from the temple with stones (16).

Celsus (first century A.D.) coined the word insania and wrote *De Medicina*, an excellent textbook, one of the first medical books to be printed (1478).

Arabic medicine dominated from about the fifth century (when it was believed the first asylums were built by the Moslems) through Maimonides (1135–1204 A.D.) in the 13th century (15). With but few exceptions, through the centuries in the Middle Ages, charity for the disadvantaged, children, poor, and sick was left to the church and its monasteries. The mildly insane were cared for at home or roamed about, and the violent were imprisoned and chained with criminals (17).

In 1247, The Star of Bethlehem priory (now the Bethlehem Hospital) was established in London and is the oldest mental hospital still in operation. Veneration of the relics of the murdered St. Dymphna (1250) brought the mentally disordered to Gheel, Belgium, where healing was reported. The acceptance of the mentally ill into private homes while undertaking the ritual cure marked the beginning of family care. Visitors to Gheel were so impressed with this form of care for chronic mental disease that they replicated the system in the United States. Gheel's family care system endures to this day.

One of the early legal rulings regarding mental illness was England's Lunacy Law, passed in 1320, stating that the property of the mad was vested in the crown (15). In the calamitous 14th century, it was believed that a hostile God punished a sinful people with a fourth round of the plague called Black Death (1388–1390). Some 40 percent of the population died (20).

As the 15th century opened, at a time when Spain was an expanding world power, an event occurred—a human response to a not uncommon scene—that established a mental hospital to protect the mentally ill from society (in contrast to the usual demand to protect society from the mentally ill). The year was 1409 and the city, Valencia. Father Jaffre witnessed a crowd of children harassing, pelting, and yelling, "Madman, madman." So stirred was the Brother in the Order of Mercy that he set about to form an association of 100 priests and 600 laypersons to raise money to buy a house in which the mad could be properly cared for. Thus the Hospital Santa Maria Del Innocents was founded. The concept of an innocent one without malice and easily fooled led to the provision of care for those not responsible for their actions (21).

With support from cities and from the king, other similar institutions were founded on the same model "for innocents" of both sexes, from any country and of any religion, in Zaragosa (1425), Seville (1436), Valladolid (1436), Toledo (1480), and Barcelona (1481). Humane care, good food, clean cells, "bath therapy," and agricultural work (forerunners of hydrotherapy and occupational therapy) made it possible to return some patients to the community (22). Spain, the cradle of institutional psychiatry, later neglected these institutions in the centuries that followed and fell behind other countries (23).

Medical psychology was at its lowest point just before Columbus set sail. The Spanish Inquisition to purge the land of unbelievers was in full fire. Demons were believed to possess those with mental illness. Women—who aroused passion in the celibate—were the cause of sin, and witches were pawns of the devil. Two Dominican German Inquisitors, Johann Sprenger and Heinrich Kramer, wrote *Malleus Maleficarum (The Witches' Hammer)* in 1488 under the authority of Pope Innocent VIII. It went through 10 editions until 1669. A raw, cruel book, it told how to recognize witches, and how to examine and sentence them by torture and burning (16).

In the year that Columbus "discovered" the New World, Juan Luis Vives, who was to lay the foundation for objective psychology, was born in Valencia, Spain. Vives, a professor of humanities at Louvain and philosopher at Oxford, wrote *De Anima et Vita* in 1538, setting forth psychological theories elaborated in later scholarly work.

At about the time of the Spanish explorations (begun in 1492 and continued for about 50 years), a courageous Paracelsus wrote *On Diseases Which Deprive Man Of Reason* (1526). It was not published until after his death. In this treatise he ridiculed the notion that demons caused insanity. He made reference to the unconscious and noted sexual factors in hysteria. In 1563, Johann Weyer (1515–1588) said witches burned at the stake were harmless, senile, or delusional women. He recorded observations of mental illness, suggested that long talks with patients were helpful, and declared the right of physicians to treat sickness of the mind. It was the latter statement which earned him the right to be known as the founder of modern psychiatry. In 1580, Montaigne vigorously protested belief in demonology. Swelling streams of new ideas in the 16th century broke the dam of religious repression. Weyer's refutation of witchcraft and devilish sexology was built upon clinical observation and a reasoned conclusion. Medical psychology was at long last divorced from theology.

In spite of Weyer's stinging indictment of clergymen who blamed innocent women, of transformation, of flying into space, of intercourse with the devil as beliefs "so absurd that they do not deserve to be refuted in more detail," 100 witches were executed in England in 1645; and in Salem, Massachusetts, in a town of 4,000 people, some 250 were accused and 22 were executed (24). Cotton Mather's thundering voice on diabolical possession drowned out the plea for reason by a Saltonstall (ancestor of a governor of Massachusetts). By 1711, the public guilt was so great over the action that a modest financial restitution was made to survivors of the condemned. But the cycle of demonic possession turns again and again and it lingers on in the 20th century.

A 19th century example of belief in demonic possession occurred in Woodstock, Vermont in 1830. Two physicians believed a lad named Corwin who had died might be reanimated as a supernatural being and suck the blood of sleeping citizens, so they exhumed the body. Finding liquid blood in the heart, they were convinced he was a vampire. They removed the heart, drove a stake through it, and buried it under a two-ton slab of granite in the village green to prevent the vampire from attacking others.

Belief in vampires and demons as the cause of illness was waning, however. By the 17th century in Europe the church lost its control over scientific thought. New ideas, advanced by Galileo, Newton, Boyle, Harvey, Malpighi, Hook, Van Haller, and Sydenham, provided a glimpse of a future in which science would be a dominant force.

Medicine in 17th century Great Britain, from which America would develop its modified version, included three groups of professions under the rubric of medical practice: physicians, apothecaries, and surgeons. Physicians were learned in the arts, studied from textbooks written in Latin, graduated from Oxford or Cambridge (the colleges had no medical school), and aspired to be accepted by the upper class as gentlemen who treated the rich. Physicians turned to the King to protect their exclusive right to make diagnoses, to recommend treatment, and to be paid for their opinion. It was Henry VIII's authority that established the Royal College of Physicians in London (1523). The College set policy, standards, qualifications, and fees for the two grades of physicians: Fellows and Licentiates (25).

Below physicians on the social scale in England were the apothecaries, whose guild was formed in 1617. It was their role to compound drugs and to carry out physicians' recommended treatment. They could also prescribe, let blood, lance boils, or pull teeth. They were paid for their drugs and services, but not for their advice (25). Surgeons, before Joseph Lister (1827–1912) demonstrated his antiseptic technique in 1865 and introduced the era of modern surgery, were the blood letters, ligators of severed blood vessels, drainers of infections, and amputators of damaged limbs.

Although fashion favored graduates of prestigious Oxford and Cambridge, more physicians were turned out by the 'new' medical school in Scotland. For example, in 50 years (1751–1800), 246 physicians graduated from Oxford and Cambridge. (Over the next 50 years, there was a 10 percent increase.) Edinburgh, in the same period, graduated 1,598; and, in the next 30-year period, there was a 300 percent increase in that number (25).

Early colonists who came to the New World were accompanied by apothecaries and surgeons. Many decades later physicians would come to America, when life was more attractive and populations concentrated in larger towns.

MEDICINE IN AMERICA: ADAPTING MODELS FOR A NEW SOCIETY

Sir Walter Raleigh had made three unsuccessful attempts to establish a colony in the New World in what is now Virginia by 1584. (The Spanish had been successful earlier at St. Augustine.) In 1620, however, the Pilgrims established a permanent colony in Plymouth, Massachusetts, to be followed in 1629 by settlements in Salem and Boston. The violently mad were restrained either at home in a strong room or in an out-building, or were manacled in jail. The mildly mad were free to roam about. Settlement laws established a town's responsibility to provide for care. The care of the indigent resident was often awarded to the lowest bidder (17).

The Hotel Dieu, the first hospital in the northern section of the continent, was founded in Quebec in 1630. It was here that the Grey Nuns operated psychiatric facilities developed between 1621 and 1697 at Montreal-Ville Marie and at Three Rivers.*

In 1658, Jacob Varrevanger, a surgeon for the West India Company, opened a hospital in New Amsterdam (a town of 1,000, later New York City) for sick soldiers who had been quartered in private families (26).

The first medical publication in the colonies (1668) described London's plague of 1665 as "God's Terrible Voice." Boston suffered smallpox epidemics in 1677, 1702, and 1721 (27).

Off-beat ideas could get one a public whipping in the intolerant Massachusetts colony. Roger Williams was banished in 1636 because of his beliefs, and founded a settlement some few miles distant that was to become Rhode Island. When its charter was granted by Charles II in 1663, freedom, religious and political, became a reality in the New World.

In 1720, Rhode Island established a commonhouse "for the punishment of rogues and to keep mad persons in," presumably for the care of those too violent to be cared for at home or to roam about. By 1730, the indigent insane were cared for in almshouses (17).

The first hospital in the colonies to accept the physically and mentally ill, both destitute and affluent, of all races and creeds (as Zaragosa's did in Spain in the 15th century) was the Pennsylvania Hospital, in 1752. Thomas Bond, ancestor of Earl and Douglas Bond, was the founder. Benjamin Franklin was Secretary to the Board of Directors.

Although medicine in America had its origins in England and Europe, its development differed in the sparsely settled New World. Illness and trauma were cared for within the family. Women were largely responsible for care of the sick and injured in the

---

* J.D.M. Griffin supplied this information taken from his Historical Notes, Canadian Psychiatric Association Journal 20:543, 1975; 25:86, 1980; 26:274, 1981; and 27:668, 1982.

home, relying on folk medicine, the help of kinfolk, and advice from others at hand. Indian healers were respected for their skills and their traditional remedies were added to the stock of herbs women stored at home. Later, women would be assisted by books: John Wesley's (1747) *Primative Physics* (28); William Buchan's (1769) *Domestic Medicine* (29); and John Gunn's (1830) *Domestic Medicine* (30). These books, written in layman's language, borrowed from the physician's limited knowledge of effective remedies, favored bleeding, purging, and blistering, and recommended commonsense approaches (31).

Pastors often provided medical care as did, for example, Cotton Mather (1663–1728) in Boston. It was he who promoted the use of innoculation to prevent smallpox (25). There were self-appointed lay healers, and no licensure laws to restrict their practice.

Physicians in the New World were held in low esteem. After all, their remedies were not very effective; they were not accessible in rural areas; and their services were costly. A trip of 10 miles over poor roads to the physician's office in town could mean the loss of a full day of labor. Starr (31) cites an example of a physician from Vermont who charged $1.00 for the visit; but he added a travel fee of $1.00 per mile and $2.00 per mile at night to go to the patient. A doctor earned about $500 per year and much of it in kind. Fees were often put on credit, and some were uncollectable.

A few aspiring physicians followed the English pattern, attending Harvard in the 17th century, or William and Mary or Yale in the 18th century for a liberal education, then going on to Leiden or Edinburgh for an M.D. degree. The better trained were concentrated in Philadelphia, Boston, or New York.

Medical education was established in the New World during the latter half of the 18th century. The Medical Department of the College of Philadelphia began instruction in 1756, and The Medical School of King's College (Columbia) in New York was founded in 1767. John Warren gave the first lectures on medicine at Harvard in 1782 and Nathan Smith, a 1790 graduate of Harvard, founded Dartmouth Medical School in 1797. General theory and treatment agreed upon, formal training was now desired. Until medical education became established, apprenticeship had been the principal form of training, with some who could afford it going abroad to study.

Nathan Smith spent three months in Edinburgh at his own expense studying their course of instruction and purchasing books and equipment. He opened a college with an entering class of two students who attended a course of lectures in a small two-story house and who did prescribed reading. A year later, they were awarded the degree of Bachelor of Medicine (M.B.). Smith had an active practice and students accompanied him on his calls. Six years after Dartmouth Medical School opened, Smith was given a salary of $200 a year on the condition that he live in Hanover. It was not until 10 years after he began that another faculty member was added.

The proliferation of medical schools followed the same pattern for some years. A professor offered a course of lectures while continuing his practice as Joseph Gallup did in Woodstock (Vermont) Medical School (1827). Gallup was one of the first two graduates of Dartmouth Medical School.

There were a few general hospitals and these were not held in high esteem; wound infections often resulted from hospitalization and hospitals were used to control contagion. The increase in the size and number of urban centers, the mobility and high turnover of population, the threats to the community suggested by bizarre behavior of the insane, the failure in towns of informal procedures that worked in the countryside, and the influx of immigrants and poor who lacked survival skills, led to a search for a social policy for care of the mentally ill in the 19th century (32).

An earlier recognition of the need for a specialized facility for the mentally ill was the establishment of the first mental hospital in Williamsburg, Virginia, in 1773. This was established before the first free public schools in that colony.

Governor Francis Fauquier appealed to the Virginia General Assembly in 1767 recommending the building of a public hospital for the care of "those unfortunate individuals who are so unhappy as to be deprived of their reason." A humanitarian action was to be taken based upon the principle that the public was responsible for providing care for those unable to care for themselves. After the House of Burgesses endorsed Fauquier's proposal, it was referred to a committee. In 1770 an appropriation was made to build, and procedures for admission and discharge were outlined. Admission was open to all who needed care. Those who could pay were charged 15 pounds of tobacco a year (33).

In 1780, in Gardner, Massachusetts, Oliver Upton and his wife bid 10 shillings for four children and sold a white man for profit. The breakup of families of the indigent was not rare, nor was indentured labor. "Strong backs and weak minds" made good farm hands. The public became aroused when shocking disclosure of wretched care of the poor was brought to their attention (17).

A world-wide humanitarian period began in Europe in the late 18th and early 19th centuries, and it took nearly 50 years for its full impact to be realized. The social philosophy emerging in the late 18th century considered man perfectable, not corrupt. The struggle of the common man for freedom and dignity, begun so disastrously in the tumultuous 14th century (and typified centuries later in the successful Revolutionary War) had its impact on the care of idiots and lunatics.

The 18th-century hospital in Paris—the Bicetre—with one or two exceptions, was no different from other places in which lunatics were confined. When confined, they were placed beside murderers and chained. Underfed and without hope of release, they were exhibited for a fee (which was pocketed by keepers) to a public who enjoyed hearing them shout and rave or who enjoyed seeing their strange mannerisms. France was in the throes of its revolutionary struggle for equality and for the responsibility of the state toward its citizens. Other voices calling for reform and humanitarian care preceded Phillippe Pinel's bold action to remove the fetters of his patients at the Bicetre in 1793. Shortly thereafter, he took over as administrator of Salpetriere where he again removed the chains, trained the attendants, advocated kindly care, light work, and exercise. To Pinel goes the credit for administrative reform of the institution of care of the insane. Many other leaders of reform in care followed: Vincenzo Chiarugi in Florence, Italy, demanded humanitarian care of the insane (1794); and William Tuke at the York Retreat (1796) set the pattern for good institutional care that served as a model for the development of similar hospitals in the United States (34).

While Pinel, a physician, played a major role in reform in Europe, it was a Quaker layman, Tuke, who had a greater influence in the New World British colony. To avoid the stigma associated with the words "asylum" and "madhouse," Tuke named the institution "The Retreat" to denote a place of refuge. The tenets held by Tuke laid the foundation for what was to be called moral treatment: the building and surrounding areas were to be as attractive and noninstitutional in appearance as possible; a family environment was to be created; employment and exercise were required for patients; patients were to be treated as guests and not as inmates; compassionate and kindly care was emphasized; and there were to be no chains, no intimidation, and no bloodletting (17).

In 1798, Jean Itard of Avignon began to study a lad of 17 who was living wild and naked as a savage. Itard set about to study and to train this youth, who was deprived of all education from birth. While he failed to educate the lad, he accepted Pinel's opinion that he was an idiot. It was Edward Seguin of Paris who continued to develop insights into the causes, nature, and treatment of mental retardation that were to influence the growth of interest in the feebleminded (17).

Benjamin Rush (1746–1813), honored as the father of American psychiatry, holds a unique place in history not for his advancement of the science of medicine and psychiatry, but for his role as champion of reforms. He was a university graduate, trained abroad in medicine, who came from a family that settled in the Philadelphia area in 1683. A patriot in the Revolutionary War with service as a surgeon in the Continental Army, he was one of four physician-signers of the Declaration of Independence. An aggressive, energetic advocate for free public schools, higher education for women, for temperance, abolition of slavery, and free dispensaries, he battled for unpopular causes that made him more enemies than friends (35).

Diseases of the mind was a special interest among Rush's many medical interests. His textbook of the subject, *Medical Inquiries and Observations upon the Diseases of the Mind*, was the first in the New World. It went through five editions and many translations and was the dominant book on the subject for nearly 70 years. A brilliant lecturer and teacher, he influenced thousands of students in the subject of mental disorders.

Physicians were rebuffed in their attempt to establish themselves as an elite group in democratic America. The public in a free society, devoid of hierarchy, retained the right to choose whatever healing method they wished to follow. As we shall see in the next chapter, many types of healers, with varied backgrounds and beliefs, competed in offering healing services: self-appointed healers; physicians who were apprenticed only; physicians who were university educated; followers of Thomson (the herbalist who franchised his method); followers of Hahnemann (the believer of "like cures like" in minute doses); and followers of Graham (the diet and exercise regimen).

The first protective legislation won by physicians was in 1760 in New York City, which was extended statewide in 1797. The law was the product of a united effort by local medical societies. To be a physician, a certificate had to be presented to the local medical society from a reputable physician, who stated that the applicant had studied for four years (for three years if the applicant was a liberal arts college graduate) and was qualified. This legislation was expanded in 1806 to state that those who practiced without the above "license" were to be denied access to the courts to collect fees (25).

As the humanitarian policies began to grow in France, Italy, and especially England under Tuke's example, America demonstrated acceptance in awakening reform. It was moral to be responsible for the welfare of others. Wealth was to be used productively. Private mental hospitals were founded with the aid of citizen philanthropy: Friends Hospital in 1817; McLean Hospital in 1818; Hartford Retreat in 1822; and Brattleboro Retreat in 1834. The medical and economic benefits of institutional care became evident under moral management. The private mental hospitals cared for all and soon the financial burden of the indigent insane became apparent.

The welfare role of the state was the subject of debate in the 1820s. Massachusetts requested a legislative study in 1820, New York in 1823, and Philadelphia in 1827. A crisis was perceived in public welfare. On the one hand poor laws were held to foster pauperism; but on the other hand, aid to the dependent poor was seen an essential right.

Horace Mann (1829) conducted one legislative survey in which he identified 289 lunatics in Massachusetts. Of these, 138 were in almshouses; 141 were either in jails, prisons, or at home; and only 10 were in mental hospitals. From Mann's advocacy emerged a state's responsibility for the care of the insane. Legislation passed in 1830 authorized the building of the Worcester State Hospital in 1833, a hospital which was to become a model for the development of many other similar institutions.

America borrowed from Europe: family care, the model for mental institutions, and reforms in the care of the insane employed humanitarian methods and scientific advances in theory, concept, and practice in medicine. America also adapted English law to its society.

America modified Europe's practice of medicine and law, and Europe's model institutions, to suit a free and open democratic society that placed barriers in the way of the creation of a physician elite. Lacking unity, medicine faced many obstacles that eroded its prestige: commonsense family folk medicine, lay and pastor healers, competing schools of medical thought and practice, cultists, and quacks. No examination for competence or exclusive licensure laws set standards. The individualistic, self-confident citizen solved problems, even those of illness, largely within the family until industrialization, urbanization, and immigration exerted pressure so great that solutions were sought in organizations and institutionalized social policy.

2

The Birth of
Organized Psychiatry
in the 1840s

Mankind never lives entirely in the present. The past, the traditions of the race and of the professions live on in the ideologies of
the present and in new changes.

—Sigmund Freud (1)

Times were changing. Railroads held promise of some day being
a joined system. Travel was still by horse and boat. The stage-
coach, with its frequent changes of four-horse teams, covered 50
miles in a day over unpaved roads. Letters, which kept people in
touch with one another, used the same leisurely routes. Industrialization was underway, pulling farm folk into towns and women
into factories. People were on the move westward into the new
country. Kinfolk and community support systems were broken (2).
Those alone in the city turned to physicians for help. Later it would
become apparent that commonsense and folk remedies were inadequate to challenge the diagnostic skills of trained physicians.

In the early 19th century, many Americans refused to accept the
physician as authoritative (3). Commonsense approaches, it was
felt, could relieve most illnesses. Women cared for the sick at
home and sought the help, if needed, of kinfolk and friends close
by. I referred, in Chapter 1, to helpful popular family medical
books that suggested useful remedies for common ailments.

Laws granting authority to medical societies to license practitioners were passed in the 1820s. New York, in 1844, revoked the

special privileges the medical professional had enjoyed. Laws for licensure only made the courts unavailable to the unlicensed to collect unpaid bills, but did not prohibit the practice of self-taught folk healers, botanical doctors, midwives, bonesetters, or nostrum peddlers.

Many could not afford professional medicine, although credit was extended and payment in kind for services was accepted. Still, many doctor bills went unpaid. However, the number of physicians was growing faster than the population, making it difficult to attract enough patients to gross a moderate income of $500 a year—the average earnings of a physician in the 1830s (3).

Of the estimated 3,500 medical practitioners in the colonies in the 1700s, more than 400 had formal training (in 1775 the ratio was one so-called doctor to 600 persons) (4). The number of physicians with training would still be only about 35 percent of the total number of practitioners in 1840 in New England, and but 17 percent in Tennessee (3).

The Revolutionary War and stimulating contact with French physicians who communicated new knowledge and techniques provided the impetus to improve medical practice. Hall Jackson's work led to Dr. John Morgan's (Director General of the Continental Army) regulations for regimental surgeons. Benjamin Rush made one of the war's most important contributions to medicine in *Directions for Preserving the Health of Soldiers*, published in a Philadelphia newspaper in April 1777. In this article he wrote, "A greater proportion of men perish with sickness in all armies than fall by the sword." He advocated personal cleanliness, adequate diet, protective clothing, and suitable campsites avoiding swamps (5).

Contagion was most dreaded by civilians and rightly so, for epidemics claimed many lives. The most common causes of death were consumption, infectious diseases, dysentery, accidents, and suicide. Maternal and child mortality was high. Children who survived and reached age 30 could expect to live to age 52–67. Cardiovascular mortality went unrecognized, and cancer was called maramus or the "decay of nature" (6).

THE RISE OF INSTITUTIONS

Care of "madness" in colonial New England drew attention only when the individual being cared for was indigent or violent. The violent were chained, imprisoned, and treated like criminals. Those who could be controlled were cared for in the home by their families. The mildly mentally ill were allowed to roam the streets. Strangers who were mentally ill were told to leave town. If they returned, they were whipped or put in stocks. As early as 1639, settlement laws to establish residence were enacted with one purpose: to identify the stranger who had no claim for support by the town.

The first law pertaining specifically to the mentally ill was enacted in 1676 by the Massachusetts Bay Colony. It empowered and enjoined the selectmen of towns to take care of "distracted" persons so they would not "damnify" others. The law also empowered the selectmen to safeguard the property of the insane and enabled the cost of their care to be paid from their estates. In 1725, madpersons and vagrants were placed in houses of correction. In 1736, the Judge of Probate had authority to direct selectmen of towns to provide proper care for the mentally ill. The "furiously mad," by 1798, were the only ones to be sent to a house of correction. The county and town poorhouses provided shelter for the poor, sick, and disabled. The undifferentiated almshouse (poorhouse) cared for all classes of dependent persons, including the insane, at public expense (7).

There were few institutions in the colonies and few people perceived a need for them. The able-bodied poor were cared for in their homes. The church saw poverty as an opportunity to do good, for charitable acts expressed Christian concern. Honest men who had fallen on hard times were deserving of help, but rogues and vagabonds were not. Crime was a sin, so the individual under the devil's power was punished by whippings and public display in stocks to satisfy the demand for retribution. Neighbors, if there was no family, cared for orphaned children. Families cared for their mad (8).

The 18th-century workhouses in the colonies incarcerated at hard labor the needy stranger and the idle poor who were able to work. Those unable to care for themselves and without family support were lodged and fed in the almshouse. The house of correction was reserved for the violently insane who could not be cared for elsewhere. These dependents were not seen as a threat to the security of society as they had been perceived in the 1600s, but were viewed more as a tax burden; and, to cope with this financial burden, an institution was the least expensive mode of care.

By 1820 institutional care was still a rarity, for there were only about 30 almshouses in 130 towns and cities.

Hospitals for the Mentally Ill

When informal procedures of management no longer were effective to provide adequate care for the growing populations concentrated in cities, mental hospitals came into being. The increase in numbers of the insane in an expanding population, as well as the humanitarian desire to improve the conditions under which they existed in undifferentiated local institutions, led to the development of the mental asylum.

Early in the 1800s general hospitals were established for the care of those disconnected from reliance on the family: seamen, travelers, the homeless poor, and the elderly living alone. It was safer to be cared for at home. Kitchen table surgery was less likely to be followed by infection than surgery in the hospital with its septic environment.

The first hospital to provide care for the insane in colonial America was Philadelphia's Pennsylvania Hospital in 1752. In 1751, Benjamin Franklin had drawn up a petition and presented it to the provincial assembly noting the increase in the number of persons "distempered in Mind and deprived of rational Facilities" who "Were a terror to their Neighbors, . . . wasting their Substance . . . to the great injury of Themselves and Families." Those who needed help, Franklin maintained, could be cured with proper treatment, such as the treatment provided at Bethlehem Hospital in London (9).

On May 6, 1751, the Pennsylvania Assembly passed an act "to encourage the establishing of a Hospital for the Relief of the Sick Poor of this Province and the Reception and Cure of Lunaticks." The hospital began in a private home until the building was completed in 1756. As had been the case in earlier workhouses and almshouses, the insane were cared for in basement cells. They were chained by the waist or ankles to a cell wall, their scalps were shaved and blistered, and they were bled and purged. It was not until 1796 that a new wing made it possible for the insane to emerge from the cellar into the light of moral treatment.

The first hospital devoted exclusively to the care of the mentally ill in colonial America was the Public Hospital for the Insane, opened on October 12, 1773 in Williamsburg, Virginia. As early as 1767, Governor Francis Fauquier pressed for action to establish a public hospital for the care of the insane. The House of Burgesses responded in 1770 by authorizing construction of an institution founded on the principle of public responsibility for the care of those who could not pay for it.

The original building was two-storied, with 12 patient rooms and the keeper's apartment on the first floor; the second floor had the same number of patient quarters, and a meeting room for the 15 citizens on the Court of Directors who met weekly and considered all applicants for admission. (The original building, which was destroyed by fire in 1885, was restored in 1985 as a museum at Colonial Williamsburg.)

James Galt, a goldsmith, became the first Keeper and thus the first mental hospital administrator. He called John de Sequeyra (a London born and Leiden trained physician) to examine each new patient and to supply medical care when needed. The original triad model of lay administrator, medical authority, and citizen board would return years later. James Galt started a family tradition of service to the Williamsburg institution that was to endure for 89 years. It was his grandnephew, John M. Galt, a physician, who was superintendent for 20 years at the Eastern State Hospital, and who was a founder of the American Psychiatric Association (10–12).

The first legislative act providing for a state institution to care for the mentally ill was passed on January 20, 1797. The act "to encourage the establishment of a hospital for the relief of indigent sick persons and for the reception and care of lunatics," called for the establishment of "a common state hospital in or near the city of Baltimore" and directed payment of $8,000 to the mayor of the city "to be applied to the establishment of the hospital." A gift of seven acres of land to the state of Maryland was made by Jeremiah Yellot of Baltimore for "a lunatic and general asylum" (7, p. 5111).

As the sum of $8,000 was insufficient, another $18,000 came from citizen gifts and from the city treasury. The building was not completed until 1808 when the City of Baltimore leased it for 15 years to Drs. James Smyth and Colin Mackenzie, to be used by them for the care of the insane as well as for the care of general medical patients. The Maryland Hospital (as it was called in 1828) required $15,400 to complete housing for 40 insane and 150 general medical patients. It became known as Maryland Hospital for the Insane (1838) and then Spring Grove State Hospital in 1896 (7, 13).

In Boston, Thomas Hancock left the city a legacy of £600 in 1764 to build a house for the care of those deprived of their reason. The selectmen of Boston declined to accept the money, as they believed there were not enough insane in the colony to warrant the erection of such a house (7). A hospital for the mentally ill was not opened in Boston until after the War of 1812. The McLean Hospital opened in 1818, one year after Friend's Hospital (1817), which had been modeled after Tuke's York Retreat (14). The first "private" hospitals were soon followed by the Bloomingdale Asylum in New York (1821) and the Hartford Retreat (1824).

A survey conducted by Horace Mann in 1829 found 289 lunatics in Massachusetts: 78 were in poorhouses, 37 in private homes, 19 in jail, 10 in the mental hospital (McLean), and the rest in a Charlestown almshouse or elsewhere. Mann's plea for reform in the public policy in the care of the mentally ill led to the opening of the Worcester State Hospital in 1833, which soon became the model institution widely copied.

In the larger cities such as New York, Baltimore, Philadelphia, and Boston, the pauper lunatics were still cared for in almshouses, houses of correction, or in a unit of the general hospital. In the year 1839, both Boston and New York opened exclusively psychiatric institutions. Boston's Lunatic Asylum, established by an act of the legislature in 1836, was built at a cost of $32,000 by inmates of the house of correction, and had accommodations for 100 patients. New York City Lunatic Asylum on Blackwell's Island accepted 197 transferees from the almshouse when it opened in June 1839 (15–17).

By the year 1844 there were 24 mental hospitals in the United States, with two more in Canada (at Toronto and New Brunswick), as shown in Table 1. Fifteen were public hospitals, six nonprofit, two proprietary, and one church operated.

The first mental hospital built on the Kirkbride plan was the Trenton State Hospital in New Jersey in 1845. T.S. Kirkbride's plan advocated a linear projection of wards in lateral wings (one for men and one for women) from a central administration building. Previous plans favored separate buildings set around a quadrangle. Kirkbride was largely responsible for the building standards (propositions) unanimously adopted by the American Psychiatric Association at its annual meeting in 1851. He elaborated his ideas in *The Construction, Organization and General Arrangements of Hospitals for the Insane,* first published in 1854 (with a second edition in 1880 by J.B. Lippincott). Kirkbride's design became the dominant one for construction of mental hospitals.

MEDICAL EDUCATION IN THE 1840S

In 18th- and early 19th-century colonial America, colleges for the most part prepared students for the ministry (20–22). The faculties of Harvard (1690), Pennsylvania (1700), Yale (1713), and Dartmouth (1769) were mostly theologians. Emphasis upon science was rare. No college in the colonies had a medical school before 1765. Medicine in rural areas (where there were no physicians) was a part-time activity for the clergy, farmers, and housewives. Of 400 physicians with training at the time of the Revolutionary War, 112 had studied at the University of Edinburgh (20). It is, then, not surprising that Edinburgh became the model for the medical schools founded in colonial America.

The first medical school in our new country was the College of Philadelphia Medical School, established in 1765. The second was King's College (Columbia) in New York, established in 1768. Harvard founded a medical school in 1783 that in a few years moved to White's Apothecary Shop until its new building was constructed (construction was completed in 1816, delayed by the War of 1812). Dartmouth became the fourth medical school in 1797.

John Morgan, co-founder of the College of Philadelphia with William Shippen, advocated the following requirements for admission to medical school: three years' apprenticeship with a reputable physician; education in the liberal arts, mathematics, and natural history; and a working knowledge of Latin. The medical school curriculum, he said, should cover anatomy, materia medica, botany, chemistry, physiology, pathology, and clinical medicine, in that sequence. Thomas Bond, at the Pennsylvania Hospital, added demonstrations of the clinical care of patients. Bond recommended, in addition to clinical demonstration, a curriculum extending over three years with an examination to be taken at the end of the course and a thesis to be written in Latin.

Table 1. Mental Hospitals in the United States and Canada
          in 1844 (20)*

Year Founded	Hospital	Location	Superintendent in 1844	Auspices
1752[a]	Pennsylvania Hospital	West Philadelphia, PA	Thomas S. Kirkbride	nonprofit
1773	Eastern State	Williamsburg, VA	John M. Galt	public
1798[b]	Spring Grove	Catonsville, MD	William Fisher	public
1817	Friend's Hospital	Philadelphia, PA	Charles Evans	nonprofit
1818	McLean Hospital	Belmont, MA	Luther V. Bell	nonprofit
1821[c]	New York Hospital (Bloomingdale Asylum)	White Plains, NY	Pliny Earle	nonprofit
1824	Institute of Living	Hartford, CT	John S. Butler	nonprofit
1824	Eastern State	Lexington, KY	John Allen	public
1825[d]	Manhattan State	New York, NY	None	public
1828	Western State	Staunton, VA	Francis T. Stribling	public
1828	South Carolina State	Columbia, SC	John W. Parker	public
1830	Lunatic Asylum	Hudson, NY	Samuel White	proprietary
1833	Worcester State	Worcester, MA	Samuel Woodward	public
1834	Cutter's Retreat (Pepperell Private Asylum)	Pepperell, MA	Nemiah Cutter	proprietary
1835[e]	Provincial Lunatic Asylum	St. Johns, New Brunswick	George Matthews (lay administrator), George P. Peters (medical officer)	public
1836	Brattleboro Retreat	Brattleboro, VT	William Rockwell	nonprofit
1838	State Hospital	Columbus, OH	William A. Awl	public
1839	Boston State Hospital	Boston, MA	Charles H. Stedman	public
1839[f]	Brooklyn State Hospital	New York, NY	None	public
1840	Tennessee Lunatic Asylum (Central State Hospital)	Nashville, TN	John D. Kelley	public
1840	Mt. Hope Retreat (Seaton Institute)	Baltimore, MD	William Stokes	church
1840	Augusta State Hospital	Augusta, ME	Isaac Ray	public
1842	Utica State Hospital	Utica, NY	Amariah Brigham	public
1842	New Hampshire State Hospital	Concord, NH	George Chandler	public
1842	State Hospital	Milledgeville, GA	David Cooper	public
1843	Provincial Lunatic Asylum	Toronto, Ontario	None	public

* Copyright 1944 Columbia University Press. By permission.

ᵃ There were only two patients housed in the basement of a private dwelling that was the temporary hospital, which moved to its new building in 1756. Wings were added five years later, allowing the mentally ill to move out of the basement. It was not until 1808 that the mental patients were moved to a separate institution, first alongside the main hospital and, in 1841, to West Philadelphia.

ᵇ From 1798 to 1808 the institution was the public asylum of Baltimore.

ᶜ The Society of the Hospital in the city of New York founded the New York Hospital in 1771, making it the second general hospital in the country. The Bloomingdale Asylum was separated from this parent hospital and later moved to White Plains, New York.

ᵈ Before 1825 New York City's insane poor were cared for either at the almshouse on Blackwell's Island or at the Bloomingdale Asylum. In 1825 a general hospital was built on Blackwell's Island connected to the almshouse, which evolved into Bellevue Hospital. In 1841, a three-story building was erected to care for the noisy and violent insane. It had room for 66 patients and often held twice that number. There was no resident physician or medical superintendent in 1844. Patients received medical care from physicians at the general hospital. It was not until 1847 that the insane were assembled from the almshouse in a new building for 260 patients. Until 1850 one nurse assisted by two convicts cared for the patients. The first medical superintendent, Moses Ranney, was appointed in 1857.

ᵉ The first care of the insane in any of the colonies of North America (except in Mexico, as noted in Chapter 1) was in New France, Canada. In 1656, Louis XIV stated his intent to build a series of general hospitals to care for the poor, helpless aged, lunatics, and idiots. To us, the term general hospitals means medical institutions. The King's action was to establish houses of "general hospitality" for the sick, disabled, and helpless. These were nonmedical facilities for compassionate care. Bishop Saint-Vallier founded the Quebec General Hospital (actually an almshouse) in 1692, which, in 1714, admitted lunatics. In 1717 "loges" were built with six "cells" for women and in 1720–1722 a similar facility was built for men. In 1694, the Hospital General de Ville Marie, also known as the Hospital General de Montreal, was founded by the Bishop and run by the brethren. The facility deteriorated due to lack of funds so, in 1747, the Sulpician Order (Grey Nuns) took over its operation. The third institution founded by the Bishop Saint-Vallier was the Hotel Dieu de Trois Rivieres in 1697. The Three River facility in New Brunswick also had detached "loges" with "cells" for the insane. It was destroyed by fire twice and was rebuilt in 1752 and again in 1806.

The first provincial asylum in Canada opened in St. Johns, New Brunswick, in 1835. At the 1905 APA Annual Meeting, T. J. W. Burgess reported that it began operating in an abandoned wooden building that had housed cholera patients. George Matthews was the lay administrator and Dr. George P. Peters was the Medical Officer in 1836, and served until the 90 patients were transferred to a new hospital in 1848. The Provincial Asylum in Toronto began operation in 1841 in an old jail building. In 1844, a commission was approved to supervise the construction of a new building. That structure opened in 1850. According to information obtained by the Canadian Ministry of Health, it was not until 1853 that Joseph Workman, M.D., was appointed as the first Medical Superintendent.

ᶠ This was Long Island State Hospital in Brooklyn. An 1824 New York law established county poorhouses for the care of the mildly insane. In 1830, three patients were sent to Bloomingdale. In 1838 an asylum and workhouse were built on a 70-acre farm in Flatbush. An 1844 law authorized construction of a new asylum (Hurd (7) could not determine when it officially opened). By 1852 it had outgrown its facilities and therefore a new building, with facilities for 178 patients, was completed in 1854. Also in 1854, the first medical superintendent—T. M. Ingraham—was appointed, at Brooklyn State Hospital.

The ideal goal, set in 1765, was not attained until about 100 years later. By 1812, medical schools began to appear in remote areas, chartered by the states to award degrees, with a faculty of two or three local physicians, a small library of books loaned from the personal collections of the faculty, a lecture hall, and one or two more rooms. Examples of schools in remote areas were the College of Physicians and Surgeons, Western District at Herkimer County, New York (1812), and the Vermont Medical Academy (1818) at Castleton, Vermont. By 1840, 26 medical schools had opened in 16 of the 26 states then in the Union. Enrollment was 2,500 students, who paid a fee to attend lectures (20).

Nathan Smith Davis, a 26-year-old physician from Binghamton, New York, became the spokesman for reform of medical education in 1843. When elected as a delegate to the State Medical Society, he urged that body to take a strong stand to raise medical school standards. It was evident that he lacked support, so he persuaded the state society to sponsor a national conference. This conference was held in 1846 with 119 delegates in attendance. Two-thirds of the medical schools failed to send a representative. A second convention was held in 1847. This time it was well attended, by 239 delegates from 22 of the 29 states.

Out of this meeting, the American Medical Association (AMA) emerged. The low state of medical education was duly noted as were "lamentable deficiencies" that "should be corrected" as well as the "failure of the states to distinguish between qualified physicians and the unqualified" (21). In its first years, the National Medical Association (which later became the AMA) did "more debating than crusading" (20). A more positive view of the actions taken by the Association is given by King (21). According to King, requirements for admission were formulated, and the two lecture series of four months each were to be expanded to eight subject areas: theory and practice of medicine; principles and practice of surgery; anatomy, physiology, and pathology; therapeutics and pharmacy; mid-wifery; diseases of women and children; chemistry; and medical jurisprudence. The course was to last six months instead of the previous four. Clinical instruction in hospitals was also advocated (few schools offered this instruction in 1847—only 16 out of 40).

Nathan Davis joined Rush Medical College in 1849 and tried to get that school to adopt the proposed plan. When unsuccessful, he left to found the Chicago Medical College in 1859, which later became the Medical College of Northwestern University. There he tested his curriculum. Other schools did not follow his pioneering venture.

In a period when the one-room school provided education for six or eight years for most children, Amariah Brigham wrote a book in 1832 intending to awaken public attention to the importance of making some modifications in the method of educating children (23). He believed the eagerness for intellectual improvement might press too hard, too early on the young with the hazard of overexcitement of the mind and overstimulation of the brain. Brigham recognized the importance of education but stressed the overlooked connections between mind and body, calling for greater attention to health and physical conditioning of the body.

Standards were not high in the medical schools of the period 1820–1850. The course of lectures given supplemented rather than replaced apprenticeship. By 1839, there were 30 medical schools with about 2,000 students (Philadelphia, 444; King's, 102; Harvard, 74; and Dartmouth, 50). In the 1840s many doctors still entered practice without any formal training or medical education (4).

The few students who wished to enter medicine had two choices open to them: serve for two or more years as an apprentice to an established physician, or attend a series of lectures and demonstrations in a medical school for a year and also serve as an apprentice. A few completed their training with a period of study in Europe. It was not uncommon for graduates to open a medical school and give a course of lectures. Psychiatry as a subject in the lecture series was a rarity until the 1870s. However, there were some exceptions: Benjamin Rush in 1812, in his role as Professor of Medicine and Clinical Practice at the University of Pennsylvania, included lectures on diseases of the mind. His book *Medical Inquiries and Observations upon the Diseases of the Mind* (1812) was the first standard textbook on mental disorders in the United States.

MEDICAL ORGANIZATIONS FROM 1780–1850

Organizations of craftsmen and artisans originated in medieval times to assure training, protect rights, and extend privileges of members. Medical organizations came into being in the late 18th century, modeled after those in England and France, where some

American physicians went for training. Amidst the Revolutionary War, Boston experienced a burst of social, political, and institutional creativity (8). In 1780 a state constitution was ratified, the American Academy of Arts and Sciences, the Massachusetts Charitable Society, and the Boston Medical Society were founded. In 1781 a bill for incorporation of the Massachusetts Medical Society was passed by the legislature. The expansion added 15 other physicians to the Boston Group and included Drs. Cotton, Tufts, and Holyoke (8). The goals of the new society were to examine candidates, to award certificates of qualification to practice, and to disseminate knowledge aided by the establishment of a library. The medical society's journal, the *New England Journal of Medicine,* was to appear in 1812.

In the 1790s and early 1800s state and local medical societies developed rapidly to protect physicians from competition by the untrained and to secure legislation for licensure.

Until the 1830s, state medical societies were moderately successful, as they could readily unite against quacks and pretenders. A decade later divisive forces developed within medicine over theory, the training required to prepare for practice, and who should control licensure (24).

There had been general agreement in the 18th century that disease was the consequence of imbalance in bodily function in its solid or liquid parts, or in systems such as the circulatory. Treatment sought to restore health by bringing the body back into balance.

Rush embraced this theory and believed that when disease manifested by fever it was due to the accumulation of bodily poisons, in the liquid parts, which caused restriction of small blood vessels. His therapy was designed to rid the body of the poisons by bleeding, purging, sweating, or by bringing the poison to the surface by cupping or blistering the skin (20).

Disagreement with both theory and practice increased and led to its ultimate collapse. Facing public rejection of bleeding and purging as favored therapy, and growing opposition from herbalists, naturopaths, and homeopaths, the medical profession united in 1847 to form what was to later become the American Medical Association.

State medical societies sought to protect the public from the untrained and the quacks by restricting the right to practice to those holding a license granted by the medical society. From 1826 onward, efforts to gain cooperation between societies in the various states had failed. By 1844, the loss of confidence in traditional medicine came to a head in New York State, when the special privileges granted physicians were repealed; a license was no longer requisite to practice the healing arts in that state (26).

Rather than fight to restore privileges, the New York State Medical Society called for the national meeting, in 1847, out of which emerged the American Medical Association (26).

THREATS TO TRADITIONAL MEDICAL PRACTICE

The threats to medical practice came from the herbalists, the naturalists, the homeopaths, the new knowledge from France (brought by doctors attached to French troops during the Revolutionary War), and the broad popular acceptance of the new practitioners who rejected healing by heroic measures such as bleeding and purging.

The threat to traditional medical practice came first from Samuel Thomson of Orford, New Hampshire (1769–1843). Following ancient traditions in China and North America, certain persons became adept at collecting herbs and roots that were found to have curative value. After Thomson's mother died under a regular physician's care, and after curing himself and his wife with botanical remedies, he lost confidence in traditional doctors. First treating only his family and neighbors, Thomson gave up his farm in 1805 to become an itinerant herb doctor. Thomson's therapy began with massive sweating, which he said made the body receptive to herbal treatment. He condemned bloodletting and chemical purgatives in favor of his natural herbal remedies. He played upon public discontent with treatments that didn't help and that made one feel worse. He advocated a do-it-yourself approach that was popular in rural areas of the new country where the wife and mother cared for the sick (25, 27).

In 1813, Thomson patented his healing method and sold rights to 137 agents all over the country to promote the system. In the 1830s the spread of his doctrines won adherents and gained followers such as Wooster Beach, who founded eclecticism, and who sought to establish medical schools and dispensaries blocked by Thomson. Botanical medicine became a powerful counterforce to traditional medicine. In New York State, 50,000 signatures obtained in 1844 secured the repeal of the restrictive privileges given to physicians.

Another threat to traditional medical practice came in the form of the naturalist movement, whose leader was Sylvester Graham (1794–1851). Graham stated that his approach cured disease through natural means: a healthful diet, regular hours of work and sleep, exercise, and morally uplifting conversation. A follower of his regimen and its healthful lifestyle would not need a physician, he said.

Natural foods, vegetarian diets, and emphasis on lifestyles have a way of recycling in popularity. Followers of Graham in the early 19th century joined followers of Thomson in opposition to traditional medicine. Graham's memory is forever preserved in the well-known cracker, all that remains of the Grahamite Houses that once were the places to go for a cure and change in lifestyle (25).

Herbalists, naturalists, and their followers were threats to traditional medical practice from without the profession; threats from within the profession came from France, Germany, and from the homeopaths.

The Revolutionary War, as already noted, brought military surgeons into contact with French medical officers, whose superior knowledge and skills were appreciated. Furthermore, facts produced from research overturned traditional theories. Along with measuring pulse and fever, the stethoscope demonstrated conditions in the chest. Statistical methods demonstrated that bloodletting was not an effective method of treatment (25). These new ideas could not be ignored as Thomson's were.

Samuel Hahnemann (1755–1843) was a German born and trained physician who, in 1790, while translating Cullen's *Materia Medica*, found the germ of his own doctrine "like cures like" ("simila, similibus curantur"). In an experiment on himself using Cinchona bark (quinine) which was an effective remedy for intermittent fever—malaria—produced symptoms such as fever, rapid hard pulse, palpitations, flushing, and thirst. When the Cinchona produced symptoms that resembled a fever and it was known to cure intermittent fever, he concluded that "like cures like." On no evidence at all, he extended this doctrine to other substances and insisted that minute doses were more effective than larger ones. He also believed no two diseases could coexist. "A disorder artificially produced by drugs would drive out the occurring disease provided the new disease was similar to the old" (24, p. 1222).

Homeopathy came to America in 1825, introduced by Hans Grom, who studied medicine in Denmark. From his New York practice, he attracted many disciples. Articles in reputable medical journals spread the doctrine of homeopathy and gained adherents. Scathing critical attacks upon Grom and his followers proved a double-edged sword for they led to examination of the clinics of traditional physicians as well as those of homeopaths. All physicians' practices were under scrutiny for evidence that "cures" in use were effective (24, 28).

While the rise of the American Medical Association was the result of threats to the theory and practice of physicians and to the loss of their licensed privilege status, the formation of the first national medical organization in America—the organization that was to become the American Psychiatric Association—had a very different origin, as we shall see later in this chapter.

THE CAUSES OF INSANITY AND ITS TREATMENT

I have already mentioned the influence for over 50 years of Benjamin Rush's *Medical Inquiries and Observations Upon Diseases of the Mind* (1812). If we are to understand the prevailing views in the 1840s about mental disorders, we must begin with Rush.

Rush believed that the mind interacted with the environment through the medium of the body. The events which aroused the passions to excess produced malfunctioning of the body and the arterial supply of the brain, which, in turn, disturbed the mind. He believed that individuals differed in their sensitivity to external events: that single persons were more predisposed than married persons, that the rich were more predisposed than the poor, and that persons engaged in certain occupations (poets, painters, sculptors, and musicians) were more predisposed to mental illness. Rush believed that mental illness was a disorder of the total person, with an origin in bodily impairment and in emotionally stressful events. He believed that preoccupation with past suffering and worry over future events predisposed one to mental illness, as did excessive withdrawal from others and injured feelings.

As early as 1789, Rush's lecture, "Duties of a Physician," expressed his views on treatment:

- Preserve a composed and cheerful countenance
- Inspire hope of recovery
- Preserve the belief that one can will to recover
- Convey that confidence and trust in the physician and his therapy enhances recovery
- Divert the patient's morbid preoccupation with illness
- Exercise the body and divert the mind with activities
- Be kind and just with patients
- Restore body equilibrium
- Convey that recurrence of the malady once cured does not mean that medicine has no power over it. (Rush cited the recurrence of catarrh, pleurisy, and intermittent fever.)
- Be aware that recovery is more certain in cases of acute mania than in what he called manalgia and amenomia

Rush's classification of mental disorders included four types:

1. Intellectual derangement (mania, manicula, manalgia)
2. Partial intellectual derangement (hypochondriases, ameno-mania)
3. Demence or dissociation
4. Fatuity (congenital, postfebrile, senile, postmanalgic)

Rush's description of manalgia resembles modern catatonic schizophrenia, and amenomia resembles paranoid states (30, 31).

American physicians also assimilated the views of European medicine along with the views of Rush. As already noted, Paracelsus, Weyer, and Montaigne rejected the belief in demonology in the 17th century. The 18th century was a period of revolt against authority, old beliefs, and traditions. Observation and biological experiments laid the groundwork for new science and a change in the mode of practice with a wave of humanitarianism as the century began. A religious awakening held man as perfectable. Man could control his life on earth. Dain believed that this philosophical change was as important as any medical discovery for the spread of moral treatment (32). The surge of optimism in a view of unending social progress fueled the fire of reform.

Three European writers profoundly affected practice in America. Phillippe Pinel wrote a *Treatise on Insanity* in 1801 (it was translated into English in 1806) in which he called for an attitude "of good feeling and consideration with energetic and moderate coercion instead of the use of chains." Samuel Tuke wrote the classic work on humane treatment, *Description of the Retreat* (1813). James Connolly instituted a policy of no restraint at Hanwell (1838–1844) that stirred a controversy in the United States (33).

Samuel B. Woodward's views on the cause of insanity were perhaps similar to those held by enlightened physicians in the 1840s. Woodward, the distinguished Superintendent of the Worcester (Massachusetts) State Lunatic Hospital, believed the following:

• The brain was the organ of the mind.
• Insanity was caused by disease of the brain—a somatic disorder that affected the physical organ but left the part of the mind identified as the soul untouched.
• Mental phenomena had natural causes.
• Abnormal behavior led to impairment of the brain; being self-inflicted, it ignored laws of life.
• The more complex the society, the greater the proportion of insane.
• Excessive stress, failure, disappointments, and losses produced insanity in the predisposed (34).

Amariah Brigham held similar views of somatic causation and accepted some of the views of phrenology. He believed that mental excitement increased blood flow to the brain, in which each faculty had "a separate and material instrument or organ" (24). He cited a case of pressure on the brain in a young man whom he treated in Hartford after a fall "through the scuttle of a store." The man had gone home but the next day was found senseless in bed. Dr. Brigham removed a portion of bone over the ear and found "a gill of clotted blood" which he removed; the man immediately spoke and recovered. In his view, the causes of insanity were whatever powerfully excited the brain, or damaged it by blows, falls on the head, inflammation, or fevers (24).

John Galt wrote a book of abstracts, *The Treatment of Insanity*, in 1846 (35). It was based upon his extensive reading of articles, many from abroad. According to these articles, mania and melancholia were treated with bleeding, cautery, and induced vomiting using antimony or hellibore. Opium was the preferred therapy to quiet patients. Open bowels (with calomel) were helpful in relieving melancholy. Galt cited a treatment for madness practiced in 1716, which employed the "juice of swallows and blood taken from behind the ear of an ass." Barley water, moderate exercise, and a long sleep were also recommended. Hypochondriasis was treated by exercise, narcotic tonic, and a clyster of mutton broth and brown sugar.

In 1841, Brigham's treatment for cerebral excitement called for topical bleeding, water falling on the head from four or five feet, a warm bath, and cotton oil with a tonic of molasses, wine gaultheria, sassafras, and tincture of aloes and myrrh.

Woodward's treatment (1842) expressed increase in self-respect, careful examination, kindness, continued attention, cold applications to the head (when the tongue was coated and the head hot), mercurial purge, moderate doses of narcotics for excitement, warm and cold baths, and a full diet. The patient was to work if able. Punishment was never given, bleeding was rarely used, and only short periods of seclusion and no muffs or waistcoats were to be used. Woodward expressed the conviction that the patient be given a full explanation of any medications used and the treatment employed. He observed that reasoning was often of little benefit at the outset of an illness but was most useful later.

Galt compared three views on the use of restraint in *The Treatment of Insanity:* 1) the Bethlehem and St. Lukes modified coercion; 2) limited restraint checked frequently by the superintendent as employed at York; and 3) the abandonment of all restraint as practiced at Hanwell. Galt believed that entertainment, reading, and exercise made the need for restraint infrequent, and believed that good attendants should prevent disturbance, not punish it. When all else failed, Galt believed that the patient should be gently escorted to his or her own room and secluded in subdued light.

Galt stated that there was no institution in the world with results superior to those obtained at the Vermont Asylum (Brattleboro Retreat). The males did farmwork, cut wood, and made shoes, while the women sewed or did needlework. Exercise and work improved the mind. The patients engaged in ball, quoits, billiards, chess, dominoes, painting and drawing, singing, piano playing, reading, and publishing a hospital journal. Patients walked, rode, fished, danced, and held parties. The importance of proper management by attendants was stressed (35).

A typical patient day at Pennsylvania Hospital was described by Bond:

> The morning bell rang at quarter to 5 in summer. Attendants then unlocked doors, that had been closed for the night. Breakfast was at 6:15 A.M. followed by a work period for all who were able. Dinner at noon was an interruption after which work was resumed with tea and a rest period at 6 P.M. Then one walked, played games, sang with the piano, or rode out of doors on a miniature circular railroad (36).

FOUNDING OF THE ASSOCIATION OF MEDICAL SUPERINTENDENTS

In the spring of 1844, Samuel Woodward visited Francis T. Stribling in Staunton, Virginia. Why did Woodward undertake the arduous journey to see the young Dr. Stribling? On his way south, Dr. Woodward stopped in Philadelphia and found that Dr. Kirkbride was away. Would one go so far without arranging an appointment? Certainly the visit to Staunton was planned, and perhaps on the way an opportunity presented itself for a side trip to Philadelphia.

Woodward's Worcester State Lunatic Hospital was overcrowded by this time and forced to expand once again. No sooner had it been built (1833) than it was forced to deny admission to one-half of the applicants. The beds added between 1835 and 1838 didn't solve the problem. The numbers of insane being neglected in almshouses and houses of correction had not declined but had increased since the opening of the Worcester Hospital. Dorothea Dix had called the attention of the Massachusetts legislature to appalling conditions in institutions in the states. As a result, still another expansion to the Worcester Hospital was authorized in 1843 (37).

Industrialization, urbanization, and immigration were changing American society. The numbers of insane were increasing faster than the population. Sheer numbers of patients threatened the small institution and its successful moral treatment. The national model asylum Woodward had created at Worcester was deteriorating under these pressures. The optimistic doctor must have been confident that standards of care could be preserved if efforts were made to solve the problem.

Stribling had toured the better known institutions when he was elected to head the Western Lunatic Asylum and had returned to incorporate the best in institutional practices in the Staunton Asylum. Perhaps Woodward met Stribling on that tour and was sufficiently impressed to seek him out.

What is known is that the two men discussed common problems and were so bouyed by the experience that the idea of an association of superintendents captivated them. They set out to explore its feasibility with Drs. Kirkbride and Awl. Annual reports of several of the founders had noted the birth of the British Association of Medical Officers of Lunatic Asylums in 1841. The wish was expressed that there might be similar cooperation in the United States. A call for a meeting in Philadelphia was sent either by Stribling or Woodward. However, when Woodward indicated he planned to stay at the Jones Hotel, young Dr. Kirkbride took over all the arrangements for the conference to be held in his home city.* On the evening before the scheduled gathering, 13 superintendents of public and private hospitals for the mentally ill were invited to be the guests of Dr. Kirkbride at his home. The meeting was held in the building now known as "The Mansion" on the grounds of the Pennsylvania Hospital (18).

At 10 A.M. on October 16, 1844, the group assembled in Philadelphia's Jones Hotel, located on Chestnut Street near 6th. The meeting was to last for four days. Those present, "The Original 13," were: Samuel B. Woodward (the meeting probably was his brainchild); Francis T. Stribling (who shared the idea of meeting together); Thomas S. Kirkbride (of the Philadelphia Hospital for the Insane); William McClay Awl (of the Central Lunatic Asylum, Columbus, Ohio); Luther V. Bell (of the McLean Asylum, Somerville, Massachusetts); Amariah Brigham (of the Utica State Hospital, Utica, New York); John S. Butler (of the Hartford Retreat, Hartford, Connecticut); Nemiah Cutter (of the Pepperell, Massachusetts, Private Hospital); Pliny Earle (of the Bloomingdale Asylum, White Plains, New York); John M. Galt (of the Eastern

---

* Additional details about the organizational meeting and of the founders and their motivation can be found in McGovern C: Masters of Madness. Hanover, New Hampshire, University Press of New England, 1985.

Lunatic Asylum, Williamsburg, Virginia); Isaac Ray (of the Augusta State Asylum, Augusta, Maine); Charles S. Stedman (of the Boston City Lunatic Asylum);· and Samuel White (of the Private Asylum, Hudson, New York).

From this assembly emerged an organization—The Association of Medical Superintendents of American Institutions for the Insane (later to become the American Psychiatric Association)—with Woodward elected as President, Samuel White as Vice President, and Thomas S. Kirkbride as Secretary and Treasurer. It was the first national medical association in the United States, organized three years after the first national psychiatric association in the world had been founded in England (the Association of Medical Officers of Asylums and Hospitals for the Insane—now the Royal College of Psychiatrists).

The group of four surgeons (White, Awl, Brigham, and Stedman) and nine general physicians sought to pool their knowledge about mental illness. In that process they would lay the foundation for a medical specialty—psychiatry—and shape the development of American psychiatry.

Pliny Earle stated the objectives of the Association as set forth in the organization's circular letter: "The medical gentlemen connected with lunatic asylums should be better known to each other, should communicate more freely the results of their individual experience; should cooperate in collecting statistical information relating to insanity and above all should assist each other in improving the treatment of the insane" (38).

Samuel White, the oldest of the group, would die at the age of 67, before he could assume the office of president. Galt, at age 25, was the youngest superintendent. Butler would be active in the association for the longest period, 46 years; followed by Earle, 41 years; and Kirkbride, 39 years, 26 of them as an officer. Brigham founded the *American Journal of Insanity*, and Ray would gain renown as a forensic expert. (See Table 2 for a summary of activities of the founding fathers and consult Appendix B for an abbreviated biography on each of the original 13.)

The asylum superintendents who accepted the invitation to meet in Philadelphia in 1844 gained a place in history; their names are remembered. Those whose local affairs kept them from attending—such as Andrew McFarland of the Concord, New Hampshire, Asylum or William Rockwell of the Brattleboro Retreat in Ver-

Table 2.   The Founders

Name	Probable Number of Years Active in APA	Officer (X) President (P)	Age in 1844	Medical Training Apprentice	Medical Training Formal	Study Abroad	Life Span	Major Contribution and Special Interests
Awl	7	X P	45	X			1799–1876	Founded Ohio Asylum and Institution for the Blind
Bell	12	X P	38		X	X	1806–1862	Politics, heating and ventilation, Bell's Disease, advisor to Dorothea Dix; with Ray, founded Butler Hospital. Resigned in 1856
Brigham	5	X	46	X		X	1798–1849	Founded *American Journal of Insanity*; administration, occupational therapy, individual therapy
Butler	46	X P	41	X		X	1803–1890	Individual patient treatment plan—legal issues, administration
Cutter	15		57		X		1787–1857	Founded successful private asylum in Pepperell, Massachusetts
Earle	41	X P	35		X	X	1809–1885	Contributor to literature (second only to Ray); fostered accurate statistics; introduced German and Austrian contributions to the U.S.

Name						Years	Notes
Galt	18		25		X	1819–1862	One of Galt dynasty of administrators; scholar (Greek, Arabic, European languages); occupational therapy; recreation; bibliotherapy
Kirkbride	39	X P (26 yr)	35	X	X	1809–1883	Administration; organization; nursing standards; hospital construction
Ray	23	X P	37	X	X	1807–1881	Renowned medico-legal expert, with more than 100 publications; introduced term "mental hygiene"; founded Butler Hospital (resigned in 1867)
Stedman	7		39	X	X	1805–1886	Charles Dickens wrote about him; politics; senior surgeon (resigned in 1851)
Stribling	30		34	X	X	1810–1874	Progressive administrator; occupational therapy; training of attendants
White	−1	X	67	X	X	1777–1845	Foremost specialist in New York; President of the New York State Medical Society; founded successful private asylum
Woodward	6	X P	57	X	X	1787–1850	Model of his institution was widely copied; national reputation; advocate of medical care for alcoholism; popularized work of Pinel and Esquirol in the U.S.; resigned as superintendent of Worcester in 1846

mont—were equally worthy of a place in history, though they joined the group at its second meeting in 1846.

Stedman, one of the original 13 members who had just been appointed Superintendent of the Boston City Insane Asylum in 1842 when John Butler left to become head of the Hartford Retreat, was made immortal by a distinguished visitor to Boston. Charles Dickens praised what he saw instead of expressing his usual displeasure about the care of the insane. Dickens had this to say about the Boston Asylum in Volume 2 of *American Notes* (1842):

> At South Boston, as it is called, in a situation excellently adapted for the purpose, several charitable institutions are clustered together. One of these is the hospital for the insane; admirably conducted on those enlightened principles of conciliation and kindness, which twenty years ago, would have been worse then heretical, and which have been acted upon with so much success in our pauper asylum of Hanwell. . . .
>
> Each ward in this institution is shaped like a long gallery or hall with the dormitories of the patients opening from it on either hand. Here they work, read, play at skittles, and other games; and when the weather does not admit their taking exercise out-of-doors, pass the day together. In one of these rooms, seated calmly, and quite as a matter of course, among the throng of madwomen, black and white, were the physician's wife and another lady, with a couple of children. These ladies were graceful and handsome; and it was not difficult to perceive at a glance that even their presence there had a highly beneficial influence on the patients who were grouped about them. . . .
>
> Every patient in this asylum sits down to dinner every day with a knife and fork; and in the midst of them sits the gentleman, whose manner of dealing with his charges, I have just described. At every meal, moral influence alone restrains the more violent among them from cutting the throats of the rest; but the effect of that influence is reduced to an absolute certainty, and is found, even as a means of restraint, to say nothing of it as a means of cure, a hundred times more efficacious than all the strait-waist coats, fetters and handcuffs, that ignorance, prejudice and cruelty have manufactured since the creation of the world. . . .
>
> In the labour department, every patient is as freely trusted with the tools of his trade as if he were a sane man. In the garden and on the farm, they work with spades, rakes and hoes. For amusement, they walk, run, fish, paint, read and ride out to take the air in

carriages provided for the purpose. They have among themselves a sewing society to make clothing for the poor which holds meetings, passes resolutions, never comes to fisticufs or Boowie knives as sane assemblies have been known to do elsewhere; and conducts all its proceedings with the greatest decorum. The irritability, which would otherwise be expended on their own flesh, clothes and furniture is dissipated in these pursuits. They are cheerful, tranquil and healthy. (pp. 626–627)

John Curwen, Secretary of the Association, wrote about the original 13 members for the approaching 50th anniversary (39). He had this to say about the founders:

Such were the men who met together to form this Association. Men of determined purpose, great benevolence and philanthropy and in every way admirably fitted for the work which they laid out for themselves.

It may not be amiss to state succinctly some of the principles which they believed laid at the foundation of all efforts for the relief and treatment of the insane. That the State should make ample and comfortable accommodations in properly constructed hospitals for all classes and conditions of the insane; and while private liberality and philanthropy might arrange for the care and treatment of a limited class, the greater portion of the insane were included in that class for which alone the State, in its capacity as Sovereign, should give all that was required for their accommodation and for the protection of the community at large. Acting on this principle they used all their influence and persuasion on the several communities of which they were residents, by their personal influence as individuals and by their writings, to obtain the fullest and most complete provision in every respect for all of the classes indicated. They were not to be thwarted in the attainment of the object by any ordinary opposition, but they persevered, many of them in the face of apparently unsurmountable obstacles, until, after the lapse of years, they had the gratification of seeing their views endorsed and embodied in stone and brick. They held firm to the opinion that "every hospital built at the public expense, while possessing every thing that can contribute to the health, comfort and restoration of its patients, should yet be plain but substantial in character, in good taste architecturally, but avoiding all extravagant embellishment or unnecessary expenditures."

All the arrangements of the wards should be so made as to give the greatest amount of light, cheerfulness and homelike surround-

ings. Studiously avoiding everything which could convey unpleasant impressions, while "abundant means for occupation, amuse-
ment, and all that comes under the head of moral treatment, should
be provided in every hospital." In the selection of a site for a
hospital cheerful surroundings and an extensive and varied pros-
pect should be sought for, and all the resources of the art of
landscape gardening should be employed to make the views on the
grounds, and the grounds themselves, as beautiful and attractive as
possible (39, p. 47).

THE ASSOCIATION'S ACTIONS DURING THE 1840S

When the Association convened for its second meeting on May
11, 1846 in Washington, D.C., they were joined by 10 additional
members: James Bates of the Augusta State Hospital, Augusta,
Maine; Andrew McFarland of The New Hampshire State Hospital,
Concord, New Hampshire; William Rockwell of the Brattleboro
Retreat, Brattleboro, Vermont; George Chandler of the Worcester
State Lunatic Hospital, Worcester, Massachusetts; G.H. White of
the Hudson Lunatic Asylum, Hudson, New York; R.S. Stuart and
John Fouderden of the Maryland Hospital, Baltimore; William
Stokes of the Mt. Hope Asylum, Baltimore; J.W. Parker of the
South Carolina Hospital in Columbia; and William Telfer of a
private institution in Flushing, New York. The tradition of holding
the Association's annual meeting in May was established at this
gathering. A memorial for the deceased Sam White was prepared
at this meeting and William Awl was elected to take White's
vacated post as Vice President.

A membership rule was formulated to admit to membership "the
medical superintendent of any incorporated or legally constituted
institution for the insane now existing on the continent, or may be
commenced prior to the next meeting, and to all who have been
medical superintendents." Where a medical superintendent did
not exist in an institution with a different organization, the regular
medical officer could attend (40).

Reports of the committees appointed two years earlier were
heard and 18 new committees were formed. Their titles indicate
the range of interests of this small group of dedicated men: treatment of incurables; relations between phrenology and insanity;
admission of visitors into patient halls; correspondence with patients; kinds of manual labor; proper number of patients in one

institution; night attendants; locked as opposed to unlocked doors at night; cottages for wealthy patients; fuel for heating; nature of insanity due to intoxication; care of insane in British Provinces; relation of menstruation to insanity; treatment of the poorer classes with the greatest economy; effects of tobacco on insanity; reading (bibliotherapy) and recreation as treatment modalities; use of water closets on wards; and construction and arrangements of institutions in warmer climates.

At the third meeting in New York in May 1848, the reports from the 18 new committees were heard. The group, after a visit, condemned New York's Blackwell Island Lunatic Asylum and recommended improvement in construction and management. Most of the changes suggested by the Association were made by the State of New York.

In another action, the group opposed political appointments and urged that the "best man" be named Medical Superintendent. Another resolve broadened the invitation to attend meetings to trustees, managers, and official visitors. During its formative period, the organization brought together top executives. It was not open to staff physicians but only to the governing group.

The areas of interest were heavily weighted with everyday administrative concerns, with some attention given to theory, causation, and treatment of mental illness. Learning together, the group sought solutions to management issues.

The difficulties of travel made possible only three meetings in six years. Railroads were independent carriers that traveled but a few miles; an interconnecting system was still to be created. Riverboats and sailing ships, and lurching stagecoaches that moved over unpaved roads, were the principal means of travel.

The group was small, the issues before them large. Reports on assigned committee topics required homework and correspondence with the use of the slow mails. It was an impressive group of talented men, dedicated to improving institution management and to improving patient care.

There were, nevertheless, missed opportunities. Already the influx of destitute immigrants was a threat to the small hospital and to individualized care. The threat to the entire system of care on which moral treatment was based was already evident. This central issue was lost in operational problems.

Hampered by the lack of a uniform classification system of mental disorders, reports were limited to individual observation.

Although the group was interested in the causes of mental illness and in its treatment, intensive study of similar disorders was not done and no encouragement was given for research. The science and practice, as a consequence, were not advanced. The founders had little comprehension of statistical methods, a deficiency which was reflected in overoptimistic reporting of the results of treatment.

The major advances were in the administrative aspects of institutional practice and in the creation of a therapeutic milieu. The small size of their asylums in their early years made possible knowledge of the individual patient, with good supervision of staff who delivered kindly, humane care. There were more mentally ill in need of care outside of their institutions than inside them. The drive to help that group came principally from outside the organization through the crusade led by Dorothea Dix. Her work seems not to have been a central concern of the group, although several Association members were her close friends and advisors. With so much to learn about mental disease and about administration, it is surprising that so few were able to effect as much change in the system as they did.

The founding of the Association represented the first organized group effort in America to bring humane care to the mentally ill. The small group of physicians—administrators sought to establish, with public support, small institutions for the mentally ill that permitted personal care, uniform standards for performance, and control by the medical superintendent. By consensus, they articulated general operating policies. Asylums were to be located in the country away from the contagion of the city, in an atmosphere of wholesome peace and calm, where there existed an opportunity to work at farming and useful tasks. The mentally ill were to be cared for by humane and compassionate attendants, and never be subjected to indignities. Diets were to be adequate, suitable recreation was to be provided, there was to be minimal use of restraints, and there were to be opportunities for religious worship. In this milieu, with support, the residual inner strength of the patient would be fostered and, in time, he or she would become well. At the outset the founders were confident that if asylum programs provided this care, most patients would recover.

3

The Formative Years: 1850–1899

Your hospitals are not our hospitals; your ways are not our ways. You live out of range of critical shot; you are not preceded and followed in your ward work by clever rivals, or watched by able residents, fresh with the learning of the school.

—S. Wier Mitchell (1)

The true objective of the association . . . is to consider the practical management of insane hospitals and all subjects pertaining thereto. . . . The chief medical officer must always have charge of all departments of administration . . . the instant a layman takes his place, the patient loses his identity as such.

—Walter Channing (2)

The sweep westward into the new country kindled the fire in which the indomitable spirit of men and women adventurers was forged. The challenge was brutal, the hardships exhausting, the dangers everpresent, but the frontier people carved a country out of the wilderness. It took strength of character and hard labor to survive. Fields were cleared, houses and barns built, land plowed, crops harvested, and the whole process defended by one's own hands. No wonder that pride in a civilization of one's own making was the result.

The years between 1850 and 1899 were ones of great growth, calamitous Civil War, flourishing of the arts, astounding scientific discovery, improvement in the clinical management of illnesses and injuries, and advances in medical education.

An almost endless flood of immigrants poured into the country at this time. The United States (with a population of 23 million in 1850) increased by 3 million immigrants during the decade of the 1850s. The number of immigrants grew after the Civil War, with great numbers coming from Ireland, Germany, and other countries in Europe. Many settled in the eastern cities, were unable to find work, and many became public charges. The fragile balance in the economics of survival made new families choose to send a mentally ill family member to an asylum.

These years were marked by expansion of mental hospitals, a crisis of criticism when asylums deteriorated, reforms with centralization of systems, and, after a decline in the influence of the Association of Medical Superintendents, its return to a position of influence after internal change. At the end of the century, psychiatry emerged as a medical specialty.

THE ADVANCEMENT OF MEDICAL SCIENCE

Medicine was developing a scientific base in the discovery of new facts, knowledge was expanding, and new tools for the improvement of diagnoses were introduced (3–7). Rudolf Virchow (1821–1902), the father of pathology, asserted that medicine was a "social science in its very bone and marrow." He sensed that the advances in science might lock the medical profession in a biophysical and mechanistic paralysis (4). Claude Bernard demonstrated the glycogenic function of the liver in 1850 and, in the same year, Hermann Helmholtz estimated the speed of nervous impulses. In 1851 Helmholtz invented the ophthalmoscope, and in 1856 he wrote a manual on optics. In 1857, Louis Pasteur demonstrated that fermentation in wine was caused by living organisms. Ignaz Semmelweiss described child bed fever in 1862. Charles Darwin's *Origin of the Species* appeared in 1859 and upset the world with his theory of evolution (which still disturbs some people more than 100 years later). The major contributions to the advancement of science in the second half of the 19th century also contributed to the advancement of knowledge of nervous and mental disorders, and came from Great Britain, France, Germany, and Switzerland.

In Great Britain, Thomas Addison (1793–1860) produced a major work on the adrenal gland; Charles Bell (1774–1842) on paralysis of nerves in the face; Richard Bright (1789–1859) on kidney disorders; James Parkinson (1755–1824) on the shaking palsy; and Thomas Hodgkins (1798–1866) on a type of leukemia that enlarged lymph glands.

In France, Pierre Broca (1861) described the third frontal convolution's responsibility for aphasia; Gustave Dax (1863) discovered the left hemisphere lateralization in language; Claude Bernard (1865) located the motor center of language; and Jean Charcot (1873) outlined the phases in the development of hysteria as well as its signs and symptoms.

In Germany, Theodore Meynert (1833–1892) demonstrated that a stimulus excited a localized area of the brain. Inadequate brain circulation produced excitement, in his view. Carl Wernicke (1848–1905) studied brain localization, described the syndrome that bears his name, and advanced understanding of loss of memory for recent events in organic brain disorders. Willem Wundt (1832–1920) advanced knowledge of sensory physiology, and in 1886, Richard von Krafft-Ebing wrote *Psychopathia Sexualis*, a masterful description of psychopathic sexuality. Emil Kraepelin (1855–1926) introduced a description of dementia praecox in 1898. In 1883, he developed a system of classification of mental disorders in his textbook of psychiatry, *Psychiatrie Ein Lehrbuch*, which he developed in subsequent editions. Josef Breuer (1842–1925) used hypnosis in the treatment of hysteria in 1882. Sigmund Freud (1856–1939), who worked with Breuer, enjoyed his most creative years (1888–1898) and developed a basis for the understanding of the neuroses.

The preeminence of France in the study of the nervous system yielded to Germany and Switzerland in the 1860s. Wilhelm Griesinger began his research in Germany on the somatic aspects of mental disorders, which he believed were always diseases of the brain. Then, as professor of medicine in Zurich (1860–1864), the second edition of his textbook *Mental Pathology and Therapeutics* appeared. This work advanced psychiatry as a medical discipline, explained the role of infectious diseases in, and the pathological anatomy of, mental illness. Auguste Forel (1897), at Switzerland's Burgholzli, contributed to brain anatomy, hospital organization, teaching, and the study of alcoholism. Eugene Bleuler

(1857–1939), director of the Burgholzli after Forel (1898–1927), coined the term schizophrenia and detailed the concept in 1911.

In Russia, Ivan Pavlov (1849–1936) experimented with conditioned reflexes, which led to the treatment known as behavior therapy.

Four of these proved to be giants among men whose contributions to science and medicine were to change the form and practice of psychiatry in America. They were Pavlov, Kraepelin, Freud, and Bleuler.

PROGRESS IN UNDERSTANDING MENTAL ILLNESS IN AMERICA

At the end of the 18th century in America, the generally held concept that all insane persons had deranged reason lost support. It became increasingly clear that often the power to reason was maintained but the emotions and will became unbalanced. This concept, called moral insanity, was conceived as occurring in individuals with an intact intellect who, although rational, sometimes committed horrible crimes. The person's capacity to adhere to society's moral precepts was lost. From this view evolved the concepts of neurotic character and psychopathic personality.

Not all American psychiatrists believed in moral insanity. Rush apparently did, as did Todd, Wyman, Bell, Brigham, and others. John Gray was one of the more influential voices raised against it. There was extensive discussion of the concept at the 1863 annual meeting of the Association, culminating in a vote (this is reminiscent of a similar vote on the subject of homosexuality more than 100 years later). Five votes were recorded for and eight against the concept of moral insanity. The discussion brought to the forefront the legal and social implications of the decision (8).

The belief in phrenology declined in the second half of the 19th century, and the conviction grew that physical damage to the brain was the cause of insanity. Phrenology, which had many adherents in the United States from 1830 on, held that the mind was not unitary but composed of independent, identifiable faculties localized in different regions of the brain. These faculties could be consciously developed. The normal or abnormal functioning of the mind depended on the physical condition of the brain (9).

The basis of the need for institutional care of the insane and justification for the Association's view that asylums should be on the outskirts of towns was another development in the understanding of mental illness. The following is a passage from the report of Edward Jarvis, Boston psychiatrist, one of three commissioners appointed by the Governor of Massachusetts:

> The associates and the scenes of home, the common affairs of the family, and neighborhood, and business, amidst which the mind became disturbed, furnish most of the ideas and suggest most of the thoughts to those who are among them; and, therefore, if an insane person is to be relieved of the thoughts and ideas that troubled him, and have a change in his mental action, he must be removed from his home and friends, and have a change in his associates and in the objects of his attention and interest (9, p. 106).

The salutary effect of separation from troubles, and the practice of moral treatment, led to the conviction that insanity could be cured. I wish to postpone consideration of the phenomenal growth of institutional care, and to focus for the moment on the major contribution of the Jarvis Report (1855).

A three-man commission (Levi Lincoln, a former Governor of Massachusetts; Increase Sumner, a member of the state senate; and Edward Jarvis, M.D.) was appointed to guide the legislature on state policy concerning institutional care for the mentally ill. Worcester's asylum, which had been a national model, was now described "as one of the poorest if not the poorest in the country" (9), and the second institution at Taunton (1854) had in no way diminished the pressure for admissions upon the state. The Commission identified 1,017 insane in the hospitals: at Worcester, 327; Taunton, 250; Boston, 200; McLean, 200; and Pepperell, 40. Nine hundred more individuals were identified as mildly insane and harmless, who could be cared for at home. Another 700 were in need of care, some 150 were in jails or prisons, and 40 were in almshouses, for whom no places were available. The figures are not as important as Jarvis' clear finding that "the problems posed by mental illness were inextricably intertwined with the broader issue of indigency and welfare" (9, p. 71). Jarvis had introduced social class and ethnic factors into a public policy discussion. (Years later these ideas would be refined in studies by social scientists.) Also contained in the report were the ideas that some have chronic and incurable illness; that the poor and those from other cultures require different approaches to treatment; and that individualized treatment in small hospitals, where close personal relationships between patient and staff were possible, was the treatment of choice.

At the 10th annual meeting of the Association in 1855, the report received extensive discussion. Bell, Kirkbride, and Ray praised it. The Association unanimously adopted a resolution commending the Jarvis Report "as the first successful attempt in America to secure entirely reliable statistics on this subject" (10, p. 94). The concern over the report was to begin a controversy about separate institutions for chronic mental patients, and a 10-year effort to develop propositional statements on national policy that was culminated in 1866.

Laboratory Development

Psychologists, who in the previous century had worked in relation to philosophy, began to study sensation and learning in the laboratory. The first psychological laboratory was founded in 1878 by Willem Wundt in Germany, and the first in the United States was founded at Clark University, Worcester, Massachusetts, by G. Stanley Hall in 1883 (11).

It was Adolf Meyer who established the first pathological laboratory in a mental hospital in America, at the Illinois Eastern Hospital in Kankakee (1895). When Meyer moved to Worcester, he started a laboratory in that state hospital in 1895. A major step toward organized research in the public system was taken in New York in 1895 with the establishment of the Pathological Institute of New York State Hospital. Ira Van Gilson was its first director and Adolf Meyer its second. Within a short span many other laboratories appeared in state hospitals before the turn of the century (12).

MEDICINE DURING THE CIVIL WAR

Though the threat of war had been present for 10 years, America was unprepared when the Civil War began in 1861. There was no plan for the delivery of medical services in the field, no hospital system, and no plan for casualty evacuation (13, 14). In June of

1861, President Lincoln appointed the United States Sanitary Commission. It was a body of 500 physicians, military officers, clergymen, and laymen. Their assigned task was to provide the Army medical department with doctors and nurses and "whatever else relates to care of the sick and wounded" (13, p. 369).

It was not until April 1862 that a Surgeon General of the Army was appointed: William A. Hammond, a young man of strength, clinical skills, and drive, who developed a medical service, founded the Army medical museum, and whose vision recommended an Army medical school and a Surgeon General's library.*

In 1863, Hammond designated "a ward be set apart in either South or Christian Street Hospital (Philadelphia) for the exclusive treatment of diseases of the nervous system" (13, p. 369). Drs. S. Wier Mitchell and George R. Moorehouse were assigned to be in charge. Later, when more space was required, W. W. Keene joined them. On this original group of three was built the foundation for the specialty of neurology in the United States. Together they surveyed the extent of malingering among military patients. They described a form of emotional disorder that they called "nostalgia," which 50 years later would be called combat exhaustion (14).

The prevailing opinion was that any soldier who failed to perform his duty in combat when he was not sick or wounded was a coward. It was policy to grant a furlough only rarely. One Army surgeon, J. Thomas Calhoun, advocated a liberal leave allowance to allow men to rest and to maintain morale as a counter to nostalgia. Nostalgia was described as a species of melancholy caused by a continuous longing for home. Calhoun noted that action in battle tended to alleviate nostalgia when hardship and danger were shared. This flash of insight would years later become the principle of identification with the group or unit, a period of respite from stress away from the battle zone, and early return to duty after illness or injury. S. Wier Mitchell developed his "rest cure" out of his military experiences (15).

---

* Hammond was promoted to the position of Surgeon General over the heads of several eligible officers. He got into conflict with the Secretary of War, Stanton, and the result was a court martial and dismissal on charges of irregularity in handling supplies. A review of the court martial in 1879 vindicated Hammond. Hammond became a leading neurologist, a professor of nervous diseases, and author of the textbook *A Treatise on Insanity in Its Medical Relations* (1871).

In the four years of war 2,600 cases of insanity were identified and 5,200 cases of nostalgia required hospital care. In addition to the concept of nostalgia, the work related to neurology, and the survey on malingering (relating it to the bounty system), the need for screening out potential mental disorders was noted—a need that was not remembered when the next great conflict again immersed the country in war.

The Civil War demonstrated the necessity for planning medical services and increased awareness of the tremendous manpower loss resulting from infection and infectious diseases. During the years of the Civil War, it was the neurologists who seized the opportunity to serve casualties and to carry out studies utilizing the war experience in order to advance knowledge.

At its meeting in May 1864 in Washington, D.C., the Association directed Charles H. Nichols, Superintendent of the Government Hospital for the Insane (St. Elizabeths), to call upon the Surgeon General and to offer the services of the Association "to assist in the care of the sick and wounded now at Fredericksburg" (13, p. 378). (The military hospital was filled with the recently wounded.) The offer was declined with thanks by the Surgeon General with the comment "should a more urgent situation arise, we will call upon you." There is no record that a call was ever made. Dorothea Dix gave an account of her observations in the field at the 1864 meeting of the Association. It was an accolade to the heroic conduct of soldiers wounded in combat.

Another matter aroused emotions at the 1864 meeting. Soldiers with mental disorders, it was said, were discharged from the army and found confused, lost, and wandering, or were released from government hospitals without supervision or an escort home when required. This prompted a letter of protest to the War Department, citing several instances of improper release. Earlier the Surgeon General had issued an order prohibiting the discharge of mentally ill soldiers on certification of disability. The reply the Association received from the War Department indicated that soldiers would be transported to the nearest asylum (or to the Government Hospital for the Insane) and would pay for hospital care at 75 cents per day.

One finding surprised the public at the time of the Civil War: rates for insanity among civilians did not increase during the war years. This was to be rediscovered as true in national disasters when all were united in a mutual effort.

PROGRESS TOWARD A MODEL IN
MEDICAL EDUCATION

The recognition and treatment of mental disorders was not taught in medical schools, save for an occasional lecture, until after the Civil War. The subject area was seldom mentioned in the schools before the 1880s. Awareness of the importance of the inclusion of information about mental disorders developed slowly following the recognition of the need for reform in all of medical education. A working model was not developed until the late 1890s when Johns Hopkins put into practice the recommended action (16).

The lack of instruction in the mental diseases was the subject of a formal resolution of the Association of Medical Superintendents in 1871:

> *Resolved:* That in view of the frequency of mental disorders among all classes and descriptions of people, and in recognition of the fact that the first care of nearly all these cases necessarily devolves upon physicians engaged in general practice . . . it is the unanimous opinion of this Association that in every medical school conferring medical degrees, there should be delivered by competent professors, a complete course of lectures on insanity. . . .

> *Resolved:* That these lectures should be delivered before all students attending these schools and that no one be allowed to graduate without as thorough an examination on these subjects as in other branches taught in the schools.

> *Resolved:* That in connection with these lectures, whenever practicable, there should be clinical instruction . . . giving the students practical illustration of the different forms of insanity and the effects of its treatment (16, p. 152).

The short-lived Association for the Protection of the Insane and the Prevention of Insanity (about which I shall have more to say later) issued a circular in 1882 that was sent to every medical school. After a preamble which re-emphasized the important role of the general practitioner in recognizing the incipient stages of mental disease, and which noted the usually imperfect diagnosis, the lack of appropriate treatment, and the need for all students to be trained, the circular urged that a chair or lectureship in psychiatry be established in every medical school and a clinic be held in a nearby asylum. To gain an understanding of why these sensible recommendations failed to achieve their purpose, we need to look further into the ferment within the medical education system.

Benjamin Rush's book, *Medical Inquiries and Observations Upon the Diseases of the Mind,* had an enormous influence on medical education. Published in 1812 (the year before his death), it was the first text on the subject in America and was to remain dominant until superseded by Hammond's and Spitzka's textbooks on insanity in 1883. "The whole development of psychiatry has been marked by man's struggles to rise above the prejudices of his age," wrote Binger (18, p. 249), one of Rush's biographers, who noted Rush's relentless struggle for unpopular causes: against alcoholism, against capital punishment, against discrimination toward minorities and for improvement of jails and prisons, for the emancipation of women, and for free and public schools. During the last decade of the 18th century, Rush began to investigate the causes and remedies of diseases of the mind. He wrote to Thomas Jefferson that he wished to read everything written before he committed the results of his investigation to writing (18). Rush made reforms in the care of patients in asylums and put patients to work at useful tasks (occupational therapy). He gave the first course of lectures on disease of the mind and on medical jurisprudence.

It was not until 1847—35 years later—that some other formal lectures on insanity would be given. In that year Samuel M. Smith was named Chairman of Medical Jurisprudence and Insanity at Willoughby University in Columbus, Ohio, the first such department in a medical school. In 1852 Edward Mead became professor in the same subject at the Cincinnati College of Medicine and Surgery. One year later Pliny Earle delivered a course of lectures on mental diseases at the New York College of Physicians and Surgeons.

The University of Michigan was, in 1837, the first American college to give science prominence over the classics. Its medical school, begun in 1850, was planned by the university and was under university control. Its faculty was paid by the university and not by student lecture fees; it was supported by the state and had a separate laboratory building for chemistry where the subject was taught as a science. Harvard lengthened its medical education from two to three years in 1871, made the medical school a department of the university, paid faculty members, made a successful drive for endowment, required premedical education, and extended the period of schooling from 8 to 27 months. Pennsylvania also made similar changes. Mr. Johns Hopkins founded the first university on the European model in the United States in 1876, in Baltimore. A modern hospital was constructed in 1889 as part of the university and its medical school, and in the 1890s had in place a revolutionary model that marked the attainment of the goal laid down so many years before: Premedical college training with a degree was required for admission to Johns Hopkins University medical school; both men and women were admitted; the medical degree course was four years long; the faculty was fully salaried; and research was expected of both faculty and students. The hospital had interns and residents. The model was soon copied by progressive schools. What was most advantageous was the diligent search made for the most outstanding faculty it could assemble. Recruited were such greats as William Osler, William Welch, William Halsted, William H. Howell, and Henry Hurd. With the development of the educational base, teaching of diseases of the mind with clinical demonstrations became a part of the medical school curriculum in some, but not all, medical schools.

EXPANSION OF INSTITUTIONS FOR THE MENTALLY ILL

Moral Treatment Lauded

Moral treatment was a major advance in the treatment of the mentally ill (5, 7, 19–21). Its application resulted in significant recovery rates for newly admitted patients. A supportive environment and compassionate interpersonal relations were held to be central in this therapy. Early case finding, prompt application of treatment utilizing social and psychological approaches, and release to the community as soon as possible were essential elements contributing to successful outcome. The familiar historical cycle of striking results from the application of a concept by a dedicated group, loss of credibility in the confusion of change, and, years later, the rediscovery of its essential truth, characterized this therapeutic modality. Moral treatment was more than what we call milieu therapy, but included it.

Moral treatment developed out of the humanitarian movement of the late 18th century in the actions of Pinel, Tuke, and others, and in a philosophy which differentiated body from soul, or brain from mind. The brain was subject to damage by injury, tumors, blood vessel abnormality, or disease. It could also be damaged by "moral" agencies: emotional stress, overwork, religious fanaticism, and self-abuse. Any stressor of a psychological nature was referred to as a "moral" cause of damage to the brain. "Moral" becomes easier to understand if we define it as emotional or psychological. In 1847, Amariah Brigham defined moral treatment as "The removal of the insane from home and former associates with respectful and kind treatment under all circumstances, and in most cases manual labor, attendance on religious worship on Sundays, the establishment of regular habits of self control, diversion of the mind from morbid trains of thought are now generally considered as essential in the moral treatment of the insane" (20, p. 1). Pliny Earle stressed an application in the asylum akin to judicious parental management of children, applied by intelligent attendants of kind disposition, with good judgment supported by firmness.

Moral treatment was introduced into the United States at Friend's Asylum in Pennsylvania by the Quakers, who modeled their institution on England's York Retreat. McLean, Bloomingdale, and Hartford Retreat all utilized moral treatment. Its proving ground was to be Worcester State Hospital (founded in 1833) under Samuel Woodward, an ardent supporter of the method. Bockhoven (19) assembled from annual reports a 20-year series of patients who had been ill for less than one year prior to admission to Worcester State hospital. There were 2,267 such individuals: 1,618 were discharged as recovered (66 percent) or improved (5 percent or more). The results in those patients who were ill for longer than one year prior to admission (there were 4,119) were that 45 percent recovered and 14 percent improved.

The records of the Hartford Retreat from the year 1834 reported that 516 patients were treated over a period of 10 years, of whom 25 percent had recent illnesses. Of the acute cases, 230, or 90.9

percent, recovered. In 263 old cases the recovery rate was 27.3 percent (21). But the top attainment was reported by William M. Awl of Ohio State Lunatic Asylum, with a 100 percent recovery rate that gained him the nickname "Dr. Cure-Awl."

Moral Treatment Discredited

One of the first voices against moral treatment, the movement that came to be known as the "Cult of Curability," was that of Isaac Ray in his 1841 Annual Report of the Maine Insane Asylum. He called the separation into "recent" and "old" cases arbitrary and misleading, and cautioned against deceptive statistics.

Dr. Pliny Earle became Superintendent of the Northampton (Massachusetts) State Hospital in 1864. Unlike his former pre-dominantly wealthy patients at Bloomingdale, nine-tenths of his 450 patients were predominantly from the pauper classes, who were transferred to the newly opened hospital from the most chronic wards of other hospitals to make room for new admissions (24). Moral treatment, which Earle had previously used, didn't produce the expected recoveries. His rates were much lower than those his colleagues reported. He began to investigate the annual reports of other hospitals. It appears that his intention was not to discredit his fellow superintendents but to demonstrate by means of his statistical studies that cures were much less frequent than commonly believed, and to stimulate the search for alternative methods of treatment for the chronic mental diseases.

Earle's 1875 Annual Report called attention to statistical inac-curacies, lack of clarity, inconsistency in the use of the term "recovered," and the practice of counting the same patient as recovered each time the patient was admitted in one year. Earle's assembled studies were published in his book *The Curability of Insanity* in 1877, and expanded in an 1887 edition. Unfortunately, his work did not have the effect he intended. The professional view, and the popular view as well, changed from optimism (in-sanity was curable) to pessimism ("once insane, always insane").

Bockhoven (19) was to show Earle's bias, and to show that the unpublished work of Park contained raw data which confirmed the recoveries of patients who had been given moral treatment during the early years. Only about 20 percent of patients required con-tinuing care in a mental hospital for chronic mental diseases. Isaac Ray also could not accept Earle's devaluation of the early results of treatment and presented a paper rebutting Earle's findings in 1879, entitled *Recoveries from Mental Illness*, read before the College of Physicians and Surgeons in Philadelphia.

What is evident is that treatment at the Worcester State Hospital by the 1850s was not working, and the hospital was described as having so many deficiencies that Jarvis recommended against investing money for renovation and suggesting that it be sold and the proceeds used to purchase a new site (9, p. 60). The deterioration in care was not limited to Worcester. An extensive survey of mental hospitals in the United States was conducted in 1885 by George A. Tucker of Australia. His findings were published in a government report, *Lunacy in Many Lands*. What he described was excessive use of restraint, reprehensible care, and neglected patients. Miserable conditions were not universal, however, and he duly noted exceptions and good standards when he found them.

One hundred years later hindsight reveals there were multiple factors interplaying to cause the breakdown of moral treatment, which had been so successful in its early years. The loss of dedicated leaders with no trained replacements was one of these factors. The champions of moral treatment, such as Eli Todd, Samuel Woodward, and Amariah Brigham, had died. Only four of the original founders lived into the 1870s. The training of a handful of assistants was inadequate to staff the hospitals that grew from 23 in 1844 to 125 in 1895.

Small hospitals afforded individualized treatment that was essential to moral treatment. As the hospitals grew in size, the individual became submerged in the mass, and the efficacy of moral treatment declined. John S. Butler wrote a book entitled *Curability of Insanity* in 1887; its purpose was to persuade the Association of Superintendents to limit the size of hospitals. Butler had been instrumental in getting the Association to pass resolutions limiting size in 1851. Large hospitals, Butler held, harmed patients by denying them personal attention and caused them to be treated like a mob in which they lost their human attributes.

The cultural differences among the patient population that resulted from massive immigration interfered with staff–patient relationships and therefore with moral treatment. The mentally ill who came from destitute immigrant families (many of whom were Irish) came from a different culture and held values unlike those of hospital physicians and staff. Negative attitudes fostered a poor response to moral treatment. As a greater number of poor were admitted, the mentally ill who were from self-sustaining native born families diminished in the case mix. As an example, at the Worcester State Asylum in 1844, of 236 admissions, 10 percent were foreign born. In 1863 the percentage of foreign born in admissions was 47 and in 1893 it rose to 67.

The resources available for intensive, individualized treatment diminished. This resulted in a deterioration of standards of care, thereby diminishing moral treatment. Public hostility toward increased taxes to support "foreigners" influenced the legislature to decrease funding. The cost of care per day that had been comparable to the cost of general hospital care fell drastically in comparison. Overcrowding, understaffing, and underfinancing doomed moral treatment.

The conceptual shift from viewing moral treatment as the central most important part of the program to viewing it as having an adjunctive role was a crushing blow to the attitude of optimism as to the curability of insanity. Influential leaders such as John Gray, Editor of the *American Journal of Insanity*, fostered this view. (It is not unlike the central emphasis today upon drugs, with social and psychological interventions seen as peripheral.)

It is indeed remarkable that the tiny band of superintendents in the Association were able to produce excellent results from the application of moral treatment in the early days. The enduring value of their understanding that psychological factors can produce behavior changes is evident to us. We also applaud their recognition that attitudes and behavior of staff, a full day of scheduled activities, work, and recreation in balance do much to prevent chronicity and custodialism.

THE DOROTHEA DIX CRUSADE (1802–1887)

No one contributed more to the growth of institutions for the mentally ill than did Dorothea Dix. She was probably the greatest social reformer in American history. A most successful social activist, she was also a master politician who catalyzed action to provide humane care for the mentally ill. She is credited as being responsible for the building of 32 mental hospitals. It was she who most influenced the policy of state responsibility for the care of the mentally ill (27).

Before the Association of Medical Superintendents was formed, Dorothea Dix's crusade was already underway, as demonstrated by the 59-page *Memorial* to the state legislature of New York (Jan. 12, 1844). Dix, having surveyed the existing hospitals at Utica and New York City, the almshouses, prisons, and jails, was able to dramatize the shocking conditions she observed and to specify corrective action. These excerpts from her report give its flavor:

- Notwithstanding liberal appropriations, large numbers are unprovided for
- These are permitted to fall into states of most shocking and brutalizing degradation
- Idiots and insane women are exposed to the basest vice
- Dungeons, totally dark, unventilated, and loathsome, emit a horrible stench, and are a dreadful place to house the insane
- They have committed no criminal offense but exist as a hideous object, with matted locks, unshorn beards, wild countenances, disfigured by uncleanness and nudity while living in loathsome filth

Miss Dix's crusade from 1840 to 1870 was aided by Horace Mann, Samuel Gridley Howe, and by her friends in the Association—especially Isaac Ray, Luther Bell, and Pliny Earle. Dix was knowledgeable about advances in care of patients, knew all of the superintendents, and advocated adoption of Association positions when pressing for a new institution. As consultant, she would select the site and even suggest a suitable superintendent. She was more than a crusader for improved care of the mentally ill. She fought for removal of the mentally ill from almshouses, jails, and prisons, and for placement in mental hospitals under humane care. She rode the crest of public desire to improve other institutions: schools, colleges, hospitals, and prisons. Above all, she insisted that humane care was the responsibility of the state.

As early as 1848, she pushed for federal responsibility for the insane. In her first *Memorial* to Congress she called for a grant of five million acres of land in the public domain, the proceeds from the sale to be set apart to create a perpetual fund for the care of the indigent insane. Five thousand copies of her *Memorial* were published. Her request died in a congressional committee. She was better prepared when she reintroduced an expanded bill requesting a land grant of 10 million acres and 2 ½ million acres for the blind and deaf.

The Association passed the following resolve in 1851 in support of Miss Dix's actions:

> That this Association regards with deep interest the progress of the magnificent project, which has been and continues to be urged . . . proposing the grant of a portion of the public domain . . . the proceeds of which are to be devoted to the endorsement of public charities throughout the country and that it meets with our unqualified sanction.
>
> —Thomas S. Kirkbride, Secretary

The Land Grant Act passed both houses of Congress in 1851, although maneuvering kept the bill in Congress until it was cleared through Miss Dix's persuasion in 1854. Six years of struggle came to naught when President Pierce vetoed the bill in 1854. He said, "The government can grant no aid for any humanitarian cause for it would transfer to the federal government responsibility for all the poor" (5, p. 178).

President Pierce did sign Miss Dix's bill to establish The Government Hospital for the Insane (St. Elizabeths). She continued her crusade in Scotland, Italy, Greece, and Constantinople, returning to become head of women nurses in the Civil War. (For a brief biography of Dorothea Dix, see (22) and Appendix C.)

INSTITUTIONAL REFORM: CONTROLS AND SYSTEMS

Criticism of asylums for the insane began in the post-Civil War reconstruction period (1865) and continued well into the 1890s. Dorothea Dix's crusade was still underway with the building of new institutions. The influx of immigrants created a change in the case mix, with more foreign than native born patients. Moral treatment had become ineffective and, as the quality of care deteriorated, chronic patients accumulated. The Association of Medical Superintendents' stand was inflexible on limiting the size of institutions, so it viewed building more institutions and increasing the number of staff as the appropriate course to follow. State governments sought to remedy deteriorating care and the loss of public confidence in asylums by monitoring, regulating, and unifying the system under state control. In the process, the superintendents lost autonomy of their institutions and the Association lost prestige. Criticism of asylum care came from other organizations, from the press, and from the public. It led to reform in institutions and in the Association, with a return of optimism and confidence at the end of the 19th century.

The crescendo of criticism of asylums occurred at a time of great change in society. The South was in economic collapse. Lincoln's intention, supported by President Andrew Johnson, was to act as though southern states had never seceded in order to restore the Union. Congress overruled the plan establishing military districts and military government in the South (troops were withdrawn in 1877). In order to rejoin the Union, each state had to adopt a new constitution guaranteeing equality to all citizens and profess loyalty to the United States. The 1866 Civil Rights Act gave all rights to Negroes. "Carpetbaggers," the Northern military presence, and the repressive repatriation of "enemy states" would build a century-long hatred of Yankees. Former slaves, often illiterate and dependent on plantation owners, were set adrift without the skills necessary to adjust in the financially ruined South, while plantation owners had no money to pay farm labor after the disintegration of the plantation system.

An economic depression that began in 1870 stifled, for awhile, attempts to increase resources to the asylums at the very time they were under attack. One strand of public criticism of the asylum system developed in 1860 when Mrs. E. P.W. Packard was committed to the Illinois State Hospital for the Insane by her husband and, as Grob (23) suggests, "by the probable cooperation of Dr. Andrew McFarland, the Superintendent." There had been exposés of mental hospitals before 1860, but this one attracted nationwide attention, as Mrs. Packard was an effective crusader. She induced the Illinois state legislature to investigate hospitals and to pass legislation to insure legal safeguards. In 1867, Illinois law protected personal liberty and established procedural safeguards by providing a jury trial in sanity hearings. Other states, such as Massachusetts and Pennsylvania, took similar action (23, 24).

In addition to criticism in the public press, British psychiatrists were critical of American superintendents who relied too much on restraint, and were critical of the custodial nature of American mental hospitals (25). Tucker, of Australia, visited most American mental hospitals between 1882 and 1883, and reported that superintendents were so overburdened with the details of management and clinical duties that they had no time or inclination for scientific studies, or even for the proper care of their patients (25, 26).

The controversy was fanned by an attack on asylum superintendents by Dr. Harvey B. Wilbur (a superintendent of a school for the mentally retarded in Syracuse, New York) before the Conference of Charities (which became a principal forum for asylum reform). He stated that newly built asylums were extravagant and unfit, trustees were perfunctory in inspections, and that superintendents were loaded down with duties but absent from their posts to be expert witnesses in court, and absent from their posts to be present at lucrative consulting practices. This left the institutions, he said, in the care of inexperienced assistants who overused restraint (13). Later Dr. Wilbur would become the first president of another group, the National Association for the Protection of the Insane, critical of asylum management.

The attack by neurologists upset the Association of Medical Superintendents the most. In 1878 and 1879, the New York Neurological Society petitioned the legislature to investigate asylums and to correct abuses (18). The National Neurological Association published in its 1879 journal an attack upon the superintendents charging isolation from the rest of medicine; failure to use outside consultants; failure to engage in scientific studies; failure to deliver promised cures; fraud in building of institutions and purchase of supplies; corruption and abuse of patients; and need for better supervision (21, 13, 27). Neurologists also appointed a committee that included George Beard and E.C. Sequin to form a new association, the National Association for the Protection of the Insane and the Prevention of Insanity (NAPIPI).

The NAPIPI was formed in Cleveland on July 1, 1880. Several members of the Association of Medical Superintendents joined this reform group, including John S. Butler, William Gedding, Walter Channing, and others. The objectives of the reform group were:

1. To thoroughly observe the clinical and pathological aspects of asylum management
2. To educate the public regarding the nature of mental illness, early treatment, and improved management
3. To press for enlightened state policy with no unnecessary tax burden
4. To attend public meetings to stimulate state supervision for protection of society and of patients

5. To protect patient rights
6. To overcome public disinterest in asylums by making asylums more like other hospitals (18, 26).

The new organization got off to a flying start, supported by the National Neurological Association, by social workers, and by many general physicians. The magazines picked up the charge: insanity was increasing, palatial asylums had failed to check the increase, and patients were neglected and abused (18).

At the 1881 meeting of the Association of Medical Superintendents, Superintendent R. Gundry of the Maryland State Hospital ventured that some of the criticism was justified, and "inner reform" could forestall drastic measures imposed from outside the Association. In response, John P. Gray stated that he favored centralized lunacy boards. He restated the Association's stand against outside "meddlers," and then decried the critics of hospitals as numbskulls and scoundrels bent on personal vengeance (5).

The defensive posture would continue for a decade and asylum superintendents would become beleaguered specialists. In spite of resolutions introduced by Isaac Ray (1875) opposing "supernumerary functionaries" with supervisory authority, reforms were made (23). Building on Massachusetts' first attempt to centralize policymaking and supervision under a Board of State Charities (1863), some 12 key states followed with administrative solutions. A single State Board of Health, Lunacy, and Charity was created in Massachusetts in 1879. No sooner were the agencies linked when pressures developed to separate them again (23). The struggles are reminiscent of 20th century cycles of separate versus umbrella systems, and centralization versus decentralization.

As a consequence of internal dissension and external pressure, the Association of Medical Superintendents was powerless to halt the advance of state management systems. "Few could quarrel with the goal of making the welfare system and its varied institutions function in an efficient and rational manner" (23, p. 81). Although policy didn't change significantly, administrative solutions introduced investigations, state control, monitoring of practice standards, common fiscal procedures, record keeping, and uniform statistical information.

The struggle to separate the care of the indigent from that of the mentally ill continued in the 1870s and 1880s. State Boards of Charities divided to establish Commissioners of Lunacy. By 1889 mental hospitals serving geographical districts were ready for the changes, stimulated by advancing medical sciences in Europe, which would shift managerial concerns to clinical issues of biology and diagnosis.

From 1865 onward the search for alternatives to care of the chronic mentally ill was a major issue for the Association of Medical Superintendents. Separate institutions for long-term care, farm colonies, and family care were introduced. In the latter half of the 20th century the problem remains and the solutions sound like the earlier ones with different labels: nursing homes, rehabilitation and sheltered workshops, and group homes.

THE DEVELOPMENT OF INSTITUTIONS FOR THE MENTALLY RETARDED

Institutional care for the mentally retarded began in the poorhouse and almshouse in America (5, 28–34). For example, in 1736, New York's Poor House, Work House, and House of Correction accepted the dull in mind along with the crippled, diseased, offenders, and insane whose families could not care for them when they were unable to support themselves, or when they were jailed for some offense. By the middle of the 18th century, law breakers were segregated in prisons or jails, and the almshouse cared for the other groups. As mental hospitals evolved they accepted some mentally deficient, in addition to mentally ill, individuals.

The period of growth of institutions for the insane occurred earlier than the period of growth of institutions for the feeble-minded or mentally retarded. The spurt in the number of asylums occurred during the years of Dorothea Dix's crusade, from the 1840s to the 1870s. Institutions for the feebleminded grew in the last 15 years of the 19th century. Both institutional systems arose in response to the humanitarian desire to correct social injustice. Asylums and hospitals grew following advances in medicine and the optimism engendered by the success of moral treatment. State schools for the retarded followed the development of concepts in education and the encouraging results of experimental trials of education and training. Both systems fostered release back to the community as soon as improvement made this practical. Each system found release increasingly difficult when the number admitted outstripped its capacity to meet individual patient or student needs. Early optimism gave way to pessimism and a conviction that most conditions were irreversible.

From the date of its founding in 1844, the Association of Medical Superintendents demonstrated a concern for the mentally retarded. Awl addressed the 1844 meeting and noted "the importance and need for asylums for the care and instruction of idiots in our country" (28, p. 1130). Others also spoke to the topic and this led to the appointment of a committee, "Asylums for Idiots and the Demented," with Awl as Chairman, and Brigham and White as Cochairmen.

In 1845 both Woodward and Brigham, in their annual reports, referred to the plight of idiots in their asylums and in the community, and called for the erection of an institution for their care. Woodward noted that training had been successful in France. Brigham noted 1,600 idiots in "a wretched state" in New York. Both influenced the legislature, in their respective states, to act. Massachusetts appointed a commission headed by Samuel Gridley Howe, and New York authorized an experimental school.

When the Association met next in Washington, D.C. on May 11, 1846, it heard the reports of its committees. Awl, when named Vice-President to replace White (who had died during the interim), relinquished the chair of the Committee on Idiots to Brigham. The report made note of a fact of history: The first public movement on the subject of an institution for the idiots in our country took place in neither Boston nor New York, "but before the Association met for the first time in October of 1844." It began, according to Awl, in the city of Philadelphia in 1844 (33).

Origins: Care of the Mentally Retarded Before 1850

Hippocrates was aware that anencephaly and cranial malformation may be found in idiots. Sparta and Rome had laws permitting the extermination of severely retarded infants (revived by the Nazis in our lifetime). It appears that ancient China and Persia were humane in their approach to the feebleminded, whereas medieval Europe sometimes saw them as sinister, evil beings—the work of the devil—or as freaks and occasionally as court "fools." The Jewish Talmud exempted the retarded from criminal responsibility, while 13th-century law in Great Britain put imbeciles under the protection of the King (36, 37).

John Locke (1632–1704), an English philosopher and teacher at Oxford, was also a student of chemistry, meteorology, theology, and medicine. He left England in 1683 to escape its intrigues and oppressive politics, living in Holland until he returned with William of Orange. He was 54 when he began to write so effectively that he captured the attention of scholars everywhere. He spoke out in defense of religious freedom, on civil liberty, on the ultimate sovereignty of the people, on personal identity, on free inquiry, on universal toleration, and on the natural rights to property and personal freedom. He said government had no right to interfere with religious beliefs not inconsistent with civil society, and asserted the right of the people to govern themselves. This great mind initiated modern concepts of the foundation and limits of knowledge. In 1693, he wrote a classic essay, *Thoughts on Education*. In this essay he emphasized that the goal of acquiring information was secondary to having a useful character, good health, and a child who was happy while being taught. Learning, he said, was facilitated when curiosity of the child was stimulated and associated with some personal experience.

In Colonial America of 1661, town officers were charged with the duty to care for the mildly insane or idiots in their homes. The idiot could earn part of his keep as a servant of the master. Locke's writing may have been catalytic to freedom lovers everywhere, but stimulated no action to educate the retarded.

It was a most unlikely character, Jean-Jacques Rousseau (1712–1778), who contributed insightful observations on education. He was an engraver's apprentice, a runaway, a wanderer, an adventurer, educated by a woman whose lover he was, a music copier, a philosopher, and a writer with no formal education, whose ideas made him a hero of the French Revolution. It was his eloquence, not his logic, that gained him attention. In 1762 he wrote *Emile*, which inspired educational reform. Rousseau said it was important to allow children to learn through the senses from which ideas originated, and to learn by doing things for themselves, unhampered by rigid external restrictions (35).

Rousseau influenced Johann Pestalozzi (1746–1827), a Swiss educator and teacher of children of the poor. Pestalozzi believed that knowledge stemmed from observation, which, in turn, stimulated development of one's innate potential. Influenced by this work, Frederick Froebel (1782–1852), a German educator, believed that a child is like a flower that blooms best when nurtured by an interested gardener. (He coined the word *kindergarten* to encompass the application of this concept.) He advocated free play, nature study, field trips, and handcrafts under permissive guidance of the teacher.

It was in this educational climate that, in 1798, a 17-year-old boy, nude and savage, living in the wild on nuts and roots, was found by hunters in Aveyron, France. The hunters brought him to Jean Itard, the Chief Medical Officer of the Institute for Deaf and Dumb in Paris. Pinel saw the boy in consultation and thought he was mentally defective and not educable. Itard postulated that his inability to use language and his savage behavior were due to lack of civilizing influences. Itard's efforts were the first serious attempts to educate a mentally retarded person. In five years the lad did improve in social behavior.

The progress of Itard's work was followed by intellectuals as well as the general public. Edward Sequin was Itard's student at this time; he would later become a powerful force for education of idiots in the United States. At the time Itard was conducting his experiment, the feebleminded were cared for in insane asylums. Esquirol advanced knowledge by differentiating idiocy from dementia. In 1824, Belhomme published an essay on idiocy while he was a physician at Salpetriere, where he became convinced that the feebleminded were teachable. In 1829 Ferrus, at Bicetre, organized a school with basic instruction in reading, writing, exercise, and, in 1832, added farm work.

It was upon this foundation that Sequin built when he began to test his ideas at Bicetre in 1839. He described his work in 1846 in his book *Moral Treatment, Hygiene and Education of Idiots* (29). The program Sequin followed in education of the feebleminded divided pupils according to ability: slow learners, intermediates, and fast achievers. Each unit of activity was geared to what the group could succeed in doing. The full day of planned work began at 5:00 A.M. and continued until bedtime after 8:00 P.M. Personal hygiene was taught, as was geometric drawing, development of all the senses, counting objects, gymnastic exercise, reading, writing, music, speech instruction, and crafts or manual labor (29). Sequin's book influenced H.B. Wilbur to try the instructional method on the feebleminded boy whom he brought into his house in Barre, Massachusetts, in July 1848.

Samuel G. Howe opened an experimental school in South Boston in October 1848, which after three years became the Massachusetts School for Idiots and Feebleminded Persons (later Walter E. Fernald State School). Sequin came to America in 1848 and was appointed the first superintendent of the Boston school (29).

Sequin visited all of the established schools. The New York school, opened originally in Albany, had been moved to Syracuse (1854) by the time of Sequin's visit. The Pennsylvania Training School for the Feebleminded at Elwyn, Pennsylvania, had been founded in 1853 (5). Sequin was advisor and consultant to all of the individuals who founded schools for the feebleminded in this country. (Sequin's son, Edward, born in 1843, figured prominently in the development of neurology in this country, in the development of the mental hygiene movement, and in the Association of Medical Officers of American Institutions for Idiots and Feebleminded Persons.)

Two other events in the development of institutional care for the mentally retarded should be mentioned. In 1818 the Hartford (Connecticut) School for Deaf and Dumb admitted several idiots for training. This endeavor seems to have had little impact on the institutional movement, unless it influenced Howe in Boston to admit idiots for trial education at his school for the blind and deaf in 1837. The second event occurred in Switzerland in the mid-19th century, when Guggenbuhl introduced institutional treatment of the retarded. Guggenbuhl believed that all retardation was a manifestation of cretinism; his promise of total cure was, however, unfulfilled. Through his treatment attempts he did make the study of mental retardation a respectable field of medicine and a legitimate educational endeavor (31).

Building on the Past: Care of the Mentally Retarded, 1850–1899

The early institutions in Massachusetts, New York, and Pennsylvania that have already been mentioned, as well as those in Ohio (1857), Connecticut (1857), Kentucky (1860), and Illinois (1865), all started as experiments to determine what education and training for the mentally retarded might accomplish. These institutions were also considered a necessary but omitted link in the public education chain and were, therefore, designated as schools. The capacity of these institutions was enlarged when physicians as well as the public became convinced that real improvement had taken place in the patient's social behavior, self-esteem, and ability to work (34). When the Massachusetts School at South Boston planned to expand onto a new site in Waverly, the report of its achievement was so compellingly written that it was widely distributed in the United States, Canada, and England under the title *On the Causes of Idiocy* (34).

Using the occasion of the Centennial Exposition in Philadelphia, seven medical superintendents met at the Pennsylvania Training School in Elwyn on June 6, 1876. The invitation to attend stated that they would "consider matters relating to the care and education of idiots and feebleminded." Present were Edward Sequin (New York), son of the pioneer in the field; Harvey B. Wilbur (New York); G. A. Doren (Ohio); Charles T. Wilbur (Illinois); H. M. Knight (Connecticut); Isaac Kerlin (Pennsylvania); and (on June 7th) G. W. Brown (Massachusetts). The group drew up a constitution, adopted the name The Association of Medical Officers of American Institutions for Idiots and Feebleminded Persons, elected officers (President, Sequin; Vice-President, H. B. Wilbur; and Secretary-Treasurer, Kerlin), and established the *Proceedings* of the Association to record their transactions. The objectives of the new organization were to influence the establishment of new institutions and to be concerned with causes, conditions, statistics, management, training, and education of the feebleminded and idiots.

When the Association of Medical Officers of American Institutions for Idiots and Feebleminded Persons was founded, there were only seven states with such facilities. Growth was slow and the group attending annual meetings was small—less than 10 for the first 20 years* (35). During the early years major concerns of the

---

* The name was changed in 1906 to American Association for the Study of the Feebleminded. In 1934 the present designation was adopted, American Association on Mental Deficiency. The transactions of the Association were recorded in *Proceedings* from 1876–1895. From 1896–1939, the official publication was the *Journal of Psycho Asthenia*, a term devised as a universal word that implied knowledge of idiocy and feeblemindedness, and that included epilepsy. The Association's official publication from 1940–1970 was the *American Journal of Mental Deficiency*, which is still published. In 1971, *Mental Retardation—MR*—recorded official business of the Association.

Association were to develop separate public institutions for the idiots and feebleminded where none existed; to explore the relationship of feeblemindedness to alcoholism, vagrancy, prostitution, and criminality; and to institute educational and vocational programs to increase self-reliance. The public never supported the Association's recommendation to sterilize the retarded as a preventive measure (although Indiana did legislate asexualization in 1907, and by 1915, eight states had laws permitting it.) With the passing of the founders, the emergence of new leaders, and the waning interest in sterilization, the struggling Association that had barely survived the disinterest of members and fiscal problems began a period of vigorous growth and expansion. There were 10,000 members of the Association in its centennial year.

In 1877, Isaac Kerlin formulated principles for the institutional care of the feebleminded:

- The feebleminded should be placed in separate institutions, and not in insane asylums, almshouses, or penal institutions.
- Idiots and imbeciles should be separated in treatment programs.
- Well organized institutional care is better than home care (34).

Kerlin adopted Froebel's kindergarten and lowered the ages of admission. He introduced music into the treatment of his patients. He was astonished to discover that some who could not read were able to learn to play by note. Doren formed a band, and Stewart had 75 percent of his students in industrial placement programs (such as shoemaking, farming, mattress making, and chair caning). In 1881, Illinois was the first state to establish a farm colony for older boys. The Boston School in its 1880 report noted "20 percent of its boys under proper supervision could work on a farm and pay for their keep" (29, p. 31). In 1881 Massachusetts purchased the Howe farm near Medfield for this purpose and later a 1,600-acre farm at Templeton.

In the 40th year of its operation the Boston School appointed Walter E. Fernald (1859–1924) to be its Superintendent. Under his inspiring leadership, the institution he built on the site at Waverly for 400 students was to become a national model for the care of the retarded, just as the Worcester Asylum had been in the 1830s for the care of the insane. Fernald was a builder, a superb administrator, an educator (he established the finest library on mental retardation in the world) constructing a model 24-hour student program, a scientist (he inaugurated the Waverly Researches in Pathology of the Feebleminded), and a consultant. Thousands of delegates, many from Europe, came to study the methods used in the school. No institution was built without Fernald's advice. He taught physicians and staff members, established (in 1891) free outpatient diagnostic clinics, started special classes in public schools for the developmentally disabled, and advocated farm colonies and separate institutions for the defective delinquents. His influence in the first quarter of the 20th century was even greater.

A period of great expansion in the number of institutions for the retarded began in 1888 when there were but 15 in as many states. By 1927 there were 73 in 43 states and the District of Columbia. In 1923 there were, in addition to the state facilities, 89 private institutions for the retarded. Only five states had no provision for the feebleminded. As the century closed (1896), L. Whitmer coined the term "clinical psychology" in connection with his establishment of the first psychologic clinic to use remedial educational methods in treating mental retardation. The institutional system of care for the retarded was firmly established at the century's end.

GROWTH OF ORGANIZED PSYCHIATRY

In the latter half of the 19th century, the Association of Medical Superintendents was forced to turn from the improvement of their small asylums to larger issues created by mental illness (5, 17, 25, 36–39). The gap widened between the goal of individualized treatment and its practice as an increasing number of persons in need of care for mental illness were identified. The "moral management" period ended at the time of the Civil War. With the exploding population came an increase in illness, insanity, feeblemindedness, dependency, and crime. Available resources were drained as all institution populations continued to rise. Almshouses, prisons, and asylums were overcrowded.

In the post-Civil War period of economic collapse in the South, a depression in the 1870s, political tensions, and the dominance of other societal concerns, the condition of mental hospitals deteriorated. The optimism as to the curability of mental illness faded in a torrent of criticism of the Association and its institutions. The outcry was to persist until the 1890s, when the era of reform began.

The disaffection with the establishment caring for the mentally ill was not confined to one state or institution. Society had little confidence in physicians in general and did not acknowledge that the medical professional possessed any special knowledge; as a consequence, society bestowed no special privilege upon medical doctors. In this regard, not much had changed since colonial times. Lay healers were still seen as equal to physicians in importance and effectiveness. Just as the religious sects multiplied (with the Mormons, Swedenborgians, Christian Scientists, and denominational splits) so did the medical sects multiply to disunite the medical profession. There were Thomsonians, Grahamites, homeopaths, eclectics, and, in the 1890s, osteopaths and chiropractors.

Medical education posed an ongoing dilemma: If standards were set high, too few would benefit, for the untrained were equally acceptable to the general public. Instead, medical schools admitted all interested students and had little influence on the competence of the profession as a whole. Top students usually chose to study for the ministry or the law. In the 1850s the Massachusetts Medical Society purged itself of "heretics" (sectarians), and court battles followed over the right to expel dissenters from traditional medicine. By 1871, approximately 13 percent of physicians and 15 out of 75 medical schools were sectarian (40).

Authority was slowly gained by physicians and solidified in the 1890s and in the early decades of the 20th century. Reforms in medical education and evidence of legitimacy in application of the new science, coupled with internal unity of the medical organizations, were key factors in winning public favor. Other factors were collective action taken to win public support, establishment of clear boundaries of competence, and building of confidence and trust with patients (40).

The last half of the 19th century witnessed the construction of 110 state mental hospitals, among them 38 new county, 2 city, and 12 church-operated or nonprofit mental hospitals. The attempt to meet the demand for care with a greater number of institutions, or by statewide management systems and governmental regulations, did not solve the problem of the increasing numbers of chronic mental patients who were unresponsive to existing methods of treatment. This problem and lack of solutions led to the Association's major concerns during the period 1850–1899: issues of policy, medical–legal issues, and political interference.

Policy

The design and planning of hospital construction, with the evolution of propositions (standards), and the details of lighting, heating, and ventilation, were the earliest concerns of the Association. At the fourth annual meeting (1849) in Utica, New York, members visited the nearby institution which had been publicly criticized as a "palace for paupers," and gave support to the idea that comfort of asylum residents was essential to proper care and treatment. Asylums, they said, should be well planned for convenience and should be attractive both inside and outside. As an example of concern with detailed standards, the Association passed a resolve in 1849 that pure air at proper temperature should be an essential element in the treatment of the sick. The best method for achieving this goal was to pass fresh air over pipes or plates containing steam or hot water (not above 212° Fahrenheit at the boiler) and that large air chambers should be located in the cellar (37). At the 1851 annual meeting, standards on construction of hospitals were adopted as follows:

- *Planning:* to be done by experienced physicians
- *Location:* in the country, less than two miles from town
- *Site:* not less than 50 acres, and 100 acres for 200 beds
- *Size:* 200 to 250 beds, maximum, with 8 wards, providing separation for sexes and allowing classification of patients by behavior
- *Fire safety:* stone or brick with slate or metal roof, iron or stone stairways with sufficient number for egress, and 10-foot-wide corridors
- *Utilities:* fresh warmed air (as in the 1849 resolve), underground drains and sewers, and gas lighting; as it was clean, safe, and economical, an adequate number of waterclosets and bathrooms, with 10,000 gallons daily water supply

- *Wards:* all patient rooms above ground, single rooms 8 × 10 in size with 12-foot ceilings, windows with movable glazed sashes framing a pleasant view from each patient quarter, parlor, clothes room, dining room with dumbwaiter and speaking tube to kitchen, and dormitory for two attendants adjacent to patient quarters
- *Design:* central administrative section with lateral wings for patients: the central section to include offices, visitor's space, and an apartment for the superintendent (37)
- *Miscellaneous amenities:* walled recreation yard, detached laundry

Public policy, articulated first in 1851, was to remain an active issue for the Association for 17 years. It was first stated as a resolve: The community has a duty to provide suitable care for all classes of the insane. Care and treatment of the insane is the responsibility of a resident medical superintendent. It is improper to confine the insane in county poorhouses or in correctional institutions (41).

In 1866, after years of discussion on the proper size of a mental hospital, and after heated arguments on the desirability of separate institutions for the chronic patient, the Association adopted the following positions:

1. Every State should make ample and suitable provision for all its insane.
2. That insane persons considered curable, and those supposed incurable, should not be provided for in separate establishments.
3. The large States should be divided into geographical districts of such size that a hospital situated at, or near, the centre of the district, will be practically accessible to all the people living within its boundaries, and available for their benefit in cases of mental disorder.
4. All State, County, and City Hospitals for the Insane, should receive all persons belonging to the vicinage designed to be accommodated by such hospital, who are affected with insanity proper, whatever may be the form or nature, of the bodily disease accompanying the mental disorder.

5. All hospitals for the insane should be constructed, organized, and managed substantially in accordance with the propositions adopted by the Association in 1851 and 1852, and still in force.
6. The facilities for classification, or ward separation, possessed by each institution, should equal the requirements of the different conditions of the several classes received by such institutions whether those different conditions are mental or physical in their character.
7. The enlargement of a City, County or State institution for the insane which, in the extent and character of the district in which it is situated, is conveniently accessible to all the people of such district, may be properly carried, as required, to the extent of accommodating six hundred patients, embracing the usual proportions of curable and incurable insane in a particular community. (42, pp. 61–62)

The vote on the last statement was nine in favor and five against. Some still felt strongly that individualized treatment, essential to the effectiveness of moral treatment, could best be carried out only in small hospitals.

New York, the state with the biggest problems, broke both the barriers in size (first at Utica) and in segregation of the chronic patients (at Willard in 1869, with 1,500 chronic patients assembled from almshouses). Similar problems were present in California, Illinois, Massachusetts, and Pennsylvania. The Association stand was seen as rigid, out of touch with reality, uneconomical, and, as a consequence, it lost credibility (5). Moreover, the public and the patients objected to the label "incurable." Opposition to separate institutions mounted until most states abandoned the practice. Wisconsin reverted to the use of county asylums when recovery did not occur within one year of admission (5).

Compromises that defused some of the argument over segregation of the chronic mental patient in a separate institution were the construction of separate buildings (the cottage plan as distinguished from the Kirkbride plan) and the use of farm colonies. Dr. Charles H. Nichols, the first Superintendent of the Government Hospital for the Insane who had served under Amariah Brigham at Utica, was probably the first to institute the multiple building concept as he modified the Kirkbride plan and constructed a separate building for "colored insane" and later a military hospital as well as other buildings (39).* However, the multiple building concept, as a compromise solution for segregation of acute from chronic patients, would be more widely applicable after an 1870 conference of Illinois officials. A comprehensive study of existing institutions was made with consensus that the "cottage system in combination with that presently in vogue is desirable" and would "increase both the economy and efficiency of asylums" (5, p. 212). The result was a group of small buildings, each having about 100 persons, grouped around a central building constructed at Kankakee—the Illinois State Hospital—in 1877 (5). Multiple buildings permitted differentiation into classes "to allow each patient the largest measure of liberty of which he is individually capable" (5).

The colony system was introduced at the State Asylum in Kalamazoo, Michigan, as a farm colony in 1885. Studies of institutions in Europe convinced some superintendents that stable chronic patients could benefit from work on a farm in a separate colony. However, the idea preceded the application in practice. The annual report of Richard Hill in 1863 at the Columbus, Ohio, State Lunatic Asylum had proposed a farm colony for the insane to be planned as a village. At the 1867 meeting of the Association, Dr. Joseph Workman of the Provincial Lunatic Asylum at Toronto read a paper entitled *Asylum for the Chronic Insane in Upper Canada*. In his paper he described the establishment of "branch asylums" about three miles from the parent institution that had

---

* Dr. Nichol's annual reports of 1856, 1859, and 1860 elaborate the concept. It is interesting to note the role Dorothea Dix played in the founding of this hospital. The Secretary of the Interior and President Millard Fillmore inspected the site and were advised by Miss Dix to choose a part of the old St. Elizabeths tract which had a commanding view high above the Potomac River. Miss Dix also negotiated the purchase of the land from a farmer. She also, knowing Association views, counseled the appointment of a Medical Superintendent. In addition, Miss Dix drafted the basic law for the establishment of the hospital. She wrote, "The title of the institution shall be the Government Hospital for the Insane and its objects shall be the most humane care and enlightened creative treatment of the insane of the Army and Navy of the United States and of the District of Columbia" (42, p. 5).

proven satisfactory (5). At the annual meeting of the Association in 1871, Edward Jarvis spoke in favor of the cottage system and aroused a difference of opinion (43).* Within the next 10 years, many institutions were to adopt plans for multiple buildings and to establish farm colonies. From 1854, when Kirkbride first published *On the Construction, Organization and General Arrangements of Hospitals for the Insane* until its expanded second edition in 1880, he was to be champion of construction and design standards for mental hospitals. The concern for standards as an activity of the Association was abandoned in 1888 when the original propositions no longer held, and the issue would not come up again for years (5).

A backward step away from the Association's strongly supported public policy advocating state responsibility for all of the insane was taken at the 1885 annual meeting. The limited capacity of asylums led to the recommendation by the Association that chronic patients be moved back to county poorhouses to make room for acute cases. The policy was put into action by state legislatures, but was a mistake and ran counter to all early strivings of the Association. It threatened "a return to wretchedness and squalor," said Pliny Earle in an article in the *American Journal of Insanity*: "It is cheaper to violate a law of humanity than to discharge a decent obligation" (44).

Medical—Legal Issues

During the 50 years beginning in 1850, the Association, largely through the work of its leading expert in medico-legal issues, Isaac Ray, made significant contributions to law as it affected the mentally ill and retarded. The more important issues addressed in this period were the insanity defense, the role of the expert witness, the relationship of mental illness to crime and suicide, the abuse of patient rights, rights of foreigners, and commitment laws. Several others among the founding fathers, as well as other members

---

* Other pertinent references to the "cottage plan" can be found in the *American Journal of Insanity*: Kirkbride 7:374, 1851; Workman 24:42, 1869; Earle 33:483, 1876; Fisher 50:1–10, 1894; and 51:160–170, 1895. References to colonies may also be found in (39) and in the *American Journal of Insanity*: Palmer 44:157, 1888 and Stedman 46:327, 1890.

as the Association grew, also were expert in matters of law and contributed to the Association's work in this area. Ray's great influence came, in large measure, through his prolific writing. "From 1820 until 1880, only one year passed without one or more volumes or original articles from his fertile pen" (45, pp. 546–547).

Ray wrote *A Treatise on the Medical Jurisprudence of Insanity* in 1838 (46, 47). It was the first discussion of the subject to appear in the United States and went through several revisions, the last in 1871. Editions were published in England and Scotland in 1839 and the book received prominent mention in the M'Naughten trial. The M'Naughten Rule that followed was issued in 1843 (47). It is not surprising that the insanity defense came under discussion early in the Association's history and that the description of trials and the insanity defense were the subjects of 10 papers in the first 10 years of the *American Journal of Insanity* (48). The first article on the insanity defense appeared in 1844, written by C.B. Coventry (Professor of Medical Jurisprudence in the Medical Institution of Geneva College). It recounted the answers of 15 English Judges to questions related to them by the House of Lords, following the citizen uproar over dissatisfaction with the M'Naughten ruling. The first volume of the *Journal* contained a report on a murder committed under an irresistible impulse with discussion of testamentory capacity and the expert witness role (45). As an example of presentation of trials, in 1849, the *Journal of Insanity* carried the account of the murder of Lydia Pinkham and her four children by her husband, who then killed himself.

Isaac Ray noted in 1850 that most states lacked statutes defining the legal relations of the insane, both civil and criminal (51). To address this problem the Association established (in 1863) the Project of Law, with Ray as its chairman. It was to be a major effort of Ray's. He collected state statutes, drafted guidelines, and, in 1868, the recommendations were adopted (43, 44, 50–52).

Project of Law Adopted by the Association in 1868

The following is an abridged version of the Project of Law:

Preamble: Recommended adoption by every state to regulate by statute, their rights and the rights of those entrusted to their care

1. Certification by one or more physicians after personal examination, made within one week; referral for admission by legal guardian, relative or friend, acknowledged before a magistrate or judicial officer to insure genuineness.
2. Order of magistrate placed insane in hospital, if dangerous to self or others, or required care and treatment
3. Insane may be placed in hospital on order of any high judicial officer after:
   a. Statement of a respectable person that a certain person is insane and his welfare, or that of others, required restraint
   b. Judge to appoint a commission to inquire and report facts and, if found suitable, Judge issued a warrant for confinement
4. The Commission of three or four (one a physician and one a lawyer) shall give reasonable notice and shall hear evidence. During the "inquisition" the person may be placed in suitable custody
5. Any high Judge may appoint a commission to investigate the condition of a patient confined in hospital on receipt of a written complaint that confinement is unnecessary; if supported, Judge shall issue an order for discharge
6. Any officer of a hospital may initiate proceeding in Sec. 5
7. Commission designated in Sec. 5 may not be repeated to same party oftener than once in six months
8. Person placed under Sec. 1 may be removed by the party who placed him there
9. Person placed under Sec. 2 may be discharged by hospital authority
10. Municipal authorities may remove pauper over whom they have custody
11. On the written statement of a friend of a patient who is losing his physical health (placed under Sec. 3) and whose mental state no longer requires confinement, Judge will investigate and may or may not order discharge
12. Persons placed in hospital may be removed by persons responsible for the payment of their expenses if acting under free will and not under operation of the law
13. Insane shall not be tried for any criminal act during the existence of their insanity
14. Commission to be appointed; if not insane, to be tried; if insane, or in doubt, report facts to Judge

15. When acquitted in a criminal suit on grounds of insanity, the jury shall declare the fact and the court shall order commitment with retention until discharge may be effected under Sec. 16

16. When the Judge is satisfied of recovery (if the crime is the only one the person has committed) he may order discharge; in homicide cases release to be by unanimous consent of hospital superintendent, managers, and court; if previous insanity, a guardian may be appointed to give bond for any damages

17. If a person is suffering from want of care or treatment, the Judge may order placement in a hospital at the expense of those legally bound to maintain him

18. Application for guardianship shall be made to Judge of Probate, with notice and hearing

19. The insane are responsible in a civil suit for any injury they may commit to person or property (conditions specified)

20. Contracts of insane shall not be valid unless for articles of necessity and the other party had no reason to suspect mental derangement

21. A will is invalid on ground of insanity if the party was incapable of understanding the nature of the transaction, appreciating value, remembering heirs, or if the party has delusions toward heirs (39, pp. 22–23).

It was during this period when the Association was developing its guidelines to state statute development that several related events took place. In 1865 the 13th Amendment to the U.S. Constitution was adopted, abolishing slavery and involuntary servitude. The 14th Amendment was adopted in 1868. This Amendment stated that those persons born in the United States or naturalized are U.S. citizens. States may not abridge the privileges and immunities of citizens. It established due process, which had to be followed before anyone was deprived of life, liberty, or property. The Amendment also established qualifications of congressmen, apportionate representation according to population, and freed the federal and state governments from any claims or reparations incurred as the consequence of rebellion or insurrection.

In the 1860s Charles Redd wrote a popular novel, *Hard Cash,* about the illegal commitment of his hero to an asylum by associates trying to get hold of his fortune. It set the stage for citizen arousal and sympathy for Mrs. E.P.W. Packard and her crusade. As I have already mentioned, Mrs. Packard had been committed to the Illinois State Hospital in Jacksonville in 1860 upon petition of her husband, Rev. Theophilus Packard. Three years after gaining her freedom, she stated that she had been sane when confined and had been the victim of a plot by her husband, who wanted to get rid of her. She launched a crusade, wrote several books about "railroading sane to asylums" that had huge sales, addressed public gatherings, and succeeded in changing the Illinois law in 1867, with Massachusetts and Iowa following. The requirement of a jury trial to prove insanity was protested as deleterious by the Association (5). While the Association protest didn't gain repeal of the laws enacted for 25 years, it did arrest their spread to other states.

Expert testimony came into sharp focus within the Association during the trial of Charles Gutteau, held in 1881 in the District of Columbia, for the assassination of President Garfield. Chapin had addressed the annual meeting of the Association on the subject in 1880. The defense held that Gutteau had an heredity taint, irrational action throughout his life, and was insane. Defense experts were James G. Kiernan (apothecary, city asylum, Ward's Island); Charles H. Nichols (Bloomingdale Asylum, New York); Charles F. Folsom (Boston); Samuel Worcester (Salem, Massachusetts); William H. Godding (Superintendent, St. Elizabeths, Washington, D.C.); Samuel H. McBride (Superintendent, Milwaukee, Wisconsin Asylum); Walter Channing (Brookline, Massachusetts Asylum); Theodore W. Fisher (Superintendent, Boston Lunatic Asylum); and Edward C. Spitzka (leading neurologist, New York). The prosecution had the burden of proving sanity and responsibility at the time of the crime. It relied chiefly on the testimony of John P. Gray, who held the defendant to be sane. The jury agreed and found Gutteau guilty (53). The spectacle of disagreement among the experts discredited the whole procedure and the profession in the public mind, as it has so many times over the years.

In 1888 Stephen Smith presented the Association's Project of Law (developed by the committee chaired by Isaac Ray) to the National Conference of Charities and urged its adoption by all states to regulate commitment. In 1890 a new New York commitment law was commended by the Association, for it specified state care for all dependent insane. The care of all the insane in institutions operated by the states developed slowly and was still incomplete (some county mental hospitals remained) by the 20th century.

Political Interference

The Association, in 1848, four years after its founding, opposed the political appointment of superintendents and asserted that the best man for the job should be sought. Soon afterward William Awl was to become a victim of politics and was forced out of his post as Superintendent of the Columbus, Ohio, institution. Matters got worse, not better, in some states. One Illinois hospital had 8 superintendents in 16 years and another 13 in 9 years. The discharge of the respected Richard Dewey, Editor of the *American Journal of Insanity*, particularly aroused the Association's ire. Employees were given jobs on patronage and were expected to contribute to party funds. Appointment to citizen Boards of Trustees was a political reward. Opposition by the Association (as in 1876) didn't stop the patronage system (43). By the end of the century political interference, while still a problem, receded as an issue in Association priority.

MANAGEMENT OF DELIVERY SYSTEMS

The Association met in the Astor House in New York City in 1848. Twenty members were present. Floor plans of several institutions were posted on the wall for study and there were exhibits of patient crafts and restraining apparatus. The members, as was their custom, visited the local mental hospital on Blackwell's Island. They were shocked by "the degradation and neglect without parallel," and with care of patients by "thieves and prostitutes." The latter were inmates of an adjacent institution recruited to care for the insane. The Association recommended abandonment of the present madhouse, use of a design at hand to build a new one, change in the system, employment of competent staff, seeking of the best available (not the politically desirable) appointees, and appropriation of the necessary funds (37, 44). This first recorded consultation by the Association on management of an institution was highly successful. Recommendations made were carried out in a short time.

The desirability of separate institutions for "idiots and demented," for "colored persons," and for "insane prisoners" were subjects assigned to the first group of committees for report in 1846, as was a study of hospital organization.

At the eighth annual meeting of the Association in 1853 in Baltimore, propositions on management of hospitals were formulated. An abridged version follows:

1. Controlling power was to be vested in a Board of Trustees (as a protection from political change and interference)
2. The Board of Trustees was to consist of up to 12 persons who had the confidence of the public, and who were intelligent, benevolent citizens. A term of three years was suggested, with one-third of the group to be appointed in a year
3. The Board was to appoint the Medical Superintendent; the Medical Superintendent was to nominate assistant physicians, steward, and matron. The Board was to supervise expenditures and general operations
4. The Medical Superintendent was to be the chief executive officer with the education, mental, physical, and social qualities essential to his position. He was to reside in or near the institution and devote his full time to the welfare of the organization
5. Qualifications were stated for assistant physicians, steward (in charge of purchases, farm, and grounds), and matron (in charge of housekeeping)
6. One supervisor was to be employed for male patient wards and one for all female patient wards
7. When more than 200 patients were admitted, a second assistant physician was to be added
8. There should be no less than one attendant to every 10 patients. (Attendants worked the daytime hours and slept in nearby rooms for availability at any hour of the night.)
9. Enough personnel were to be available to give enlightened treatment. Employed staff was expected to be kind, benevolent, educated, actively vigilant, and in good health. Enough money was to be provided to hire good people
10. The Superintendent was to be responsible for patient safety, fire protection, and night watch (44, pp. 217–222)

In 1870 the practice was begun to call on each member to report on the conditions of institutions and plans for new ones in his home state. This practice was followed for a number of years. The Illinois proposal to develop an institution on a "village plan" in the model of a small town was discussed in 1877. Later it was implemented in Kankakee (Illinois), Toledo (Ohio), and Craig Colony (New York). Although the idea had been introduced by Butler in 1865, farm colonies were opposed by the Association, and in 1866 a resolution was put forth by a committee that opposed the colony model. The Association did approve a farm worker's building on the grounds of the Kankakee Hospital in 1877. By the end of the century separate colonies for working patients became a reality.

As noted earlier, the first mental hospital in the United States at Williamsburg, Virginia, had an active, appointed Court of Directors. Later Maryland and the District of Columbia had a Board of Visitors, and New York a Board of Managers, while the rest of the states had Boards of Trustees. In corporate institutions Boards were charged with the management and affairs of the institution. In states, the Board Members were selected by the Governor from its best citizens (noted for business ability, public service, or philanthropy) and were representatives of the commonwealth to oversee institutional affairs (44). Board members received no pay and only received expenses for official duties. For example, in Vermont's Brattleboro Asylum, trustees selected and bargained for the land, drew up contracts, and looked after the details of construction.

Gradually the management functions were wholly entrusted to the Medical Superintendent. In some states the control of institutions went to the dominant political party that exerted pressure on employment, the use of favored banks, and upon purchase of goods. Efforts to correct the evils of political patronage led to paid state boards of control. Massachusetts called its controlling body the Board of Insanity and New York named its board the Commission on Lunacy. Others had State Boards of Charities. At the start they were limited to inspections, recommendation, and advice. Later they became responsible for providing a consolidated budget. Throughout the 19th century and well into the 20th, the Superintendent of the institution had the dominant authority over management and over all clinical care.

INTERNAL AFFAIRS OF THE ASSOCIATION

Objectives

Stribling wrote to Curwen (37) indicating that his recollection of the purpose of those called to assemble in Philadelphia, as planned by Dr. Woodward and himself, was to pursue "all that concerned the interests of the insane; the organization, management, etc., of institutions for the benefit of this afflicted class." Stribling said, "It was deemed but reasonable that the noble cause would be materially promoted by some arrangement to convene at stated periods for consultations, etc. with those in charge of such institutions."

At the annual meeting in 1883, which was attended by three surviving founders—Thomas Kirkbride, Pliny Earle, and John Butler—Callender, the 10th Association president, delivered an address, *History and Work of the Association of Medical Superintendents*. He stated that the purpose of the organization was "broad and continental in scope" and "for the promotion of the usefulness of hospitals for the insane and the project of general meeting of all engaged in the care of that afflicted class" (39, pp. 1–32).

At the 1889 annual meeting, J.B. Chapin, President of the Association, formulated the objective of the organization "concerning all the interests of the insane and the organization and management of institutions for the benefit of the afflicted class" (54).

Organization

The organization, while it was small (less than 30 attended an annual meeting for 20 years, less than 100 on its 50th anniversary, and 153 at the end of the 19th century), had no constitution, and had a simple structure under three officers: President, Vice-President, and Secretary-Treasurer.

The work of the organization was carried out by committees that varied in the number of members and in productivity. Nonproductivity of committees and other elements of the Association is a contemporary problem, as it was in the 1880s, when the Association abolished all existing committees and in 1882 reorganized work under eight new ones:

1. Annual Association necrology
2. Cerebro-spinal physiology
3. Cerebro-spinal pathology
4. Therapeutics of insanity
5. Bibliography of insanity
6. Relation of eccentric disease to insanity
7. Asylum, location, construction, and sanitation
8. Criminal responsibility of the insane

The realignment of committees was a failure and was abandoned in 1885, for it destroyed and weakened member participation and initiative (44).

Reorganization of the Association was proposed in 1891 and a committee appointed to develop a constitution. The first constitution was adopted in 1892. A governing body called the Council was created; classes of members were defined (active, associate, and honorary); and authorization was given for the proceedings at meetings to be published in *Transactions*. These innovations began in 1894, coincident with the Association's 50th anniversary, and were discontinued in 1920. The name of the Association was changed in 1893 to the American Medico-Psychological Association.

Annual Meetings

Only the first three meetings were held at two-year intervals. As has already been mentioned, the tradition of meeting early in May began in 1846. Annual meetings were held starting in 1849 and continued each year with but one interruption (1861) during the Civil War.

After the 1854 meeting, Isaac Ray wrote to Thomas Kirkbride, "as nature abhors a vacuum so do I abhor that utter non-communication which frequently follows such a pleasant reunion of friends as we enjoyed last week. . . . If our yearly conventions had accomplished nothing more than to make us acquainted with one another, and with other institutions besides our own, creating feelings of personal regard and mutual sympathy, I should think they had not been in vain" (28, p. 122).

Kirkbride served as president for eight years (1862–1870) and Charles Nichols for six (1873–1879). Other early presidents served three to four years until 1882, when the one-year term of office for president was established, and it was determined that the retiring president would deliver an address. Callender was the first to give such an address in 1883.

At early meetings the purpose of the program was to hear and discuss the reports of committees; formulate resolutions or propositions; learn of new treatments; debate current issues; examine exhibits; and visit nearby institutions, suggesting action to improve them. The first original paper was presented by Luther Bell (1849) on what came to be known as Bell's Mania. On rare occasions the members met with the President of the United States when the annual meeting was in Washington, D.C., as in 1854 and 1866. In 1855 the Association met in the Massachusetts Senate Chambers and in those of the Boston City Council (37).

Callender (39) stated at the 1883 annual meeting that the Association, operating as it did without an arbitrary code to which members must abide, gave the "largest liberty of individual opinion. No personal controversies have marred the proceedings." Overlooked by Callender were the marked differences of opinion, as in use of restraint, size of institutions, and separate farm colonies. Perhaps the first major discord during an annual meeting occurred in 1855 when John M. Galt, writing in the *American Journal of Medical Sciences*, referred to another member (Luther Bell) without naming him, "one of New England's institutions under control of one of the most pernicious tinkers of gas pipes," and made other caustic remarks (46).

For over 50 years membership was limited to medical superintendents of institutions for the insane in the United States and Canada. Early guests were invited to attend who had an interest in the field, such as members of Boards of Trustees and legislators. Later, provisions were made for the continued membership by superintendents who left their posts, as did Awl and Stedman, of the founders. It was not until 1884 that assistant physicians were admitted to membership if they had five years of continuous service. After the adoption of the first constitution (1892), assistant physicians became Associate Members. As we noted earlier, the number of members grew slowly along with the expanding number of mental institutions. Ninety-eight persons attended the 50th anniversary meeting in Philadelphia, and in 1899, 153 members and 23 guests were present in New York City when Henry Hurd became the 26th President.

The first meeting to extend an invitation to guests to attend the session was the meeting held in 1899. Henry Hurd (44), defending against the many criticisms made over the years, said there had been "sufficient refutation of the imputation that the course of the Association has been characterized by an illiberal exclusiveness and that its membership was a mere self-protecting guild and not an open and candid organization for the promotion of sciences" (44).

The reorganization of the Association in the 1890s and the concomitant institutional reforms ended the inertia which had characterized the Association's behavior. Dunton (49) alleged that Association meetings had become "slumberous affairs" with "little life or activity" until Henry Hurd became secretary in 1892 and played a major role in revitalizing the Association. Hurd activated member interest, secured good speakers for the annual meeting, and, by example, motivated officers to do good work.

Amalgamation

The American Medical Association, as noted earlier, was founded in 1848. Pliny Earle had been active in its organization. An amalgamation of the Association of Medical Superintendents with the AMA was discussed in 1853, and the decision was to not merge. The matter came up again at the 25th annual meeting, held in Toronto in 1871. Dr. Curwen had been appointed the year before to attend the AMA meeting in San Francisco. After due consideration of his report, it was agreed by both associations that such a union was not wise (44). A merger with the Association of Medical Officers of American Institutions for Idiots and Feebleminded Persons, which had, in 1876, developed in a similar model with many common traditions, was deemed inadvisable in 1926 (33).

CLINICAL CONCERNS AND ADVANCES IN CARE

A shift in the Association's interest from predominantly administrative to clinical issues was evident in the latter half of the 19th century. While construction of hospitals, their size, and financial support continued to be important themes for discussion, more attention was given to the causes of insanity, its treatment, relationships to medical illness, and to alcoholism, among other topics. It was a period of burgeoning knowledge of the brain and nervous system, of sensory physiology, and of the sciences led by Darwin, Pasteur, Lister, Koch, Roentgen, and others.

At the 10th annual meeting of the Association held in Boston in 1883, Edward Jarvis (who was an important innovative molder of opinion in the Association) presented his survey on the number of insane in Massachusetts, drawing attention to the relationship between poverty and insanity, which became the foundation for later studies on social class in mental disorders.

It was also in 1883 that John Gray was appointed Superintendent of the Utica State Hospital, succeeding the deceased Amariah Brigham as Editor of the *American Journal of Insanity*. Gray's influence upon American psychiatry was considerable. Insanity, in his view, was always due to physical causes, and his search was for evidence of brain pathology.

Restraint

At the first annual meeting in 1844, the members adopted the resolve that "it is the unanimous sense of this convention, that the attempt to abandon entirely the use of all means of personal restraint is not sanctioned by the best interests of the insane." Publication was held up at Kirkbride's request when Brigham suggested changes and until the Chairmen of the Committee on Restraint could approve a revision. As it finally appeared, the resolve read: "The entire rejection of every species of restraining apparatus, under all circumstances, is not sanctioned by the best interests of the insane." Restraint and its use, or total abolition, were to be debated at several annual meetings. In 1857, the care of the violent patient in a strong room, in detached buildings, or with mechanical restraining apparatus, led to opinion opposed to strong rooms and in favor of restraining devices (44).

At the annual meeting in 1874 there was discussion of the appropriate use of restraint and of the Utica Crib bed (44). The reader, unfamiliar with restraining apparatus, will require some description. The Utica Crib was a bed with sides and a latched top that opened. Strong rooms were rarely padded, but usually were made up of a seamless space with a strongly screened window, a thick door with a peephole, and a canvas-covered mattress on the floor. Camisoles were canvas jackets with blind sleeves, with laces that tied in the back. Wristlets of canvas or leather fastened arms to a belt. Patients could be tied, arms and legs, to strong chairs fastened to the floor. Sheet restraints tied arms, body, and legs to the bed frame.

In 1883 Callender called attention to the "vexing problem of restraint and the calamitous accidents which occurred when it was not in use" (39, p. 84). Also noted as improper were chairs fastened to the floor.

It was about this time that labor and exercise were advocated as a means of reducing the need for restraint. In 1885 Fletcher, in Indiana, and G. Alder Blumer at Utica, New York (and Editor of the *American Journal of Insanity*) declared the end of the era of restraint by burning restraint apparatus in a public bonfire before an applauding crowd of onlookers, with superintendents officiating as high priests (5).*

Training Attendants and Nurses

At the founding meeting of the Association in 1844, the importance of training attendants of the insane was recognized; the assignment of Dr. Kirkbride's committee on organization was to produce a manual for training. McLean Hospital began training nurses in 1882. Buffalo was the first state hospital to train nurses (1886) followed by the provincial hospital in Kingston, Ontario (1888) (44).

Programs of Therapy

Earlier, I described the interpersonal relationship important in moral treatment and the objective of early release from the hospital. Meeting patient needs through individualized treatment, nutritious food, labor, exercise, and recreation were a part of the regimen in the early years (1833–1838) as reported by Woodward and Butler. John Gray's treatment (1855) stressed rest, adequate

---

* The use of restraint did not end in the 19th century. In 1905 Zeller and McFarland abolished the use of restraint briefly at the Peoria (Illinois) State Hospital. In the first half of the 20th century English open hospitals abolished all restraint as Connolly had advocated 100 years earlier at Hanwell. Open hospitals appeared in the United States in the 1950s. In the 1980s seclusion rooms and leather wristlets that restrain arms to a belt at the waist are still in use, despite powerful medications that control most violence.

diet, proper room temperature, ventilation, and greater freedom for patients. Occupational therapy (with a crafts exhibit) was featured at the 1848 annual meeting in New York City, and its evolution was described in the *American Journal of Insanity* for July 1880. Recreation became an area of committee interest at the second meeting of the Association (1846) and included such activities as excursions, slide shows in the evening, and rides on miniature railroads.

Religion was important, as indicated by chapels and chaplains being the subject of one of the original (1844) committees. Worship services on Sunday, a daily morning chapel service, and the saying of grace at meals was the practice in the 1860s, in a society that placed "In God We Trust" on its coins.

Hydrotherapy was a subject discussed at the 1854 annual meeting, with a new continuous bath proposed for the treatment of acute insanity. The therapy was recommended for use over a period of 6 to 18 hours for its sedative effect. Several members present at the Association's session were opposed to its use. Also in 1854, J.H. Worthington reported on "Construction of Baths and Utility of Warm and Cold Bathing in the Treatment of Insanity" in the *American Journal of Insanity* (7). Hydrotherapy developed in the 20th century and its use has persisted into the 1980s with the hot tub fad.

Medication was the subject of discussion both in 1870, with the focus on the use of chloral hydrate, and in 1874, with the focus on hypnotics in the treatment of insanity. Opium was introduced after the Civil War and cocaine was favored for a time until its addictive properties were demonstrated in the 20th century.

The relationship of insanity to physical ailments was a subject presented at the 1851 annual meeting. The relationship of tuberculosis to insanity was discussed in 1888. Care of tuberculosis patients in mental hospitals was discussed in 1894, with an emphasis on separation, disinfection, and safeguards to other patients. The Rest Cure for mental illness, introduced by Mitchell, advocated separation from stresses of home and the work place to rebuild energies.

Alternative to Hospital Care

At the 1860 annual meeting, Jarvis suggested an idea ahead of its time, namely that homes in the community might benefit quiet patients who could not return home because of trouble there. Physician supervision of patients in that setting might, Jarvis thought, enhance recovery. The prejudice toward private institutions present among Association members extended to the use of private homes; the recommendation was rejected.

In 1882 outpatient and aftercare clinics were introduced, and after 1885 (as a result of reports from visitors to Gheel, Belgium) family care was introduced into practice in Massachusetts, as Stedman reported at the 1889 annual meeting. The family care program included 113 patients who showed improvement.

The Patient Environment

Charles Dickens' complimentary description in his *American Notes* (1842) of the Boston City Asylum is one of the most lucid portrayals of the patient environment as it existed when the Association was founded. In Callender's (1883) presidential address, he contrasted bad with good patient environments. The bad environments were characterized by long corridors, scanty furnishings, absence of pictures, noise, and confusion. The good environments were characterized by attractive wards, brightly colored walls, draperies, pictures, and comfortable surroundings, as in a home. Foremost in importance, Callender said, was the attitude of staff. Attendants should be companions, not keepers of the insane.

Early in the Association's history the puritan heritage was manifest in the support of comfort for patients, but not luxury. Good design, adequate space, good lighting, good ventilation, enough washrooms and toilets, and safety were essential.

Reform: The Worcester Plan

Adolf Meyer's "Worcester Plan," formulated in a letter (55) in 1895, reviewed the current practices at Worcester and recommended changes to incorporate scientific investigative methods. Meyer noted that support for libraries and laboratories was given, but the number of staff physicians and their knowledge was woefully inadequate. Records were perfunctory accounts in jargon: "deluded, noisy, untidy, disturbed, etc. and lacking essential evidence of delirium, dementia, and physical and neurologic disorders." He deplored the way physicians spent their time: after an hour in the day and a "small hour" at night treating patients, they spent most of their time compounding drugs, answering letters, and writing reports. As an immediate remedy he suggested employing a pharmacist and stenographers. Next, he suggested a clinical conference on all newly admitted patients to demonstrate collection of essential evidence, followed by adequate recording of information essential to diagnosis, study of the disorder, and treatment.

To get better physicians Meyer demonstrated the value of a competitive examination and suggested a reasonable wage. Every intern or assistant physician should be motivated to acquire training to recognize the value of collecting information in a manner useful for clinical investigation, to be motivated toward self-improvement, and to use every opportunity to that end; and, if ability and ambition were lacking, he "is not fit for the position" (55, p. 13).

The emphasis on values, attitude, support of the administrator, the selection of the best available men or women for training, the availability of support personnel, intensive study, superior motivation, the case conference model for teaching, correct information gathering, and recording data useful for scientific investigation were elements Meyer believed in. If practiced they would not only improve patient care and form the basis for research studies in mental disorders, but also introduce the reform so strongly urged by the neurologist critics.

Catalyst to Change

At the 50th anniversary meeting of the Association held in Philadelphia in 1894, the retiring president, Curwen, used the occasion to relate the history of the Association, reviewing the progress of treatment and the development of mental hospitals.

The invited guest speaker was Silas Wier Mitchell, who had national reputation as a neurologist and who was internationally known for his "rest cure."* Mitchell was over six feet tall, graying hair parted in the middle, bearded, elegant in dress, dignified, and with charm and force that he projected upon those about him.

---

* See Beverly Tucker's description of the man and his works in reference (56). A biography was published on the 100th anniversary of his birth by Anne Robeson Burr, entitled *Wier Mitchell: Life and Letters*. New York, Deerfield and Co., 1929.

Dr. Chapin had asked him "to speak boldly with no regard to persons." He did just that and his provocative oration became a high point in the history of the Association. To prepare himself, Mitchell surveyed 30 well-known neurologists and asked their opinion about asylum management, faults, and suggested changes.

Mitchell, in his address, said boards of managers "do not know their business and do not know what they ought to know." He objected to the name "asylum" and to superintendents being "farmers, stewards, caterers, treasurers, business managers and physicians . . . Some of you," he said, "are cursed by that slow atrophy of the emerging faculties which is the very malaria of asylum life . . . Upon my word," he added, "I think asylum life is deadly to the insane" (56, pp. 84, 85). He stated superintendents ought not live and sleep in their hospitals (57).

"We neurologists think you have fallen behind us, and this opinion is gaining ground outside of our own ranks and is in part at least, your own fault. . . . Where are your careful scientific reports? You live alone, uncriticized, unquestioned, out of the healthy conflicts and home rivalries which keep us up to the mark of the fullest possible completeness" (1).

Mitchell criticized the absence in the records of physical studies, neurological examinations, and often medical examinations. He deplored politics in institutions. "There is another function which you totally fail to fulfill . . . to preach down the idea that insanity is always dangerous, to show what may be done in homes, or by boarding out the quiet insane and to teach the needs of hospitals until you educate a public which never reads your reports and is absurdly ignorant of what your patients need" (5, p. 280). Mitchell placed his emphasis upon extramural treatment of insanity but leveled his most forceful criticism at the lack of scientific spirit and competent original research (56).

Having made his critical points, Mitchell acknowledged that progress had been made toward sober administrative responsibility and turned toward the following suggestions for change. He believed there should be:

- Intelligent assistant physicians with periodic vacations to keep them from going stale on the job
- Superintendents to keep alive scientific curiosity of staff
- More trained nurses
- No barred gates, no locks or bars

- Fewer restraints
- Attractive wards and buildings close to the city
- Occupational therapy and recreation
- A varied diet
- Rewards to personnel for excellent performance

Mitchell's listeners were tolerant but responded defensively at first, with a spate of articles in medical journals refuting his charges. There was a solid basis for Mitchell's criticisms (44). His speech voiced the aspirations of psychiatrists, and particularly the younger ones present. The challenge to change was met in the years ahead with renewed interest in scientific investigation and improvement in patient care.

EMERGENCE OF THE PROFESSION OF PSYCHIATRY: A SUMMARY

The period 1850–1899 was one of discovery and advancement of science (58, 59). Brain anatomy and localization were studied, as were lateralization in the hemispheres, sensory physiology, and pathological sexuality. It was a time of ascendency of institutions with rational reforms of workhouses, jails, prisons, almshouses, and asylums. Institutions increased in number at a rapid rate. The cycle of innovation and humanitarian reform begun by the founders lasted for about a generation until 1870. The success of moral treatment was accompanied by enthusiasm and optimism of practitioners and in the positive public perception of the institutions.

Rough spots on the road of change became apparent as the cycle turned. First doubt, then open criticism induced pessimism in the 1880s. Both the Medical Superintendents and the Association came under attack. Demand for reform in the 1890s was insistent and heeded. The cycle began again.

From the inception of the Association, its members were recognized as consultant experts with special knowledge. With better educational opportunities and instruction in medical schools, the knowledge base expanded and the "alienists" (as they were called) emerged as professional specialists. At the end of the century the need for laboratories, medical libraries, and scientific inquiry was recognized and the foundation laid for the work in this area in the 20th century.

The Association's achievements between 1850 and 1899 might be summarized as follows:

- Growth in number and growth in influence, as specialists with reasoned policy statements emerged from study by committees
- Impressive results of moral treatment
- The development of administrative guides for hospital construction, heating, and ventilation
- Standards (propositions) for organizations and operation of asylums
- A suggested model for state lunacy laws
- The establishment of mental illness as a clinical and didactic course for all medical students
- Policy statements such as state responsibility for care of the insane of all types
- Improved management functions
- Application of treatment advances
- Influence upon other health or health related organizations

There were, as I have mentioned, problems and missed opportunities. Some of the major ones seem to be:

- The lack of development of a theoretical foundation for practice
- The absence of scientific research and original research, actively pursued as a goal as in European centers, with almost no perception by the Association of its absence
- The decline in the effectiveness of moral treatment and the deterioration of the mental hospitals; these problems were not major concerns of the Association
- Little if any involvement in the public health movement (1872) and in such mandated policy as denial of admission to immigrants (1891): "all idiots, insane persons, persons likely to become public charges and those with loathsome or dangerous contagious diseases" (23, p. 168)
- A major policy error (1885) that sent mentally ill patients back to poorhouses
- The lack of involvement of the Association in the development of military psychiatry during the Civil War. (One member was on active duty, one offer of service was made, and one policy statement was made concerning released military personnel.) The war seemed out of the Association's scope of concern, but

not out of the neurologists' (who were concerned with nostalgia, wounds and nerve injuries, and pain relief).

- Major reform in the delivery of care came from outside the Association through the work of Dorothea Dix. Some Association members were her advisors and the Association did support her efforts at the federal level.

The Association fostered information exchange among members, enhanced their problem-solving skills, improved the structure and organization of institutions, debated controversial issues, and, more importantly, rediscovered the patient in the new challenges of clinical management.

Important to the emergence of the medical specialty of psychiatry was the ability of the Medical Superintendents to survive the challenge of the shifts in control from independent, autonomous institutions to centralized state systems. Other challenges to the organization came from both the neurologists and from within, resulting in reorganization and change. The Association emerged from its battering with more power as a medical specialty, with public support in the use of its hospitals, and with adoption of many of its recommended policies and standards to advance the field of psychiatry.

4

Psychiatry as a Social Force: 1900–1949

Psychiatry can and should speak in positive words to a frightened and chaotic world, speak a message derived from its hundred years experience in dealing with the mentally sick on the basis of the non-violent code.

—Edward A. Strecker,
Presidential Address,
APA Centennial, 1944

A new year is greeted with the anticipation that things will be different—the old gives way to the new. As 1899 clicked over into 1900, this sense of anticipation was heightened: it was not only a new year, but a new century.

The nation's mood in 1900 was one of confident optimism. As the country consolidated its expanded territories, it seemed to be bursting with energy and eager to face the future. The optimistic mood might have been shattered had the people of the nation known the cataclysmic events that the next 50 years would bring. In the next 50 years there would be a revolution in transportation and communication, two global wars, the extermination of 6 million Jews in Europe, the development of synthetic fiber and plastics, advances in science culminating in the beginning of the atomic age, and, in response to these events, social reforms with organizations and movements serving as change agents. These were but a few of the discoveries and events that would affect the lives of every individual in the 20th century.

An innovation in transportation developed inauspiciously in a bicycle shop run by Wilbur and Orville Wright of Dayton, Ohio. The Wright Brothers successfully flew their air machine at Kitty Hawk, North Carolina, in 1903. Development of the airplane was sufficiently rapid to permit combat engagement in the first World War (1914–1918). The jet engine was invented in 1937 and the jet airplane in 1942. Ten years later jet engines powered commercial air carriers.

A skeptical press noted strange experiments with rockets in 1919 in Worcester, Massachusetts, by R. H. Goddard. The public was totally unaware that the rocket was the first blast toward the space age. The V series of rockets based upon Goddard's experiments were introduced by the Germans in the bombardment of Great Britain in World War II. In the second half of the 20th century rockets developed into the mighty missiles that made exploration of space possible.

Telephone and telegraph usage grew rapidly after 1900. The former expanded into private homes making it possible to call firemen, policemen, or physicians whenever necessary. In 1900 R.A. Fessenden of the United States transmitted human speech via radio waves, and Marconi sent a radio message from Cornwall to Newfoundland.

THE ADVANCES IN SCIENCE

The amazing developments in science in the first half of the 20th century may be illustrated by the short span of time between the articulation of theory and its application (2, 3). Max Planck formulated the quantum theory, and Albert Einstein the theory of relativity, in 1900. Only 40 years later the cyclotron would be invented (1940); the Manhattan Project to develop an atomic bomb (with top priority and richly funded) would be underway (1941); the first atom would be split (1942); the first atomic bomb would be exploded in New Mexico (1945); and two bombs would wipe out Hiroshimo and Nagasaki, ending the war with Japan (1945). The atomic age was underway.

In the first 10 years of the century the completion of the Panama Canal was made possible by the eradication of yellow fever; vaccination of the entire U.S. Army against typhoid was undertaken in the attempt to stop the death of soldiers from the disease; allergy was described; H. Cushing studied the pituitary; the electrocardiograph was invented; chromosomes and blood groups were identified; and tissue and fiber were discovered. Radioactive substances and the ultraviolet lamp became medical tools.

The vitamins were discovered in 1912 (Vitamin D in 1932), followed by hormones and enzymes. Their synthesis and that of insulin (1937) and quinine (1944) made the treatment of disease more specific.

Alexander Fleming isolated penicillin in 1928 but it was not until the 1940s that it was to be in general usage, along with streptomycin in 1943, neomycin in 1949, and other antibiotics. These substances were to revolutionize the treatment of infection and make possible the prevention of syphilis.

Insecticides were introduced in 1924. Worldwide acceptance of this boon for eradication of pests was immediate and use was massive. The poisons got into the food chain, decimating the bird population. Nitrates in widely used fertilizers, emissions of factories and automobile exhausts, and the spillage of industrial chemicals into waterways contaminated the environment.

Although the artificial heart was invented in 1936, its first use in humans was to be delayed for some years. Eyeglasses, hearing aids, false teeth, and wooden legs, common aids to bodily function, were to change with the aid of reconstructive dentistry and surgery. Audiometry developed and the urgency of World War disabilities led to greatly improved hearing aids for the deafened. Amputees were aided by prostheses designed to greatly increase functioning.

The first computer (1942) was a novelty too big to be a concern of the average person, who, indeed, scarcely noted the invention of xerography (1946) or the transistor (1947). All three inventions would, however, change the average person's life more than the invention of the ball point pen, which was readily accepted as a truly practical discovery in 1938.

The invention of the electron microscope in 1949 would enlarge the vision of anatomists and bring new insights into how the body functions. Cortisone was also discovered in 1949. In that year the world population was 2.2 billion, an awesome figure that accelerated the interest in population control—for the gains in public health, in longevity, and in the conquest of disease could be wiped out by a mass of humanity and a despoiled earth.

MOVEMENTS AND ORGANIZATIONS

The Progressive Movement

Social reforms to raise the standard of living began with public arousal over the issue of child labor and introduced the "century of the child." Exploitation of children—7- to 10-year-old children working 10 hours a day in mills, mines, and factories—was featured in the news. Less than a dozen states in 1900 had laws prohibiting child labor. The public shame led to the formation in 1904 of the National Child Labor Commission. By 1915, 33 states had moved to require children to go to school until the age of 16 (1). Children began to be seen as children and not as small adults; child development, adolescence, and behavior of children and youth began to be studied and grew into a movement.

Social movements begin with a dedicated group of individuals who have identified some misery and set out to relieve it in order to improve the human condition. The issues range from those of special interest groups to a collective social concern. The Progressive Movement brought together groups with different agendas but with a shared optimism at the start of the new century that advances on all fronts could change society. By purposive action, they believed, events might be shaped to achieve their goals.

Progressive action established the first Workmen's Compensation Law in Maryland in 1902 and the first Minimum Wage Law in Massachusetts in 1912. Socialists had favored health insurance as early as 1904, but a group of social progressives at the center of the Progressive Movement—the American Association of Labor Legislation (AALL), founded in 1906—won an uneasy alliance with the American Medical Association in support of health insurance. The drive to initiate health insurance failed when the Progressive Party (the Bull Moose Party), led by Theodore Roosevelt, lost the election of 1912 to Woodrow Wilson. Roosevelt supported social insurance including health insurance.

Progressive thought had an impact upon psychiatry. Progressives held that "evil and pathological behavior flowed from the immoral circumstances in which individuals lived" (4, p. 109). The solution was to transform the environment. A consequence was to push psychiatric thinking beyond "the physiological and biologic roots of mental disease" (4, p. 109). The "social and intellectual currents" led the profession (which was almost entirely based in mental hospitals) to accept new ideas and to search for knowledge that led beyond the boundaries of their institutions (4, p. 109).

The Social Hygiene Movement

Another of the many movements that began early in the 20th century was the Social Hygiene Movement. Its limited focus can be determined from the name of the initiating group—the American Federation for Sex Hygiene—founded in 1910. This later became the American Social Hygiene Association, which promoted public awareness of venereal disease, its mode of spread, and its prevention. The Association fostered sex education, established free venereal disease clinics, and encouraged early diagnosis and treatment, including treatment of the sexual contacts of the patient. An unsuccessful attempt was also made to restrict prostitution. Like the Progressive Movement, the Social Hygiene Movement had an impact upon psychiatry: syphilis was, at that time, a major cause of mental disease requiring hospital treatment.

The Movement to Eradicate Tuberculosis

Pulmonary tuberculosis (also then called consumption or phthisis) had been known to exist for centuries. It was the unchallenged "Captain of the Man of Death" in the 19th century (4). Benjamin Rush believed in 1800 that he could cure phthisis with opium, an animal diet, and his routine heroic measures. Lemuel Shattuck, in 1830, said, "This dreadful disease is a constant visitor to all parts of our Commonwealth but creates little alarm because it is constantly present" (3, p. 202). The blind spot for a major public health problem persisted until the 1880s. A fall in the death rate from tuberculosis was noted in 1850 and the decline continued for another 25 years. Some part of the decline may have been due to a shift to conservative medical treatment.

Public apathy toward consumption ended abruptly when Robert Koch identified the tubercle bacillus in 1882. Within a short time, studies of patient sputum revealed the bacillus; coughing transmitted it to another; a disinfectant added to the sputum cup would kill the bacillus; and a mask worn stopped the spread during coughing.

Edward Trudeau, a physician, contracted tuberculosis, and went to practice in an isolated Adirondack mountain area. There, in 1884, he founded the Adirondack Cottage Sanatorium at

Saranac Lake. It was the first hospital devoted to the treatment of tuberculosis in the United States.

By 1902, two types of tubercle bacilli were identified, human and bovine, with proof that the latter caused the disease in humans. In that same year Maryland established a commission on tuberculosis with William Welch, M.D., and William Osler, M.D., as members, among others. Out of this group emerged the National Tuberculosis Association in 1904 (3).

The Association set as its goals education of the public in the mechanism of spread of tuberculosis; elimination of diseased cattle from the herd; pasteurization of milk; and the creation of private, municipal, county, and state sanatoria. By 1917 every state and territory had its local tuberculosis association.

In 1910 the sale of Christmas seals became a major fund raising effort for tuberculosis associations. They were introduced with the help of the American Red Cross, and later the National Tuberculosis Association took over the stamp sales.

Sanatorium care, case finding, good diet, rest, and outdoor exercise caused a decline in death rates from tuberculosis. By the second half of the 20th century chemotherapy helped close the tuberculosis institutional system with its 100,000 beds (5). A dramatic and highly successful movement brought tuberculosis under control, eliminated the "hunchbacked child," and abolished an institutional care system. The control of tuberculosis was important to psychiatry because tuberculosis had been significantly present in mental institutions.

While the aforementioned movements affected the practice of psychiatry, two movements—the Mental Hygiene Movement and the Psychoanalytic Movement—had a profound effect.

The Mental Hygiene Movement

Clifford W. Beers (1876–1943), the initiator of the Mental Hygiene Movement, was a businessman recovered from a mental illness (6). In 1900 he made a serious suicide attempt and was institutionalized for a depressive illness. He spent the next three years in three Connecticut mental hospitals. During the latter part of his illness he was elated and filled with grandiose plans for reform; he spent two years after his release deliberating how best to initiate action. Impressed with what *Uncle Tom's Cabin* had accomplished, he set about writing an autobiographical account of his illness and recovery. When the manuscript was completed, he sought criticism from psychiatrists, psychologists, and others whose opinion he valued. His book, *A Mind That Found Itself* (published by Longmans in 1908), was no ordinary expose of brutal treatment. While it indicted the treatment system, it offered a plan for improvement. The book was a literary success: it attracted favorable attention worldwide and by 1935 it had gone through 22 editions.

William James (the psychologist who wrote the Introduction to Beers' book), Adolf Meyer (who suggested the use of the term "mental hygiene"), and others advised Beers to establish a demonstration organization. Beers did so, establishing the Connecticut Society for Mental Hygiene in 1908, with himself as Executive Secretary. By February 1909 Beers and his distinguished colleagues founded the National Committee for Mental Hygiene. Its mission was to improve the care and treatment of mental illness, and its goals were to raise standards of care, disseminate information to the public for the development of humane and intelligent attitudes toward the mentally ill, encourage research, and organize preventive services. It took a few years for the organization to acquire the resources needed to function. Henry Phipps donated $50,000, and the Rockefeller Foundation and the Commonwealth Fund contributed money for major association projects. The employment of Thomas W. Salmon in 1915 as the first Director of the National Committee for Mental Hygiene was a master stroke.* His administrative skills, planning ability, and dynamic leadership quickly brought the Committee to the forefront.

The climate in which the Progressive Movement thrived encouraged social concern for women, children, and minority groups. Alleviating human misery was seen as primary prevention when it could reduce the incidence of distress and thereby prevent a disorder from developing; secondary prevention could reduce the duration of the disorder by early treatment; and tertiary prevention

---

* Thomas W. Salmon became President of the American Psychiatric Association from 1923–1924. He was the first person who was not a mental institution superintendent to be so named. The collaborative relations between APA and the National Committee for Mental Hygiene were evident in the placement of the first permanent APA headquarters in the latter's offices in New York City.

could decrease the complications accompanying a disorder. It was in the framework of primary prevention that the Mental Hygiene Movement targeted its effort toward children, in the hope that later psychological and emotional illnesses might be prevented. In 1915, a survey of schools revealed emotional and behavioral problems in children with no existing resources for treatment. The drive to provide such resources set off the child guidance movement. Similar concerns led to the establishment of mental hygiene clinics in prisons and in industry.

The Committee journal, *Mental Hygiene*, appeared as a quarterly in 1917, with Frankwood Williams as Editor. Beers met with Clarence M. Hinks (8) and stimulated the founding of the Canadian National Committee for Mental Hygiene in 1918. In 1928 Beers formed the American Foundation for Mental Hygiene to serve as a financing organization. By 1936, there were 50 state and local mental hygiene societies and 30 societies in other countries. Beers' dream had been realized. Several international conferences on mental hygiene were convened (the first in Washington, D.C., with 3,000 persons in attendance, was held in 1930) (7, 8).

State and local organizations were to prove vigorous advocates of the mentally ill in the struggle to secure resources to upgrade institutional care. The National Committee for Mental Hygiene diligently pressed for legislation favoring the mentally ill. Later the National Association for Mental Health would play a major part in the Joint Commission on Mental Health and Illness to insure the implementation of the Commission's recommendations through nationwide action in leadership conferences.

The National Association for Mental Health, NAMH, as the successor to the National Committee for Mental Hygiene, was to be a part also of the Joint Commission on the Mental Health of children and a partner with APA in the Joint Information Service, which published an outstanding series of studies in books on aspects of mental health practice (8–11).

The Psychoanalytic Movement

The Psychoanalytic Movement had an enormous influence upon psychiatry, medicine, and society. To psychiatry, psychoanalysis contributed theory: of libido, the unconscious, incest, narcissism, guilt, transference, and countertransference. Psychoanalysis made it possible to interpret dreams, to uncover the antecedents in childhood of adult neurosis, and to understand mental mechanisms and the use of symbols. It provided a treatment of the neuroses (including neuroses that developed under the stress of war) and a technique for psychotherapy. It enriched the fields of psychiatry, psychology, and social work (12, 13). Psychoanalysis influenced all of medicine by making the psychological components of illness understandable, leading directly to the development of psychosomatic medicine. It brought into the open the need to deal with sexual problems (14).

The impact of psychoanalysis upon society and American culture was even greater than its impact upon medicine, for it affected all aspects of life and human values. It influenced the average lay person's thinking in many ways—for example, behavior disorders and mental illness came to be viewed as the result of inability to surmount or to successfully adapt to the difficult and disturbing conditions of life. Maladaptation came to be viewed as being rooted in the development of the individual and was seen as the result of a series of attempts to adapt (15).

Psychoanalysis brought into focus the importance of the relationships between children and parents and significant others to personality development and character formation. Psychoanalysis had an influence upon sociology, anthropology, philosophy, education, criminology, religion, art, and literature.

The foundation upon which psychoanalysis was built was laid early. Aristophanes, Greek dramatist and poet, described free association as a method of understanding human problems in *The Clouds* in 423 B.C. Charcot, Beckterev, Bernheim, and Forel studied hypnosis, out of which psychoanalysis grew, in the 19th century. Others, such as Janet, Jung, and George Beard, contributed to the knowledge of the unconscious and of neuroses.

The winds of change were blowing at the end of the 19th century. Victorian sexual morality, which held that open display of sexuality was disgraceful, was giving way to concern about venereal disease, sex offenses, illegitimacy, and birth control. Even with this change, however, Freud's sexual theories aroused uneasiness and passionate opposition (16).

Sigmund Freud (1856–1937) worked for some seven years in neurophysiology, contributing to the microscopic anatomy of the pons, the emergence of nerve ganglia, aphasia, and the medicinal value of cocaine. In 1895, Freud collaborated with Breuer on *Studies in Hysteria*. Not long afterward he became convinced that sexual factors were important in the causation of neurotic disorders. This led to a break with his friends and to a period of eight years of working alone without any disciples (17).

The year 1900 marked the appearance of Freud's widely read book, *The Interpretation of Dreams*. His first followers were attracted in 1902, the year Freud founded the Wednesday Psychological Society as a small informal forum in which to discuss ideas. By 1908, this weekly meeting grew to become the Vienna Psychoanalytic Society, with 22 members.

In 1904 Freud's successful and popular book *Psychopathology of Everyday Life* was published. This was also the year in which Freud became internationally recognized. Freud's Libido Theory was formulated in 1905. By 1908, the first psychotherapeutic clinic under medical school auspices opened at Cornell University. Morton Prince presented the first course on psychopathology at Tufts University in 1908, and James J. Putnam gave public lectures at Harvard endorsing the psychic treatment of neuroses (16). Also in 1908 the first International Congress on Psychoanalysis was held in Salzburg. The second Congress met in Nuremburg two years later (17).

On the occasion of Clark University's 25th anniversary in 1909, G. Stanley Hall, its President and America's leading experimental psychologist, invited Freud to give a series of lectures. Among the early supporters who attended the lectures were J.J. Putnam, Adolf Meyer, A.A. Brill, Carl Jung, William James, and Ernest Jones. Freud, uncomfortable with ailments, disliked America; but it was in the United States that psychoanalysis found its strongest support. In Europe, academic approval was essential to the promotion of ideas, and there greater stress was placed upon "nature over nurture." In the United States, where academic approval was less important, acceptance by such national figures who dominated the field as Adolf Meyer and William A. White led to instruction in theory and technique in the principal training centers (16).

Freud published his 28 conversational-style lectures, *A General Introduction to Psychoanalysis*, in 1910 (it was translated into English in 1920). The years 1910–1912 constituted a period of opposition, abusive dissent in Europe in response to Freud's concepts, and a time when close associates such as Alfred Adler,

William Steckel, and C.G. Jung withdrew from the circle of disciples to develop their own schools with their own followers.

A.A. Brill founded the New York Psychoanalytic Society, the American branch of the international association, in 1911, with J.J. Putnam as its first President. Three months later, the American Psychoanalytic Association, with eight members, came into being in Baltimore on May 9, 1911. In 1912, the *Psychoanalytic Review,* edited by William Alanson White and Smith Ely Jelliffe, began regular publication. The *Psychoanalytic Quarterly* appeared in 1932 under the editorship of Lewin Feigenbaum, Frankwood Williams, and Gregory Zilboorg (17).

In May of 1914, at the 70th annual meeting of what was then the American Medico-Psychological Association, the first paper was presented on Freud's work: "A Criticism of Psychoanalysis," by Charles W. Burr of Philadelphia. The formal discussants joined in a scathing denunciation of psychic causation of dream analysis and of sexual psychogenic factors. William Alanson White gave the first public defense of psychoanalysis in rebuttal. White created a new staff position in 1914 at St. Elizabeths Hospital, where he was the Superintendent, to devote all of his time to the psychoanalytic psychotherapy of hospitalized mental patients (18).

There was an unsuccessful move to disband the American Psychoanalytic Association in 1919 and to merge it with the American Psychopathological Association. The not-so-hidden agenda was to free psychiatry from the domination of the "pope in Vienna."

In the 1920s many Americans went to Vienna for psychoanalysis. Among them were Lawrence Kubie, Bert Lewin, Clara Thompson, Clarence Oberndorf, and Abraham Kardiner. Gregory Zilboorg was analyzed in Berlin by Franz Alexander.

When William Alanson White became president of the American Psychiatric Association (1924–1925) his leadership assured the place of psychoanalysis in psychiatry. In 1925, the American Psychiatric Association and the American Psychoanalytic Association began meeting at the same time and place. This arrangement lasted for 50 years until 1974, when the APA met in Detroit and the Psychoanalytic Association in Denver (meeting in the same place at the same time resumed in 1986). Beginning in 1934, psychoanalysis also had its own section in the APA annual meeting program. Winter meetings of the Psychoanalytic Association began in New York City in 1923 and have continued to the present.

Training of analysts was formalized in 1925. By 1932, Psycho-analytic Institutes had been established in Boston, Chicago, New York, Washington, and Baltimore.

When Hitler began to burn books (including those on psycho-analysis) and to persecute Jews, refugee analysts came to the United States from Germany, Austria, and Hungary. The addition of leaders such as Sandor Lorand, Paul Schilder, Otto Rank, and Sandor Ferenczi added strength to the movement in this country.

On Freud's 80th birthday in 1936, the American Psychiatric Association named Freud an Honorary Fellow. Two years later when the Nazis invaded Austria, Freud reluctantly fled to London where he died in September of 1939.

By 1940 the United States had become the world center of psychoanalysis. Debates on the merits of psychoanalysis attracted overflow audiences at American Psychiatric Association annual meetings during the 1940s. Analysts dominated the field of child psychiatry, and in the 1950s they dominated medical education, holding the majority of chairmanships in departments of psychia-try. The Psychoanalytic Movement weathered splits and rivalries within its ranks, withstood virulent attacks from medicine, but finally lost preeminence in psychiatry in the 1970s with the shift to biological dominance.

The Development of Child Psychiatry

Child psychiatry had its origins in Europe,* but its concept, as well as its growth, was wholly American (20). The pioneer builder and promoter of the model interdisciplinary team in a child guid-ance clinic was William Healy (1869–1963). He became inter-ested in the abandoned and traumatized children appearing before a judge in a Chicago court. With funds from a Chicago phi-lanthropist, and after extensive travel around the country during which he discovered only two examples of such a clinic (one in Philadelphia under Lightner Whitmer—a children's project estab-

---

* The early work of Esquirol (1836) in mental deficiency, of Griesinger (1845) in methods of education elaborated by others, and of Emminghaus (1887) in a systematic overview of the development of the mind of a child are examples of these origins. In 1905 Binet and Simon developed psychometric testing and the Intelligence Quotient, which they revised in 1908 and 1911 (19).

lished in 1905—and one at the Vineland, New Jersey, Training School under Henry H. Goddard), Healy returned to Chicago to found the Juvenile Psychopathic Institute in 1909, which later became the Illinois Juvenile Research Institute (20, 21).

The model for child mental health care expressed society's obligation to treat emotionally deprived children and children with behavior disorders. In practice, the Institute served the court for the evaluation and diagnosis of juvenile delinquents. The evaluation was done by a collaborating team of psychiatrists, clinical psychologists, and volunteer home visitors (forerunners of the psychiatric social workers who were trained at the Boston Psychopathic Hospital under Mary Jarrett and at Smith College in 1918 after World War I).

After teaching at Harvard during the summers of 1915 and 1916, Healy moved with his psychiatrist wife, Augusta Bronner, to Boston to become director of the Judge Baker Guidance Center. It was an independent agency providing treatment to children and consultation to social agencies. Not only was the Judge Baker Guidance Center a center for professional study and the model that by 1950 had spread to most cities in the United States, but it was also the model that would be adopted later by community mental health centers.

The National Committee for Mental Hygiene under the leadership of Frankwood Williams, George S. Stevenson, and Milton Kirkpatrick pressed to establish clinics similar to those of Dr. Healy's in all U.S. cities. In cooperation with the Commonwealth Fund in 1922, funds were made available for start-up and for training fellowships (the latter continued until 1946 when it was taken over by the National Institute of Mental Health).

Organizations in the Field of Childhood and Adolescent Psychiatry

The American Orthopsychiatric Association came into being in 1924 to meet the need for a forum where professionals from all mental health disciplines could exchange views on common problems. Its founders were William Healy (the organization's first president), David Levy, Lawson G. Lowrey, Herman Adler, Bernard Glueck, Karl Menninger, George S. Stevenson, and others. When the American Orthopsychiatric Association was founded only child psychiatrists, social workers, and clinical psychologists could be members; but this soon widened to include all workers in the mental health field concerned with both adults and children or adolescents.

As a result of an informal meeting in 1940, and with the stimulation of the National Committee on Mental Hygiene and the Commonwealth Fund, a voluntary standard-setting organization was created—The American Association of Psychiatric Clinics for Children (1945), with H. Frederick Allen as its first President. By 1947, it was determined that 26 child guidance clinics met the formulated standards (22).

The formation of the American Academy of Child Psychiatry was suggested first in 1947 to enhance the identity of child psychiatrists. The organization was founded in 1953, with George Gardner as its first President. It began as an elitist organization and embraced those who were diplomates in child psychiatry of the American Board of Psychiatry (1957). In the 1960s the organization expanded to permit all child psychiatrists to join (21).

Another significant strand in the evolution of child psychiatry emerged out of the institutions for the mentally retarded—the school clinics. As early as 1891, Walter E. Fernald, at the state school for the retarded at Waverly, Massachusetts, initiated an outpatient day for the diagnosis of children having difficulty in school. By 1915 mental clinics were started in Worcester, Massachusetts, which met once a month. Soon thereafter, such clinics were started in other cities in Massachusetts. Massachusetts established free school clinics in 1919 (22).

In the very early years of the National Committee for Mental Hygiene, William Alanson White stated that childhood was "the golden period for mental hygiene" (23). Books and pamphlets were developed and a quarterly journal, *Understanding the Child*, was started in 1931. However, these had little impact on educational programs in the schools. An attempt was made in 1931 to bring mental hygiene concepts into the schools. In 1932 attention was focused on the need for teacher training and for manuals and lesson plans to help students gain insight into emotional problems.

H. Edmund Bullis, who had been Executive Officer of the National Committee for Mental Hygiene, accepted, in 1940, the invitation of Mesrop Tarumianz (Director of the State Society for Mental Hygiene and Superintendent of the Delaware State Hospital) to develop an experimental program in the Delaware school system. This program was developed under the auspices of the

Delaware Mental Hygiene Society with a grant from Mrs. Henry Ittelson. Weekly classes under the "Bullis Plan" on human relations enjoyed wide popularity for a time (24).

Psychology

Psychology, with its roots in philosophy, found its first application in the field of education. As early as 1890, mental tests were developed to help identify the retarded. It would be 20 years until the Binet-Simon test made these efforts reasonably reliable. The first psychological clinic was established in Philadelphia in 1896 by Lightner Whitmer, where the focus was on educational problems of the individual retarded child. Whitmer coined the term "clinical psychology." At about this time Adolf Meyer, at the Worcester State Hospital in Massachusetts, was teaching psychology to staff physicians and giving a course in abnormal psychology at Clark University.

The Juvenile Psychopathic Institute in Chicago, established in 1909, employed psychologists under William Healy who had been influenced by the functional psychology of William James and the dynamic views of Freud (25). The model of a therapeutic team (with psychiatrist, psychologist, and what was to be a psychiatric social worker) was imitated as child guidance clinics sprang up around the country.

The Worcester State Hospital and the Boston Psychopathic Hospital in the 1920s and 1930s became centers for training and research, attracting psychologists who would become leaders in the psychiatric field. After World War II, the National Institute of Mental Health (NIMH) financed training for clinical psychologists and other mental health workers, which greatly increased their numbers. The Veterans Administration hospitals were the principal setting for training in clinical psychology.

The work of experimental psychologists such as the animal experimentation of Lashley and Liddel, begun as early as 1913, was ignored by writers of textbooks in psychiatry for about 40 years. Pavlov (1849–1936), a Russian physiologist who won the Nobel Prize in 1904 for his work on the digestive glands, developed a theory of reflexes, and from this, a mechanistic concept of conditioning and learning. J.B. Watson advanced behavioral psychology and B.F. Skinner laid the groundwork for operant conditioning that paved the road to behavior modification in psychotherapy. Territoriality was studied in song birds, social dominance was studied in the pecking order of hens, and Harry and Margaret Harlow studied the attachment to mother and surrogate mother in the behavior of monkeys (26).

The American Psychological Association was founded in 1892, but it was to be many years before its section on clinical psychology was created (27).

Psychiatric Social Work

Psychiatric social work developed in the United States from four roots. Richard Cabot of Boston (1868–1939) collaborated with social workers. Adolf Meyer's wife, Mary Brooks Meyer (the first psychiatric social worker) made visits to patients' homes and places of employment to aid in the understanding of environmental problems faced by hospitalized patients. William Healy employed volunteers to perform a similar function in the child guidance clinic in order to understand the problems of parents and the home environment. Perhaps the cooperative effort of Elmer E. Southard and Miss Mary C. Jarrett at the Boston Psychopathic Hospital was the most crucial, for it led to the establishment of the Smith College School for Social Work. The concept of psychiatric social work was first made explicit in Southard and Jarrett's book *The Kingdom of Evils*, published in 1922 (8, 9, 28).

Psychiatric Nursing

Psychiatric nursing started in the United States in 1882, nine years after professional nursing began (29). In that year, Dr. E.S. Cowles organized the first program for training nurses in the care of the mentally ill at the McLean Hospital in Belmont, Massachusetts. By 1914, there were 8 basic schools of nursing in mental hospitals and in 20 years there were 64 more. There were about 1,200 state accredited nursing schools in 1945, and of these, more than 65 percent offered a course in psychiatric nursing. Forty-five percent had a 2- to 16-week affiliation (most had 12 weeks) in psychiatric nursing in a mental hospital. In the 1940s, postgraduate training in psychiatric nursing was offered. Many nursing specialists were in administrative or teaching posts. Later basic training of nurses in mental hospitals was discontinued and training encouraged in a college course leading to a degree (30).

Occupational Therapy

Occupational therapy emerged as a profession in 1918, and has a history that extends as far back as the time of the first mental hospital. Pinel, at the beginning of the 19th century, considered work fundamental in the treatment of the insane and noted its use in one of the oldest asylums at Saragossa, Spain. The first regulation of insane asylums in France (1857) specified work as a means of therapy for patients, and mandated that the end product of work belonged to the institution (31).

The philosophy of American mental hospitals was that work was therapeutic for patients; schools for the retarded established colonies as training-grounds for farmhands or houseworkers. The *American Journal of Insanity* had a number of articles in its early issues devoted to "work cure" through the use of occupation. George E. Barton originated the term "occupational therapy" in the 1900s (32).

Susan Tracy's book, *Studies in Invalid Occupation* (1910), was the first formal presentation of occupational therapy in this country. World War I demonstrated the restorative value of occupation, which led in the year 1918 to the founding of four schools for the training of occupational therapists: Milwaukee-Downer (now Lawrence University); Philadelphia (now the University of Pennsylvania); Boston (now Tufts University); and St. Louis (now Washington University).

In 1917, the National Society for the Promotion of Occupational Therapy was incorporated. The name was changed in 1922 to the American Occupational Therapy Association. In that year it published the *Archives of Occupational Therapy.* After three years, it became *Occupational Therapy and Rehabilitation*, and in 1947 the *American Journal of Occupational Therapy.*

Pastoral Counseling

Pastoral counseling had its origin in the mental hospital. Carl Jung's *Modern Man in Search of Soul* (1933) was the inspiration for Anton T. Boisen, who started the religion and psychiatry movement. On his recovery from mental illness, Boisen wrote *The Exploration of the Inner World* (1936). At Worcester, he and his followers—Carroll Wise, Seward Hiltner, and others—established a training course for chaplains. Training in psychiatry and counseling techniques led to standard-setting and an accreditation process.

It would take us too far afield to describe even briefly the origins of organizations within the field of psychiatry that reflect the broad interests of the members of the American Psychiatric Association, such as social psychiatry, law, industry, and other subspecialty interests. I shall, however, note two developments from the many: the Group for Advancement of Psychiatry (GAP) and the American Medical Association's (AMA) activities in mental health.

Group for the Advancement of Psychiatry

The Group for the Advancement of Psychiatry emerged out of an informal group called together by William Menninger during the annual meeting of the American Psychiatric Association in Chicago in May 1946 (33). After the initial meeting and one held the following night the organization was born, with William Menninger elected as President and Henry Brosin as Secretary. Within a day a substantial number of leaders in psychiatry had been invited to pay $5 and become members of the organization with the presumptuous title The Group for the Advancement of Psychiatry. Motivated by what they perceived as a lack of response by the American Psychiatric Association in support of the military during the war, GAP members perceived the remedy to be the restructuring of the APA. A sense of urgency to begin the task without delay led the group to introduce the following day at the annual APA business meeting a rival slate of councilors to those proposed by the Nominating Committee. It is believed this was the first time in APA history that such a challenge was made. All three of the GAP slate of councilors were elected. (In the next four years, three of four presidents elected were GAP members and the fourth a GAP sympathizer.) Dominance in the governing council and in APA leadership aided the restructuring process.

The second action led by GAP was to press for the creation of the position of Medical Director, to be held by an outstanding psychiatrist. The third action was to press for an APA Reorganization Committee. The latter committee was formed and made recommendations that were adopted over several years, such as the process that led to the formation of the Assembly, which truly changed the structure of the APA.

GAP's loose organization, operating under a Steering Committee with working committees (each composed of members selected not for political reasons or prominence but for their expertise in areas selected for study) became a model for organization committees in the psychiatric field. Members, in addition to being experts in the areas of their committees' interests, had to demonstrate their willingness to devote their time and money to advance the field. Committees met for six days a year, members worked at home between meetings on the assigned project, and read critically all committee reports. This was at a time when APA committees met briefly for one or two days once a year and seldom produced anything tangible.

The American Medical Association

The American Medical Association in 1846 tried to persuade the Association of Medical Superintendents to merge with it. Efforts failed again in 1870. In 1854, the AMA conducted a study of insanity in the United States. For 12 years (1865–1877), delegates from AMA attended APA's annual meetings, and for a time in the 1870s both organizations met in the same place at the same time (35).

In the latter half of the 19th century the AMA House of Delegates issued policy statements in the form of resolutions: on restraint (1878) (that restraint was essential and not a violation of rights to personal liberty, and that supervision was necessary to insure appropriate use of restraint); on the need to collect facts in census data on the incidence of insanity and idiocy (1880); on the establishment of a psychophysical laboratory in the Department of the Interior (1901); and on inclusion of mental hygiene in public health programs, and in public education in schools (1914).

Not until 1930 did the AMA create a Committee on Mental Health. The Committee's first report, presented in 1931, called for more training in psychiatry for medical students and physicians; interns in every mental hospital; research in psychiatry; education of the public; and care of the mentally ill along medical rather than legal lines (34). The final comprehensive report presented in 1933 added comments on the needs of the profession, on administrative and legal issues, on prevention of ill health and promotion of good health, and called for closer cooperation between general physicians and psychiatrists (34). Also in 1933, an important step in collaboration between AMA and APA was taken in the establishment of the American Board of Psychiatry and Neurology, which will be discussed in detail later.

A resolve of AMA's House of Delegates (1937) expressed gratitude to the benefactors of research in psychiatry: the Rockefeller Foundation, the John and Mary R. Markle Foundation, the Josiah Macy Foundation, and the Scottish Rite of Free Masonry.

As early as 1944 the AMA's House of Delegates endorsed a recommendation of the AMA President "for a comprehensive study of the mental health of our people by all branches and professions" (34, p. 496). This action would lead to a joint national conference on mental health with APA as cosponsor in 1953, to AMA support of legislation for a national study, and to APA–AMA action to form the Joint Commission on Mental Illness and Health in 1955.

The AMA, in 1951, reestablished after 20 years its Committee on Mental Health. This action was cause for alarm by APA's Medical Director, Daniel Blain, who feared AMA might invade the program territory of an expanding APA. As a safeguard, to insure cooperative and complementary action instead of rivalry, Walter Barton was appointed liaison to the AMA Council on Mental Health. Barton served for 20 years in that role. The AMA Council thrived under such outstanding leaders as Leo Bartemier, Dana Farnsworth, John Donnelly, Loren Smith, Hamilton Ford, Julius Richmond, Lindsey Beaton, Stuart Knox, Rogers Smith, and others. Relationships with other physicians were improved and outstanding work was done by the AMA mental health group in alcoholism, drug abuse, mental retardation, and the impaired physician. The presence of a strong, active AMA Council on Mental Health made it unnecessary for the APA to launch programs in the areas addressed by the AMA.

The American Board of Psychiatry and Neurology

The American Board of Psychiatry and Neurology was established on October 20, 1934. Franklin Ebaugh, in 1931, advocated setting standards for the training of psychiatrists as well as a certification process to assure the clinical competence of psychiatrists. To develop an organization to conduct these activities, joint planning was carried on in 1933 by appointed representatives from three associations. The APA named Clarence Cheney as Chairman, and Franklin Ebaugh, C. MacFie Campbell, Adolf Meyer, and William Alanson White as representatives. The AMA appointed Walter Freeman as Chairman, and George W. Hall, J. Allen Jackson, Edward G. Zabriski, and Lloyd Ziegler as representatives. The American Neurological Association (ANA) named J. Ramsey Hunt, Henry A. Riley, and I.S. Wechsler. The Board as finally constituted in 1934 consisted of the following directors:

For APA: Meyer, Cheney, Campbell, Ebaugh
For ANA: Singer (President), Cassamajor, Pollock, Zabriski
For AMA: Freeman (Secretary), Hall, Jackson, Ziegler

Those with 15 years of specialization who graduated before 1919 were certified (grandfathered). The first examination was held in 1934. Freeman served as Executive Secretary until 1948, and Francis Braceland filled that role until 1951 when David Boyd was appointed. Boyd held the post for 20 years. R. DeJong served in an interim capacity until the appointment of Lester Rudy in 1972.

Child psychiatry was added as a subspecialty area for certification in 1959 and pediatric neurology in 1968, the year that written examinations were introduced in basic neurology and psychiatry.

With the expanding number of candidates to be examined in 1975, the Board of Directors was increased to 16 (8 psychiatrists and 8 neurologists). The APA nominated five psychiatrists and the AMA three. The ANA nominated four neurologists, and the American Academy of Neurology named two, as did the AMA. Residency programs were reviewed by a joint board of psychiatrists, neurologists, and AMA designees to insure that standards in training were met. The majority of psychiatrists and neurologists sought certification as soon as they were eligible.

Neurology in America

The history of American neurology was intertwined with the history of psychiatry in the United States, though neurology developed in Europe. Neurology developed in Germany under Moritz Romberg (1795–1873), in France under Amand Duchenne (1806–1875) and Jean Charcot (1825–1893), and in England at the National Hospital Queen Square in 1860 under C.E. Brown-Sequard and Hughlings Jackson (1835–1911) (35).

The first American book on neurology was written by an APA founding father, Amariah Brigham: *An Inquiry Concerning the*

Diseases and Functions of the Brain and Spinal Cord (published by George Adkard, New York, 1849). The father of neurology in America was S. Wier Mitchell of Philadelphia (son and grandson of a family that produced seven physicians in three generations). Mitchell was physiologist, neurologist, author of 19 novels and 7 books of poetry. During the Civil War, Mitchell was appointed to the Christian Street Hospital in Philadelphia for central nervous system disorders. From that experience he wrote, with Morehouse and Keen, *Gunshot Wounds and Other Injuries of Nerves* (published by Lippincott, Philadelphia, 1864) and *Inquiries of Nerves and Their Consequences* (35). *Fat and Blood,* about the treatment of neurosis with rest cure, was a widely read and popular book. Mitchell wrote a textbook on neurology, *A Treatise on Diseases of the Nervous System* (published by Appleton, New York, 1871). Mitchell's bold criticism of psychiatry at the 50th anniversary celebration of the APA, where he was the featured guest lecturer in 1894, can be found in the *Journal of Nervous and Mental Diseases* (21:413–437, 1894).

When the American Neurological Association was founded in 1875, S. Wier Mitchell was its first President. There were 35 charter members. Neurology journals were originally joined with psychiatry, as in the *Journal of Nervous and Mental Diseases* (1874) and *Archives of Neurology and Psychiatry* (1919). Today, the official journal of the ANA is *Annals of Neurology* (1977); the official journal of the American Academy of Neurology is the *Journal of Neurology* (1951).

By the 1960s, at the height of psychiatry's psychodynamic period, there was a move to split the American Board of Psychiatry and Neurology in two: one for neurology and one for psychiatry. The Board withstood the pressures and in the 1980s, psychiatry's interest in neurophysiology and neurochemistry, and neurology's concern with cognition and emotion, have brought the two specialties closer together in shared interests.

National Institute of Mental Health

The founding of the National Institute of Mental Health (NIMH) in 1946 was an event that was to profoundly affect the field of psychiatry and mental health. Prior to World War II the Division of Mental Hygiene of the United States Public Health Service began to plan for an organization within the federal government to support research and education on the etiology, prevention, and treatment of mental disabilities in the U.S. Army (36). The advent of World War II caused the plans to be shelved, which were revived at the end of the war in the National Mental Health Act (1946).

The new federal institute thrived under the outstanding leadership of Robert H. Felix, its psychiatrist Director. Grants were made in support of research and education of four major professional groups: psychiatry, clinical psychology, psychiatric social work, and nursing. Federal funds made it possible for medical schools to develop strong departments of psychiatry, and to finance training in research and in academic careers. Clinical services were strengthened and Hospital Improvement Grants opened up new avenues.

Within 25 years, NIMH had dramatically increased mental health manpower and the number of psychiatrists. In 1963 NIMH was to develop the Community Mental Health Center program. Beyond a doubt, the federal role in aid to psychiatry, through its agent NIMH, was the most powerful force in the advancement of psychiatry.

THE WAR YEARS

Psychiatry was extensively involved in both the world wars but the contribution of organized psychiatry, as represented by the American Psychiatric Association, was minimal. The APA's lack of leadership and constitutional, procedural, and traditional obstacles enabled other organizations and individuals to demonstrate the importance of psychiatry in the military. The dormant posture of the APA in national affairs was to lead to reorganization and revitalization of the Association in the postwar period.

World War I (1914–1917)

Europe was tinder dry, spoiling for a fight, when the spark of an assassination set off the conflagration. The Crown Prince of Austria, Archduke Francis Ferdinand, and his wife, went in June 1914 to observe military maneuvers in Bosnia-Herzegovnia, a small state under Austrian domination. Bullets fired by Serbian terrorists killed the royal couple on June 28 (37).

A disastrous war followed soon after this tragic event, with Austria declaring war on Serbia in August 1914. The decaying Ottoman Empire joined by declaring war on Russia and its ally, France. Germany invaded Belgium, which brought Great Britain into the fray, with the Allies pitted against the Central Powers. Italy couldn't decide which side to enter until 1915, when it joined the Allies.

Soon battle lines became more or less fixed in an exhausting man-killing stalemate of trench warfare. The European death dance stirred American emotions. The choices were to "fatten on old world follies," a position favored by bankers and investors; to "give all aid short of war," advocated by such leaders as T.R. Roosevelt and Senator Cabot Lodge; or to "ignore and be neutral," abdicating the role of world leader that the U.S. wished to become (37). Woodrow Wilson (1865–1924), former President of Princeton University and Governor of New Jersey, was elected President of the United States in 1912 and reelected in 1916 with the slogan "He kept us out of the War."

When the ocean liner Lusitania, with more than 100 Americans aboard, was torpedoed by a German U-boat in May 1915, popular opinion (which had supported aid to the Allies) began to favor aggressive retaliation. Munitions sent were often sunk by submarines ordered to sink all ships regardless of nationality.

After Britain cut the transatlantic cable, Germany relied on code messages. The British cracked the codes. Britain revealed a decoded message Germany sent to its Ambassador in the United States. The communication stated the wish to keep the U.S. neutral, but if that was not possible, it would form an alliance with Mexico (with whom the U.S. was engaged in border skirmishes), and give it support with the intent to return to Mexico Texas, New Mexico, and Arizona (38). President Wilson finally broke off diplomatic relations with Germany in January 1917, and several months later asked Congress to declare war on the Central Powers "to make the world safe for democracy." After a lengthy debate, Congress declared war on April 6, 1917. One month later the Selective Service Act was passed, requiring all males between the ages of 21 and 31 to register for military duty. Trainees began to pour into 16 huge base camps (38).

With the declaration of war, the deficiencies in American medical education in both neurology and psychiatry became evident. Plans were made to lessen the deficit. Six weeks of intensive instruction were made available at seven centers (Boston Psychopathic Hospital, Mendocino State Hospital in California, New York Neurological Institute, Philadelphia General Hospital, Phipps Psychiatric Institute in Baltimore, Psychopathic Hospital in Ann Arbor, Michigan, and St. Elizabeths Hospital in Washington, D.C.). Bloomingdale Hospital in White Plains, New York, prepared psychiatric nurses, and Smith College trained psychiatric aides (39).

Eight hundred thirty-one APA member-psychiatrists served in the armed forces of the United States (430 served in the U.S. and 264 served overseas). There were far too few properly trained neurologists or psychiatrists to care for the 69,394 neuropsychiatric casualties (of which 5,000 were neurological) (40).

In 1916 the foresight of the National Committee for Mental Hygiene (under the leadership of its director, Thomas W. Salmon) led to the appointment of a commission (under Steward Patton, Pearce Bailey, and Thomas Salmon) to study the psychiatric problems of men fighting the Mexican Border War, as well as those problems of men from Canada and Great Britain, already at war. In March 1917, the Surgeon General called a conference to hear a report on the commission findings. The commission findings stated that the incidence of neuropsychiatric disabilities could be reduced by screening at the induction centers. Without elimination of the unfit, the economic burden would be high, morale would be affected, and needless human suffering would be permitted (39). These findings would be applied as American soldiers entered World War I.

Strecker (39) stressed the value of the induction examination in keeping the psychiatrically fragile out of the Army. He noted that of 2,000,000 troops sent overseas, only a small number (4,039) developed neuropsychiatric disability; and of these, 3,181 had been sent overseas in spite of the psychiatrist's recommendation "that they were not fit for military service of any kind." There was also substantial agreement with original examination findings at several points in the military review of soldiers who developed mental disorders, according to Strecker (39). This conviction that proper screening at induction centers would eliminate psychiatric problems in the armed services would prove disastrous in World War II and account, in part, for the lack of planning for psychiatric casualties.

As early as 1914, "shell shock" became a major medical problem. Trench fighting, fatigue, exposure, and the use of high explosive shells were factors seen as causative. "Shell shock" was recognized as a psychological state and not a blast injury. Salmon noted that a very high percentage of men were salvageable for return to duty if treated promptly in forward areas (41).

As a result of psychiatry's role in World War I, many lessons were learned. Some of these were:

- Screening at induction centers eliminated the grossly mentally disordered and deficient who were unfit for military duty.
- Medical education of all physicians should include basic training in psychiatry and neurology.
- Psychiatrists should be involved in the planning for care of neuropsychiatric casualties that developed in combat (about 70,000 cases).
- Combat stress produced mental illness in the normal as well as in the predisposed.
- Attitudes and behavior of the treatment-givers influenced therapy.
- Treatment should be given as soon and as close as possible to the point where the breakdown occurred. (Base hospital 117, with 1,000 psychiatric beds, returned 60 percent of its casualties to duty in 14 days).
- There should be an expectation of early return to duty.
- Rest, food, assurance, suggestions, exhortation, and ventilation of feelings were effective therapeutic agents.
- Psychiatrists should be assigned to each division and as triage agents during combat.
- Every base hospital should have at least a 110-bed psychiatric unit, and all army general hospitals in the U.S. should have a 30-bed psychiatric unit.

The men who served as consultants to the Surgeon General of the Army developed a superior system for the use of psychiatry in military service (Salmon, Patton, Bailey, Adolf Meyer, and William A. White). Most productive were Thomas Salmon (assigned to the American Expeditionary Forces) and Pierce Bailey (assigned to the

Zone of the Interior). Theirs was largely an effort of individual leadership, working without the support or guidance of the American Medico-Psychologic Association.

Another incident merits comment, for it stimulated a recommendation from psychiatrists. At the end of the war, President Wilson noted the necessity for a general association of nations (a League of Nations) and the need for mutual guarantees of political independence and territorial integrity for both great and small nations. With the signing of the Armistice in November 1918, Wilson sought a basis for an enduring peace. A shift of the balance of power in Congress from Democratic to Republican dominance caused the Senate to fail to ratify the Versailles Treaty by seven votes. Wilson went on a national tour to mobilize popular sentiment for passage of the Treaty. Pushing himself to exhaustion, Wilson suffered a stroke in September 1919, the effects of which endured beyond the expiration of his term as President on March 4, 1921 (he died in 1924). During Wilson's incapacity while still President, he was shielded by Col. House, the Secretary of State, and his private secretary. It was Wilson's wife who decided whom the President might see. Official messages and matters of state were settled and documents signed under the supervision of these three persons. It is alleged that the President at times was unable to comprehend the nature of issues and was incapable of exercising judgment. Decisions were made for the President by the protective members of the inner circle. The constitutional mechanisms provided for succession were not applicable because of the attending physician's assurances of recovery. Much later—in 1973—the Group for the Advancement of Psychiatry would address the issue in a report which stated that it was imperative to formulate a plan to cover such a contingency in the future (42).

World War II: 1939–1946

Events Leading to Global War

The effort to build a peaceful world after World War I was as unsuccessful as the attempt to prevent that war had been. The Council of Ten, which drafted the peace treaty after World War I, was led by four men: Wilson, Clemenceau, Lloyd George, and Orlando. Wilson, the idealist, brought his 14 points, which included: openly negotiated pacts, freedom of the seas, removal of economic barriers, evacuation of occupied territories, reduction of armaments, and a League of Nations. Clemenceau of France sought punishment of the Germans as his principal goal. Lloyd George and Orlando placed national interests as their top priority (43). Behind the facade of an openly negotiated Treaty of Versailles (1919) and the support for and establishment of the League of Nations, secret treaties were made, and alliances once again forged, that were to lay the foundations for World War II.

A dream of world unity accompanied the formal signing of the Treaty of Versailles in May 1919. On the national scene that year in the United States, the 18th Amendment ushered in the prohibition of alcoholic beverages, with the popular slogan "See America Thirst." Its consequence was a drop in the rate of alcoholism at the price of general disrespect for the law. Speakeasies and bootleg liquor were commonplace, while mobsters built a lucrative industry based upon public demand.

Herbert Hoover, who had fed America and its allies during World War I as the Director of the Food Administration, after the war's end demonstrated a high level of American management skill as head of the American Relief Administration, with organized distribution of food to starving Europeans including revolutionary Soviets.

Margaret Sanger had been jailed for writing the book *Family Limitation*, about birth control (1915). In 1919, four women were arrested and jailed for six months for picketing the White House as advocates of women's suffrage.

Warren G. Harding won the Presidency by a landslide in 1921, with an ambiguous posture on the League of Nations and a promise to "get back to normal" with removal of war-time controls. His administration was one of scandal and corruption. The friends he appointed, "The Ohio Gang," used their high office for personal enrichment. Fraud, bribery, and other scandals emblazoned newspaper headlines. The Department of Justice became a mockery of justice by accepting bribes to allow liquor to be sold. Naval oil reserves were stolen and sold for a profit, as were supplies intended for Veterans Administration patients. When Harding died of a heart attack in August 1923, Calvin Coolidge became President (1923–1929). Coolidge was isolationist in foreign policy, against federal handouts and farm subsidies, and in favor of economy in government with tax cuts. His dry humor and frugal ways became legendary. A noteworthy event with the highest hope for success was the signing of the Kellogg-Briand Pact in 1928 to outlaw war.

Herbert Hoover followed Coolidge as President (1929–1933). He continued the policy of drastic economy in government with a balanced federal budget. Two months after he took office the stock market crashed, with a $30 billion paper loss. The Great Depression was underway with massive unemployment. By 1932, one-fourth of the work force was idle, mortgages were foreclosed, and industrial production fell to one-half that of 1929. Legislation was passed to aid businesses and farms facing mortgage foreclosures, to provide loans to states to feed the unemployed, and to expand public works. Hoover became the scapegoat for the world-wide depression and he was soundly defeated by Franklin D. Roosevelt (President from 1933–1945).

Roosevelt, who had been Secretary of the Navy, suffered paralysis from poliomyelitis in 1921. In spite of his handicap, he maintained his political stature, serving as Governor of New York from 1928 until 1932. FDR as President was a charismatic and able leader, who swung into action to combat the wreckage of depression. On inauguration day (March 4, 1933) he declared a bank holiday, closing all banks. This was followed by an avalanche of alphabet agencies such as the TVA, NRA, WPA, and more. An all-out effort to overcome fear of poverty and helplessness, and to dispel the humiliation of seeking handouts, was successful with a return of confidence and an upswing in the economy in 1935. The U.S. was preoccupied with its search for economic recovery and determined to stay out of foreign wars.

Europe at this time was in chaos. Wilson's dream of world unity collapsed as strong leaders emerged, reviving imperialism by rallying followers to take pride in their nation. One such leader, Adolf Hitler, became Chancellor of Germany in 1933. In that year he had written *Mein Kampf,* announcing his intention to restore Germany to its rightful place as a world leader, and proclaiming Aryan supremacy.

Hostility was projected onto Jews. They were marked for easy recognition, hunted, imprisoned, and used as human guinea pigs and slave laborers. Some 10 million Jews were imprisoned, and six million were exterminated in a barbarous holocaust.

While Hitler's stormtroopers marched in Berlin and harassed Jews, the U.S. celebrated the repeal of prohibition with the passage of the 21st Amendment, and Americans sang "Happy Days Are Here Again." Germany repudiated the Versailles Treaty on March 16, 1935 and annexed the adjacent industrial valley on February 27, 1936. Neville Chamberlin, Prime Minister of Great Britain, rushed to Berlin in September 1938 to try to avert war and returned proudly proclaiming a negotiated "peace in our time." Germany formed an alliance with Italy, and Japan joined the "Berlin Axis." Japan had seized Peking in 1937 and war with China was already underway. Chiang Kia-Shek joined forces with his opponent Communist leader, Mao Tse Tung, to drive out the common foe. Citizens of the U.S. sympathized with the victims of aggression although this sympathy was accompanied by determined isolationism that led Roosevelt in 1937 to denounce the reign of terror and international lawlessness without naming Germany, Italy, or Japan, saying "let no one imagine America will escape."

The act that ignited the international conflagration was Germany's lightning strike against Poland on September 1, 1939. England and France declared war but had no success in stopping Germany, as that country overwhelmed Holland, Belgium, Norway, and all of France. England retreated behind its protective channel waters to defend itself as a confident Hitler invaded Russia.

In the U.S. in 1939, Congress enacted the American Neutrality Act and the President endured protests for his arbitrary action to transfer 50 over-age destroyers to Great Britain. When Roosevelt defeated Wendell Wilkie in 1940, he was able to win passage—as vital to the defense of the U.S.—of the Lend Lease Act to send ships, munitions, and commodities to Great Britain and China. In October 1941, German submarines attacked ships close to U.S. shores and sank American ships in the Atlantic. The shooting war began as U.S. destroyers took defensive action.

Ignoring the warning of the Chinese Ambassador Hu Shih as well as United States intelligence reports, an unprepared United States was jolted by the Japanese attack on Pearl Harbor in December 1941 while negotiations were underway with Japan in Washington. The United States declared war on Japan, and Germany and Italy joined the Axis and declared war on the United States.

With the destruction of the U.S. Pacific fleet in that dawn attack on Pearl Harbor, Japan swept over China, Hong Kong, Singapore, the Phillipines, and the Pacific Islands. It was near the end of 1942 before Australia and the United States halted the advance of Japan in Asia. About the same time the United States and British forces landed in North Africa to stop the "Desert Fox," Rommell, in his conquest of the northern part of that continent. Slowly the Axis forces began to fall back. The U.S. occupied Sicily and gradually rolled back the Germans after the collapse of Italy. A masterful campaign led by Douglas MacArthur and Chester Nimitz pushed the Japanese back island by island in the Pacific war zone.

It was June 6, 1944—"D Day"—under the Supreme Allied Command of Dwight D. Eisenhower, when 535 ships carried the invading army to the shores of France under a protective naval bombardment with total command of the air. By July, the armies broke out of St. Lo and captured 35,000 German troops. By August, Paris was liberated and by September the Allies were in Germany.

In April of 1945 Mussolini was dead and Hitler committed suicide as the Russians, British, and Americans encircled Berlin; FDR died of a cerebral hemorrhage. Germany surrendered unconditionally on May 7th, 1945.

An atomic bomb was first exploded as a test on July 1945 in New Mexico. Japan refused a call to surrender in July. In August, Hiroshima and Nagasaki were devastated by two atomic bombs that killed 140,000 persons. It was estimated that the invasion of Japan, scheduled to begin in November, would cost 750,000 American and 1 million Japanese lives. That awesome sacrifice was made unnecessary by the tragic elimination of the people of those two cities; for Japan surrendered on September 2, 1945.

The war had an enormous impact upon U.S. agriculture, industry, labor, education, and communication. It touched the lives of all citizens, children as well as adults. When they entered into the military, 8,700,000 men left the work force. Some 92,000 in the Women's Auxiliary Corps released more men for combat duty. This marked the beginning of a shift of women to jobs outside the home. Many women worked in the munitions factories and filled the vacuum left by men in the armed forces. Two-thirds of all U.S. industry shifted to the manufacture of war supplies. Fifteen hundred ships were built, and 15,000 landing craft, 123,000 airplanes, and 53,000 war tanks were completed. The war is estimated to have cost $100 billion and marked the beginning of a staggering national debt. Taxes were raised and millions of people who had never paid before became taxpayers. Aliens were registered. Tragically, Americans of Japanese extraction were interned in camps. There was also censorship of the media (37).

The global war mobilized 63 million persons. Eight and one-half million military personnel were killed, and perhaps 35 million more persons died as the result of the war. Approximately six million Jews were exterminated by the Nazis. Two and one-half million individuals were wounded; many were left with handicaps. Fifteen million tons of shipping were lost and 7½ million prisoners taken. Millions more were made homeless in the destruction of cities.

It is little wonder that a search for an enduring peace and the outlawing of war as a means of settling disputes was begun in Moscow on October 30, 1943, among the Soviet Union, United States, Great Britain, and China. Senator J.W. Fulbright had proposed the development of international machinery with enough power to impose sanctions.

Planning an international structure was carried out at Dumbarton Oaks, near Washington, D.C. (August 21–October 9, 1944). Solidarity, security, and terms of peace with partition of Germany were pledged by Roosevelt, Stalin, and Churchill at Yalta (February 4–11, 1945).

The United Nations emerged from these negotiations with the hope that, through its creation (by the signing of the charter in June 1945), the dream of peace might become a reality (44).

Psychiatry's Role in World War II

The same lack of preparedness that characterized the military also characterized the medical departments of the armed services in the planning for psychiatric casualties. Forgotten were the lessons learned from World War I. The recommendations contained in Volume X of its Medical History were not remembered, except for the conviction that better screening at induction might eliminate the problem of psychiatric casualties. It was necessary to rediscover the need for division psychiatrists, psychiatric units in general hospitals, and special programs of treatment for the mentally ill. Once again it was not the psychoses that caused the major problem, but breakdown under stress.

The necessity for psychiatric services in the Armed Forces became evident from the record of experience in World War II:

- 1,875,000 of 15 million examined were rejected as unfit for military duty by reason of neuropsychiatric disorders.
- 1,000,000 admissions to army hospitals were for neuropsychiatric disorders, representing 850,000 individuals. This was a rate of 45 admissions per 1,000 troops, and comprised 6 percent of all admissions to hospitals. Seven percent of these admissions were for psychoses, 64 percent for neuroses, and 29 percent for personality disorders, mental retardation, and other conditions. Forty percent of admissions occurred overseas and 60 percent occurred in the United States.
- Of the 850,000 persons admitted to hospital, 380,000 were medically discharged and 130,000 were administratively discharged.
- 2,400 physicians served the army in neuropsychiatric capacities. Of these, 992 were physicians given a three-month course of training in psychiatry. They were assisted by 400 clinical psychologists, 700 social workers, and many more nurses (45).
- $1 billion was spent between 1923 and 1940 by the U.S. government for the care and treatment of World War I veterans with psychiatric disabilities. In 1940, three out of five beds in VA hospitals were filled with neuropsychiatric patients.

Between World War I and World War II, the Army had assigned psychiatrists to Army general hospitals and to aviation medicine beginning in 1921. In 1930 a 200-bed psychiatric unit with both open and closed wards was built at Walter Reed Army Hospital in Washington, D.C. Psychiatry was taught in the Army Medical School. Emphasis was upon the role of the psychiatrist at screening and induction. Psychiatrists were eliminated from divisions in 1940. There was no involvement of psychiatry in planning for casualties or in planning for mobilization in 1939. No criteria to detect neuropsychiatric disabilities had been developed for use in selection at induction, and no facilities had been planned for the care and treatment of psychiatric casualties, in spite of the findings recorded in Volume X of the World War I History of the Medical Department (46). When the U.S. entered World War II there were only 35 psychiatrists in the regular Army, four of whom were board certified.

In February 1942, the Surgeon General of the Army, J.S. Magee, appointed Col. Madigan as head of the Neuropsychiatric Branch of the Professional Services Division. In April 1942 he brought Malcolm J. Farrell to be his deputy. At the time there was no information on the incidence of neuropsychiatric casualties. Farrell asked the APA for a list of suggested psychiatrists to head the Neuropsychiatric Division in the Surgeon General's office. From that list, Roy D. Halloran was selected in August 1942. He had been Superintendent of the Metropolitan State Hospital in Boston. Halloran brought his staff into the Surgeon General's office: J.W. Appell for prevention, liaison, and special services; Walter E. Barton for reconditioning, occupational therapy, and rehabilitation; and William H. Everts for neurology (42).

In November 1943 Col. Roy D. Halloran, Director of the Neuropsychiatric Consultation Division, died suddenly of a heart attack. A series of fortuitous events led to the selection of a great leader to replace Halloran. William C. Menninger had been appointed as psychiatrist to the 4th Service Command. The commanding general had little use for psychiatrists. When Menninger made his formal call upon reporting for duty, the commander was working on his stamp collection. Menninger, an avid collector, won instant approval when his expertise in stamps was recognized. Menninger turned a dismal, boring dinner party for the visiting Surgeon General into a rollicking song fest with his piano playing. Top ranking medical officers gathered at a dinner to welcome the newly appointed head of psychiatry in the Army and were ready to give support to Menninger after he told a humorous story about a young bull who was properly humble among older and more experienced bulls.

General Menninger, in command of the Neuropsychiatric Consultation Division, extended the prestige and power of psychiatry in the Army. This was accomplished by changes in structure of the Surgeon General's Office, with broadened scope of action, through communication, extension of training activities, and the introduction of new programs.

In October 1943, War Department Technical Bulletin 203 presented the first dynamic diagnostic nomenclature for psychiatric disorders. It reflected psychoanalytic concepts of personality development and presented mental illness as stress reactions manifested by symptoms. This nomenclature was later to be adopted by the American Psychiatric Association as *DSM-I*.

Contributions of Organized Psychiatry to World War II

The American Psychiatric Association and other psychiatric organizations took preparatory steps to make their members, the public, and the armed forces aware of the potential role of psychiatry before the United States entered the war as a combatant.

In 1938, trustees of the William Alanson White Psychiatric Foundation prepared a report on the place of psychiatry in the armed forces, and its journal *Psychiatry: Journal for the Study of Interpersonal Processes* covered this topic in an article and in an editorial in February 1939. At the APA's annual meeting in May 1939, a Committee on Military Mobilization was appointed to confer with the appropriate governmental departments on the utilization of psychiatrists. In October 1939, the Southern Psychiatric Association adopted a resolution on psychiatry's role, and appointed a committee to report on utilization at its next annual meeting. The National Research Council created a Subcommittee on Neuropsychiatry (chaired by Winfred Overholser, Superintendent of St. Elizabeths Hospital and Secretary of APA from 1941–1946) (47).

In the middle of October 1939, the APA Committee on Military Mobilization (with Steckel as Chairman and F.W. Sleeper, A.H. Pierce, W.J. Otis, and S.W. Hamilton as members) met with the Surgeons General of the Army and Navy. One outcome of the meeting was a list of those psychiatrists available for military duty based upon a survey made by the APA of civilian psychiatrists (47). The Committee also sponsored a discussion of military psychiatry at the annual meeting in May 1940, inspected psychiatric practice in Canadian armed forces, and conferred with Selective Service (45). Also, in October 1943, the Southern Psychiatric Association sent a resolution to appropriate federal agencies, stressing the importance of psychiatry in a national emergency. The Southern Psychiatric Association reported the action taken at the APA annual meeting in May 1940. Points made in the resolution were:

- Psychiatrists can aid in selection and training of military personnel and in the maintenance of morale.
- Criteria for selection of inductees should be formulated with the aid of psychiatrists.

A committee of the William Alanson White Psychiatric Foundation was established in June 1940. Its report, published in October 1940, was the basis for Medical Circular No. 1 (November 1940) of the Selective Service and was sent to 6,400 draft boards. It was a primer on how to detect the mentally disturbed and how to recognize personality defects (46).

In 1941, Dr. Harry Stack Sullivan (affiliated with the William Alanson White Psychiatric Foundation and Psychiatric Consultation to Selective Service), along with other psychiatrists, conducted two-day seminars on screening for psychiatric disability in nine major cities for draft board physicians. In spite of screening efforts many were being discharged from the armed services for neuropsychiatric disabilities. This led to a directive to abandon the draft board examination in favor of a single examination at the induction center (it was this change, opposed by Dr. Sullivan and by others, that led Dr. Sullivan to resign his post. Raymond Waggoner replaced him in 1943) (47).

The National Research Council Committee (with Overholser as Chairman, and F. Ebaugh, Adolf Meyer, Foster Kennedy, Tracy Putnam, H. Steckel, and J. Whitehorn as members) advised the Surgeon General's office of the army to:

- Revise the army standards of examination
- Assign a psychiatrist to each division and a consultant psychiatrist to each corps
- Assign clinical psychologists to work with psychiatrists and initiate training in psychiatry for physicians
- Hold inductees for five days of observation (nine percent broke down on the first day of service)

The Surgeon General's office of the army declined to implement the recommendation (46).

Alexander Simon (psychiatrist at St. Elizabeths Hospital) and Margaret Hagen (American Red Cross field director) studied 400 admissions for neuropsychiatric disorders (soldiers, sailors, and coastguardsmen), and discovered that one in four had been hospitalized prior to induction. Their report cited the case of a man, hospitalized five weeks after induction, who had a 10-year history of schizophrenia and residence in four different mental hospitals. D.J. Flicker, an army psychiatrist, also called attention to the need for records of previous hospital treatment at induction (47). This led to pressure upon Selective Service by the National Committee for Mental Hygiene to make such histories available. Although a directive from Selective Service was issued in December 1941, it failed to produce records, probably because a mechanism for payment was not included. Implementation did not occur until 1943, when the National Committee for Mental Hygiene employed a full-time liaison officer, Luther E. Woodward, to work with Selective Service to organize history-taking, and, with the aid of volunteers, to gather medical histories.

At the annual meetings of the American Psychiatric Association, the contributions of psychiatry to the armed forces were prominently featured. Simon and Hagan's work at St. Elizabeths on the need for medical records at induction was reported in 1942. At the 1942 meeting of the APA, a resolution was prepared for the Surgeons General noting that the Army and Navy were not utilizing the resources of psychiatry and were "shockingly unappreciative of the lessons learned in World War I." The resolution was forcefully presented to the military by A. Ruggles as Chairman and Strecker and Parsons as committee members (45).

In the spring of 1943 Dr. Strecker, President of the APA, was named psychiatric consultant to the Secretary of War for the Army, Air Force, and Surgeon General of the Navy.

The APA annual meeting held in May 1943 featured Col. Halloran and Lt. Col. Farrell presenting significant developments in the Army: establishment of mental hygiene units at replacement centers; psychiatric sections in station and general hospitals; treatment; and morale building. J.M. Murray of the Air Surgeon's office reported on flying stress, and Rogers Smith reported on group neuroses in Marines at Guadalcanal. Bartholomew Hogan gave a stirring address that brought the audience to its feet with a graphic portrayal of stress reactions, self-sacrifice, and extraordinary behavior of the ship's crew when the aircraft carrier "Wasp" was torpedoed and sunk at Guadalcanal (Hogan was Senior Medical Officer of the "Wasp") (45).

Albert Deutsch called the steps taken by the APA to give leadership and direction to the psychiatric aspects of military service "hesitant and uncertain" (47). He blamed the APA for permitting the army to forget the lessons learned in World War I (47). W.C. Menninger, Francis Braceland, and Robert Felix, as noted elsewhere, called upon the APA to give active support to the military. The involvement of APA as just cited was not great enough to offset the perception that the Association failed to provide the desired leadership, and that other organizations were more effective in producing change.

Lessons Learned from World War II

World War II taught us a number of things about the role of psychiatry in the military. Organized psychiatry has a continuing responsibility to insure that the military services have a psychiatric presence, making them aware of the experience of the past, keeping them abreast of current trends, and ensuring that they are capable of planning for the future. Our past experience has taught us that the armed forces require a psychiatric team, composed of psychiatric nurses, social workers, clinical psychologists, occupational therapists, and rehabilitation personnel. Planning for psychiatric services should insure the team's availability.

World War II exposed the inadequate training of physicians in psychiatry. Medical education, we have learned, should include psychiatry in the basic training of all physicians. When qualified psychiatrists are in short supply, intensive training of physicians in psychiatry can produce acceptable substitutes. In addition to medical education, education of the general public about psychiatric illness and its treatment is essential to the creation of a climate of acceptance of the potential of psychiatry.

We have learned from our World War II experience that induction screening has limited value in detecting those who will break down under the stress of military service. The incidence of psychiatric casualties in World War II was twice that of World War I in spite of a rejection rate that was five times greater (45). We have learned that the *most essential element in effective screening is the medical history of previous hospitalizations and treatments*. The elimination at induction of the overtly mentally disabled is the desired goal. More difficult to detect are those unable to absorb training or tolerate stress. The extremely high cost of breakdowns in the service and soldiers' continued dependence on veterans' benefits suggests the value of a five-day observation at induction.

We have learned that officer selection and training has an important relationship to troop performance and morale, a factor in stress tolerance. Stress tolerance levels vary widely. Separation from the security of the family causes some to break down (nine percent on the first day of service) (48). Others could not tolerate loss of control of their lives in the Army hierarchy, with the Army's disturbed sense of equality and highly organized compulsory routine (42 percent of soldiers broke down during the first six months of training). Some became ill from the fear of personal injury, of being pinned down under fire, or after prolonged combat exposure without relief (45). As an alternative, our experience has taught us that some who are unlikely to tolerate combat stress can be placed in service jobs using vocational skills. For those who developed psychiatric disorders, group therapy proved a useful therapeutic modality.

Troop morale (valued aim and purpose, sense of competence, a belief that one matters to the group) we learned, is enhanced by competent officers, a defined tour of duty, and a period of rest and relaxation. This also aided in the tolerance of stress, as did group, rather than individual, replacements.

The availability of psychiatrists in mental hygiene clinics, in divisions, and in station and general hospitals was deemed essential for the detection and treatment of early stress reactions and illness.

Treatment of acute disorders in forward areas during World War II resulted in a high proportion of returns to duty (60 percent returned to duty with their unit in two to five days; of the 40 percent remaining, approximately one-third were salvaged for non-combat duty in the area; the rest were evacuated) (45).

Grinker and Spiegell (49) described the dynamics of stress reaction that contributed to vulnerability to breakdown and developed abreaction as a technique in therapy. Brill and Beebe (50) reported on a follow-up study of war neuroses, showing a greater number of neuroses in those with only an elementary school education as opposed to higher education, and in those who were older (there were twice the number of neuroses at age 34 than at age 18). The rate of neuroses was higher in combat regiments compared with those in quiet sectors.

Our experience has taught us that early ambulation after surgical procedures, and reconditioning exercises, maintain strength and hasten convalescence. Rehabilitation for severe physical disabilities is essential, along with awareness of the very great role of the emotional overlay as a factor in learning to live with a handicap.

The development of special hospitals for the treatment and rehabilitation of the blind, the deaf, the amputee, and the paralyzed set a high standard for the nonmilitary organizations to follow after the war. Too many closed ward psychiatric beds were built during the war. Most psychiatric disabilities were treatable on an ambulatory basis.

We have learned that in the total war effort there is a place for those not fit for combat. Even those of very low intelligence could perform in the Pioneer Corps. Many skilled tasks and laborious jobs can be filled satisfactorily by those who are unable to tolerate the stress of combat.

CHANGE IN PUBLIC OPINION AND SOCIAL POLICY

The gradual disappearance of a frontier society in America, with its shift of millions from rural to urban living, had geographic, economic, and psychological implications. Frontier society encouraged and rewarded individuality, ingenuity, and even eccentricity. The acceptance of nonconforming behavior gave way to rejection of deviance. Crowded housing, compact neighborhoods, new kinds of jobs, and competition for them brought less tolerance of deviance. No longer could one act out one's eccentricities and still find acceptance. The emotionally unstable, those unable to adapt, and those with no marketable skills were trapped in a lower class, frustrated in the struggle for equality (51).

As I have noted, social welfare movements emerged to combat poverty, delinquency, and disease, with prevention as a primary goal. Voluntary organizations directed their efforts toward tuberculosis, child welfare, social hygiene, and mental hygiene. A protective government sought to safeguard the mother, to nurture the child, to provide schools, to guide physical and emotional growth, to guarantee a job or support, and to bring security to the aged (52).

Rennie and Woodward (53), of the National Committee for Mental Hygiene, summed up the lessons learned in two global wars in a manner that seemed applicable to all persons in society:

- Satisfactory interpersonal relationships and environmental factors are important to health and stability.
- Good leadership contributes to morale.
- Prolonged exposure to (combat) stress upsets even the normally stable.

- Family, job, and community attitudes exert forces affecting morale and personal adjustment.
- Long separations have important effects upon marital partners.

During the first half of the 20th century religion lost power as a stabilizing anchor for life. The swift advance of science brought hope that human wisdom would solve the problems of all people. A warring society is a sick society. An attempt was made in 1928 to outlaw war. In 1933, the good neighbor policy was articulated to encourage hemispheric solidarity. On the domestic scene, the 18th Amendment (1919) inaugurated prohibition, in the hope that this would solve the problem of alcoholism.

The 19th Amendment (1920) gave women the right to vote. The aged were protected under social security in 1936. Employment was stabilized and compensation given to the unemployed, and an attempt was made to build interracial understanding.

At the start of the century life was perceived as a struggle for survival. The unfit had to be weeded out to make room for the more capable; this would strengthen the nation. Thus, social Darwinism reinforced the Protestant work ethic (54). The patient with a mental disorder was an object to be observed, classified, and confined. During the 50-year span the individual emerged, an experiment in the development of a unique person. This person was a unit of society—capable of adapting to and of changing his or her environment. The concept of mind–body unity, a whole person integrating cultural and social factors, laid the foundation of the advancement of psychiatry.

Some of the first studies of public opinion and social attitudes were started in this 50-year span. Bogardus (55) in 1925 advanced the concept of social distance in relation to ethnic groups. Allen (56) assessed public attitudes toward the mentally ill in 1940. He found the public to fear, stigmatize, and reject the mentally disordered. Ramsey and Sief (57) showed, in 1948, that the public was moving toward a more humanitarian and more scientific attitude toward the mentally ill (58).

Other generally held opinions during this period were:

- Early intervention in childhood could prevent major disability later in life.
- Education was a favored route to the development of mental health.

- Hereditary predisposition and psychological conflicts early in life made some individuals more vulnerable to environmental stress in the process of growth.
- Everyone has a breaking point under stress.
- Stress is reduced with the provision of jobs, housing, and economic security. Major mental breakdowns are less likely when stress on the individual is diminished.
- Early ambulation after disease or injury preserves bodily function and hastens convalescence.
- Rehabilitation of the handicapped maximizes the capacity for social functioning.
- Mental patients are expected to contribute labor, if they are able to do so, to routine operations of the hospital in which they are confined in order to reduce the cost of their care to society. Productive work fosters relationships with others, diminishes the deterioration fostered by idleness and rumination, and builds work habits that favor adjustment after leaving the hospital.
- Women have a larger role in society outside the home, in the professions, in the work force, and in the military, than they had as wives and homemakers.
- Discrimination against racial or ethnic groups, when allowed to go unchallenged, leads to shocking consequences (such as slave labor, experimentation on humans, and even extermination).

In the first half of the 20th century the United States emerged as a world power. Bursting with energy and optimism, the people of the nation believed they had "saved the world for democracy" through victory in the first World War. The shattering effect of the Great Depression followed by a second global war brought human suffering into focus. Gradually, confidence in the ability to solve problems was restored.

5

Psychiatry Advances as
a Medical Speciality:
1900-1949

The goal of medicine is peculiarly the goal of making itself unnecessary: of influencing life so that what is medicine today becomes mere commonsense tomorrow.

—Adolf Meyer (1)

From the end of the 19th century to the first half of the 20th, the diagnosis and treatment of medical conditions markedly improved. This was especially true for diseases caused by micro-organisms such as syphilis and toxic infectious disorders, dietary disorders such as pellagra, and hormonal disturbances such as thyroid deficiency (2).

As I have already mentioned, Paracelsus (1492–1541) and Johann Weyer (1515–1588) started the first revolution in thought about mental disease in the 16th century. Paracelsus, rebelling against authority, decried the teaching of ancient as well as contemporary belief in planetary influence and demons. It was Weyer's careful case studies that began descriptive psychiatry. He denounced the Inquisition and its conviction that individuals were possessed by demons. Weyer believed that mental illness should be treated by physicians and he demonstrated cures by psychological means. He earned the title of "Father of Psychiatry" for his beliefs and actions. Descriptive psychiatry extended into the 20th century as "Kraepelinian psychiatry." Emil Kraepelin (1856–1926) classified, described, and sorted out mental disorders, differentiating dementia praecox from manic-depressive disease.

The second revolution in psychiatry was to begin early in the 20th century as a consequence of the work of Sigmund Freud (1856–1939). His theories would bring new insight into the psychological origins of mental disorders and introduce a therapeutic technique.

As the century began, mental disorders were viewed as either organic (with a demonstrable physical basis) or functional (without evidence of a physical origin). Unlike the earlier period of descriptive psychiatry when theory bore no relation to clinical treatment, the excitement that followed each new discovery in this period led to application in therapy. Before I cite examples, let us look at the prophetic utterance in the presidential address of Peter M. Wise, delivered in 1901. He said that the laboratory and clinical experience led "to the conclusion that the vitalizing element of cell integrity depends more upon chemical processes than upon structure and that we may have marked digressions from the normal without structural change . . . and have no traces in the structure in the non-living tissue discoverable at least by present technique" (3, p. 79).

Most psychiatrists followed the organic tradition up to the Second World War even while incorporating the contributions of Freud and Meyer into their practice. Perhaps the most significant breakthroughs for organicists was the discovery in 1911 by Noguchi of the organism that caused syphilis—treponema pallidum. When Wagner Von Jauregg demonstrated the germ's sensitivity to heat from the fever produced by malaria in 1919 (for which he won the Nobel Prize in 1927), a new treatment for central nervous system syphilis was born. St. Elizabeths Hospital was the first to use the new therapy in 1922, and developed a strain of malaria that was in general use. Later, electricity in diathermy was introduced to generate internal heat when the patient was wrapped in blankets.

The discovery of vitamins (1912–1927) led to their application in therapy. Thomas Spies' (2) study of pellagra (diarrhea, dementia, and death) began in the 1920s. The disorder was found to be due to a dietary deficiency that could be treated successfully and prevented with the use of nicotinic acid and a diet rich in the vitamin.

The introduction of sulfa drugs and penicillin during World War II made possible the prevention and treatment of the toxic infectious psychoses once frequently presenting as delirium in mental hospitals.

ADVANCES IN THEORY

Freudian Theory

The theories of Freud led beyond descriptions of mental disorders and the focus on mental content, to a study of the forces acting upon the mental apparatus. It suddenly became possible to gain insight into the origin of symptoms.

Freud's theory of personality structured the unconscious into id, ego, and superego. A dynamic interaction of subjective needs, perception of the environment, and integration of a plan to gratify needs controlled behavior. The interplay between the repressed and repressing forces took place in the unconscious, with every neurotic symptom representing a compromise between the repressing forces of the ego and the superego and the id, the repository of the repressed (4). Symptoms were related to unconscious memories excluded from the consciousness by repression when strivings were incompatible. This was a wholly new conception of mental topography (5).

Freud's theory of instincts postulated driving forces for life (eros—love, survival) and toward death (thanatos—hate—destructive and disruptive). Libido theory embraced all the various forms of sexual and sensual excitation derived ultimately from the body's erotogenic zones and from specialized sensations such as vision (6). Displacement to unconscious objects or regression to earlier aims could occur. Sexual evolution took place in phases. Arrest in development could occur at different phases. Much more than sexual intimacy was included in the concept of libido; tolerance and respect for others was seen as a form of love, as was self-love (narcissism) or oral pleasure and substituted objects (such as love of horses or love of nature) (7).

The method Freud developed to reach the unconscious, called psychoanalysis, involved free association, dream interpretation, and awareness of the therapist and patient interaction (transference and countertransference). This is not the place to recount all the theories that streamed from the psychoanalytic movement. They did, however, lead to a dynamic concept of personality development and to new insights into human behavior.

Freud's theories were not readily accepted, even in America, where psychoanalysis flourished. I can recall attending presentations by psychoanalysts at APA annual meetings in the 1930s and 1940s. The often acrimonious debates between such luminaries as Franz Alexander and Abraham Meyerson attracted crowds. One could see Adolf Meyer seated in the front row, and hear him calm a stormy session. It was heady stuff for a young psychiatrist.

Psychosomatic Theory

Psychosomatic medicine, the study and treatment of those conditions related to the interaction of psychic and somatic functions, had strong support from psychoanalysts. Theory held that psychological disturbances arose in several different ways: from structural tissue damage, from disorders of brain function, from medical complications resulting from maladaptive behavior, or from emotional disorders manifested by somatic symptoms (8).

Before World War II, Flanders Dunbar wrote *Emotions and Bodily Changes* (1938), providing an overview of the subject. Later Edward Weiss and O. Spurgion English published a textbook with clinical applications: *Psychosomatic Medicine* (1943). Some of the other early contributors to psychosomatic medicine and its theory were the psychoanalysts Felix Deutsch, Theresa Benedek (who studied the sexual cycle in women), Franz Alexander, Thomas French (who studied peptic ulcer and asthma), Harold Wolff (who studied gastric disturbances), Stanley Cobb (who studied arthritis and mucous colitis), and Roy Grinker, Sr. (who studied anxiety and stress).

By far the most influential psychiatrist to promote psychosomatic medicine was Adolf Meyer (1866–1950), for he dominated the field for 50 years. His commonsense psychiatry had wide appeal. Meyer incorporated some of Freud's psychological insights into his theory that each person is a unique psychobiological whole. This construct was the consequence of the interaction between biological, psychological, sociological, and cultural forces. His postulated reaction types and descriptive language did not endure, but his concept of psychobiologic unity did (1).

Meyer did not write much, but as a superb teacher, he was a molder of the men and women he taught. They spread his views widely. Meyer was President of the APA (1927–1928), a pervasive force in medical education, and a change agent in improving mental institutions. In one of his few articles, Meyer said treatment and study must be undertaken "with respect to the unique whole of *personhood*, with due attention to specific needs of human physics, chemistry and biology" (9, p. 105).

Other Contributions to Theory

There were many other contributions to theory during this period. I shall simply mention some of them, since they were not as closely related to the growth of thought, at the time, within the American Psychiatric Association as those just noted.

A theory was formulated at the University of Chicago that was based on some revolutionary experiments. As a result of his experiments, Ivan Pavlov (1927) developed a theory of conditioned reflexes. Pioneers in animal experimentation, K.S. Lashley (1913), H.S. Liddell (1919), B.F. Skinner (1930), H.F. Harlow (1932), and F.F. Fulton (1935) developed theory on individual and group response to isolation, deprivation, lack of mothering, learned behavior, and effects of brain lesions on behavior. The theory formulated at the University of Chicago based on these experiments was as follows:

> whole living organisms function not simply as sums of their parts but subserve new emergent functions; organisms mature by differentiation of primary undifferentiated structure functions; living boundaries are semipermeable and permit control of input and output; structure of whole organisms exist in gradients under central control or regulation; Jackson's final common pathways carry many processes from divergent internal sources to achieve near-identical actions; and living organisms maintain homeostasis within a healthy range under conditions of moderate stress. These propositions were precursors of what Ludwig Von Bertalanffy (1968) was to describe much later as *general systems theory** (10, p. 4).

---

* Reprinted with permission of the author and the publisher, from Grinker Sr., RR: Fifty Years in Psychiatry: A Living History. Springfield, Illinois, Charles C Thomas, 1979. Copyright 1979 by Charles C Thomas.

In 1928, Emil Kretschmer (1888–1964) introduced the theory of biotypography in *Physique and Character.* William Sheldon in the United States carried on the work relating body types (mesomorph, ectomorph, and endomorph) to personality characteristics.

Sir Archibald Garrod suggested in his Croonian Lecture (1908) that inborn errors of development could be responsible for interference with normality in childhood. In the 1950s many inborn errors of metabolism were discovered (phenylketonuria, galactesemia, ceruloplasm deficiency, hypoglycemia, and tryptophan defect). Early identification of the error often made correction possible with normal child development.

In 1949, Barr and Bertram described chromotin masses in resting cells that led to exciting study of chromosomes and their causative role in mongolism, in Klinefelter's syndrome, and in gonadal dysgenesis. In 1932, Walter Cannon set forth a theory of homeostasis (the theory that an organism has a tendency to maintain within itself constant conditions necessary to perpetuate its life). In 1956, Hans Selye proposed a theory of stress (the theory that there are neurogenic and hormonal influences upon bodily organs in response to intense external stress).

In addition to advances in theory, advances in record-keeping influenced the development of psychiatry.

Epidemiologic data collection made possible analyses of the incidence and prevalence of mental disorders and of mental deficiency. Vital statistics, derived from central registration, were not widely available in the United States until the 1900s (11). The earliest American settlements kept a record of deaths. In the 17th century the Massachusetts and Virginia colonies followed the English custom of keeping records of births, christenings, weddings, and burials. Lemuel Shattuck of Boston succeeded in getting a law enacted in Massachusetts in 1842 requiring central registration of births and deaths. Edward Jarvis, in 1855, collected data on the number of insane and idiots in Massachusetts. Comprehensive analyses of incidence and prevalence of mental diseases and retardation awaited the studies of H.B. Elkins (1927), Neil Dayton (1940), B. Malzberg (1940), and the reports emerging from the Joint Commission on Mental Illness and Health, *Epidemiology and Mental Illness,* in 1960 (12, 13). During the 1970s and 1980s statistical reports were issued periodically by the National Institute of Mental Health.

ADVANCES IN DELIVERY SYSTEMS

The 50 years from 1900 to 1949 marked the move away from total reliance on mental hospitals for service delivery to the use of psychopathic hospitals, psychiatric units in general hospitals, ambulatory care in clinics, the doctor's office, and the use of alternatives to hospitalization for the chronic mentally ill.

Certainly the most significant advances in service delivery in the first half of the 20th century were the development of psychopathic hospitals and psychiatric units in general hospitals.

Psychopathic hospitals

Psychopathic hospitals, or institutes of psychiatry, were founded in the second half of the 19th century in Europe either at universities or with private support. The first institute of psychiatry in the United States was shaped on the European model. It was known originally as the Pathologic Institute of the State of New York (founded in 1896) and was the first medical institute to include in its study the psychosocial sciences. When Adolf Meyer succeeded Van Giesen as its Director in 1902, he moved the institute to the grounds of the Manhattan State Hospital on Ward's Island and changed its name to the New York State Psychiatric Institute (14). It was in 1929 that it moved again to 168th St. in New York City, to become a part of one of the world's great medical centers under George Kirby as Director.

Albert M. Barrett, one of Meyer's protegees, went to Ann Arbor to open a psychopathic unit at the University of Michigan. Although authorized by the state legislature in 1901, the formal opening for patient treatment in the new state Psychopathic Hospital was delayed until 1906.

There emerged on the Boston scene, between 1906 and 1911, a psychiatrist named G. Vernon Briggs. He was a pugnacious crusader who antagonized superintendents of the mental hospitals, blasted apathy and entrenched institutionalism, and was the fearless adversary of anyone who opposed his views. Briggs came into prominence in 1906 when, shocked by the practice of locking the mentally ill in jail over the weekend until court convened again on Monday, he led a dramatic battle to remedy the situation that squashed all opposition. In 1909, he began to fight for an outpatient department for the Boston State Hospital to be placed adjacent to Harvard Medical School and the Peter Bent Brigham Hospital. He envisioned the facility as one that would admit all classes of the mentally ill for examination, provide treatment, conduct research, and offer instruction for students, as well as provide training and education for physicians and investigators; its outpatient facilities would discharge patients early and follow their progress in aftercare, and offer consultation to those who desired it. Briggs is remembered for the Briggs Law, a landmark act passed in Massachusetts in 1921, which requires an impartial psychiatric examination of those accused of a serious crime or of those who are recidivists. The state Department of Mental Health was empowered by this act to name the examiners, making the "battle of the experts" rare in Massachusetts (15).

The Trustees of the Boston State Hospital were authorized by Senate Bill 412 in 1901 to establish a facility "for the first care and observation of mental patients and the treatment of acute and curable mental disease." It was Briggs' vigorous pursuit of action that brought the new facility into being in 1912. Henry P. Frost (Superintendent of the Boston State Hospital) said of the new psychopathic department of the hospital, "It represents advanced ideas in the care, treatment and study of mental diseases" and it was to make "public provision for the voluntary mental patient without stigma of insanity, outpatient service for the poor who need instruction and counsel in mental hygiene" (16, p. 308). Frost proudly noted the appointment of Harvard's Professor of Neuropathology and State Pathologist to be the first Director, Elmer E. Southard (APA President, 1918–1919). It is not surprising that the new facility—a general hospital for psychiatry—"reaching out into the community a helping hand to borderline and incipient cases" soon became the independent Boston Psychopathic Hospital (16).

On the occasion of the 60th anniversary of Sheppard and Enoch Pratt Hospital, Dr. Edward N. Brush, its Superintendent, presented to the audience Adolf Meyer, the Director of the newly established Henry Phipps Psychiatric Clinic at Johns Hopkins University (1913). Brush said the opening of the new facility was "a welcome ally . . . in the campaign to restore those who have succumbed to the stress and strain of life" (17, p. 28). Medical staff members from Sheppard and Enoch Pratt spent one day each week at the outpatient department of the Phipps Clinic.

Psychopathic hospitals, modeled after those in New York, Michigan, and Boston, developed in other parts of the country (in Iowa, 1920; in Syracuse, 1930; and in Galveston and Illinois, 1931). Perhaps the most notable of these was the Colorado Psychopathic Hospital in Denver (1925) under Franklin G. Ebaugh.

Psychiatric Units in General Hospitals

Psychiatric units in general hospitals in the U.S. date back to 1753 at the Pennsylvania Hospital. The Insane Pavilion at Bellevue was established in 1879, and wards in the Philadelphia General Hospital in 1890. It was not until the opening of the 20th century that they were rediscovered as a setting for treatment, and not until the 1930s that the units became widespread.

In 1900 J. Montgomery Mosher provided a blueprint for the psychiatric unit that was to open in New York at the Albany Hospital in 1902. Mosher outlined the following goals for the new facility: 1) care for acute mental illness; 2) standards of care equal to those applicable in general medical wards; 3) treatment close to the community without the stigma of mental hospitalization; and 4) training for interns and residents (18,19).

At the APA annual meeting in 1901, D.R. Brower presented a paper entitled "The Treatment of Acute Insanity" in which he advocated the free admission, without legal commitment (as was the case for other general hospital patients) to a special psychiatric ward. The idea did not meet with general approval of the members present. Brower, undismayed by the reception given his paper, predicted that such wards in general hospitals would undoubtedly be established. At the same 1901 annual meeting, Henry C. Baldwin of Boston made a plea for the establishment of an institution for the treatment of alcoholism, to be connected with general hospitals located in cities. This idea was favorably received (20).

After the Henry Ford Hospital in Detroit opened its psychiatric unit in 1924, the number of similar wards in general hospitals began to grow. By 1932, 112 of 4,309 general hospitals had psychiatric units (19). By 1978, a survey of 6,321 general hospitals found psychiatric units in 1,025, and found that 2,241 general hospitals provided some sort of psychiatric service (such as patients with mental disorders commingling with others, partial hospitalization, emergency evaluations, or alcohol and drug treatment services) (21).

A big push toward increasing the number of psychiatric units was given by the Veterans Administration after World War II, when it formulated the policy that all of its general hospitals would have such a unit.

Ambulatory Care and Private Practice

Ambulatory care and the private practice of psychiatry evolved long before the facts recorded here; these are the later signs of the evolutionary process. The physicians who became superintendents of asylums (and members of the Association of Medical Superintendents of American Institutions for the Insane) had their interest aroused by the problems of caring for the insane whom they saw in their practice. Dispensaries for medical patients existed in the latter half of the 19th century. A few of them provided ambulatory care for the mentally disordered. In 1867 the Philadelphia Orthopedic Hospital had a clinic for the mentally ill. In the 1870s the nerve clinic in the Boston Dispensary accepted patients with mental disorders, as did the neuropsychiatric department of Alexion Brothers Hospital in St. Louis, the Pennsylvania Hospital (1885), and the Germantown, Pennsylvania Dyspensary (1895) (22).

Placement of patients in family homes (family care) in the community began centuries ago in Gheel, Belgium. In 1250, after investigation of the cures brought about by a ritual held at the church where the remains of the venerated St. Dymphna were buried, the mentally ill came from all over Europe in such numbers that they were placed in the homes of townspeople. A tradition was established and kept alive in Gheel for over 700 years, of accepting mental patients into the family home. Visitors from the U.S. reviewed the system with enthusiasm. Massachusetts adopted family care in 1885, as did New York, Maryland, and Michigan. Ontario, Canada, soon adopted family care as well. About 6,000 patients in the U.S. were in family care in 1950 (23, 24).

Development of Alternative Forms of Care

I have already noted the rise in *outpatient care* of children at the Institute in Chicago and subsequently at the Judge Baker Guidance Center in Boston. Clinics for adults followed soon after the establishment of these clinics. By 1935, 373 outpatient departments were identified—281 of these served patients discharged from mental hospitals (68). Psychoanalysts began seeing patients, and as their numbers increased, so did the office practice of psychotherapy. From a slow beginning in the 1920s, private practice gained momentum in the 1940s and 1950s. By the 1950s, 23 percent of 1.7 million patient care episodes were cared for in outpatient treatment, and 77 percent in inpatient treatment. At the start of the century all patient care episodes were treated in institutions (66).

Two other extramural facilities emerged in the 50-year period. The first *day hospital* in the United States began to function at Adams Nervine in Boston (1935). Patients with psychoneuroses were believed to recover more swiftly with a full day of treatment while they continued to live at home. Kerbikov, in Russia, described a comprehensive program of community psychiatry that was established to meet a critical shortage of beds in 1918 with district dispensaries and a day hospital in the 1930s (24). D. Ewen Cameron's (24) Montreal Day Hospital (1948) demonstrated the value of day hospitals (25).

The *halfway house* barely got started as part of the delivery system before the 1950s, but from that time on it has thrived. Its utility was recognized in England as early as 1871 (27), and by 1879 women who were discharged from the mental hospital, and later men, were placed in cottage lodges. Boston State Hospital from 1934–1937 placed 8 to 10 women in a large dwelling as a treatment facility (the City Mills Project). Spring Lake Ranch in Vermont and Gould Farm in Massachusetts were early halfway houses (24).

The first *social club* for ex-mental patients was started in the U.S. by Abraham Low in Chicago in 1937, though it was Joshua Bierer in England (1944) who stimulated their development. Dr. Low's club brought patients together to extend his unique method of treatment into the community (in 1962 there were 250 Recovery Inc. "clubs" in 20 states). The oldest clubs that have followed a more conventional model are the 1947 outpatient clinic group (OPC) at Menningers, and Club 103 of the Massachusetts Mental Health Center (1949). The most widely known club and the most copied organization is Fountain House in New York City (1948). It provides outreach, by invitation, to ex-mental patients to participate in a full daytime volunteer work program and evening social activities. It establishes and maintains relationships, offers assistance in job training and placement, help in obtaining welfare assistance and other agency contacts, and does much to smooth re-entry into community living (24).

Development of Mental Hospital Care

Mental hospitals in the 50-year span, after an initial improvement over earlier conditions, slumped to a disgracefully low point during World War II and improved again after 1949. Pressures to change the geographical isolation of mental institutions developed near the end of the 19th century. Neurologists such as Spitzka were critical of the superintendents as early as 1878. According to Spitzka, the institution heads were seen as efficient business managers wholly without scientific works (26).

Another neurologist, S. Weir Mitchell, blasted superintendents out of their complacency in 1894 and thereby led them to put their mental hospitals in order. In 1884, Dr. C.K. Clarke had already taken some steps in that direction at the Kingston Asylum in Canada. He tore down airing court walls, established meaningful factory-type work programs such as quarrying, cutting stone, and building under supervision. George Zeller in 1905 made such radical changes that he was ousted in three years and his innovations abandoned. Zeller, at the Peoria State Hospital (Illinois), removed all iron bars, doors, and gratings, opened wards, instituted the eight-hour day, and assigned women to work in male wards. Patients were responsible for themselves and worked at useful tasks (28).

Less dramatic improvements were underway in most mental hospitals. Attendants formerly worked long hours from early morning; they awakened patients, helped them dress and wash, took them to breakfast, and cared for them until night, when patients were put to bed. It was common practice for attendants to sleep nearby in an apartment on the ward. Then a night shift was added, and day attendants slept in an employee's building. The Kalamazoo (Illinois) State Hospital went on a three-shift schedule in 1907, and other Illinois hospitals followed in 1916 (29).

Food (stated as excellent by standards of the day) was meager, and the diet poorly balanced from a nutritional perspective. Although congregate dining rooms date back to 1885, most hospitals served food in ward dining rooms. Food prepared in central kitchens at a distance reached the ward distribution point in less than optimal condition. The cafeteria, introduced in mental hospitals in 1922, and spread by William A. Bryan's advocacy in 1936, remedied the situation (30). Food then reached the consumer in peak condition, a choice could be offered, and in smaller space, with a scheduled flow, several seatings were possible during the meal hours.

Mental hospitals grew larger and their population expanded at a faster rate than that of the United States. In 1890, the population of the U.S. was 63 million, and the number of mental patients in hospitals and asylums was 74,000; in 1940, the population of the U.S. was 131.5 million, and in 1941 the number of mental patients in hospitals and asylums had jumped to 473,000 (29). In the late 1940s the Association's standards were ignored as limits set for size were exceeded with huge 7,000- to 12,000-bed hospitals. Overcrowding, understaffing, and underfinancing were the consequences of expansion and tight budgets. The size barrier was broken on the grounds of economy in overhead. State control tightened during the first 20 years of the century under a board, commission, or department governing the mental hospitals in each state (73).

Veterans Administration mental hospitals held to a size limit of 2,200 patients. The VA also contributed to better hospital design (the "Hahn-type," so named after Paul Hahn, M.D., the chief planner) that was the model used in the post-World War II expansion of the VA mental hospital system.

There were many poor mental hospitals during this period and a few that were better. St. Elizabeths in Washington, D.C., was one of the better hospitals under a great leader, William Alanson White (Superintendent from 1903–1937), who developed the first psychological laboratory (1907), added the first clinical psychotherapist (1917), organized a medical and surgical branch approved for internships (1920), first used malaria as a treatment for general paresis (1922), set up a nursing school, established occupational therapy and social work units, and made significant contributions to research (31).

Another model for mental hospitals was the Worcester State Hospital in Massachusetts, with one of the best documented historical records (32, 33). William A. Bryan (Superintendent from 1920–1940) achieved national prominence as an administrator. His vision of good mental hospitals is laid out in *Administrative Psychiatry* (30), the first, and now classic, work on the subject.

Bryan reorganized the hospital into two parts, one for acute care and one for chronic continued care; established clinics in the general hospitals of the community (1923); organized traveling teams for assessment of children in schools; organized a medical and surgical service under specialists attending from the community; offered training to interns and to students in nursing, occupational therapy, and social work; started the first training in pastoral counseling under Rev. Anton T. Boisen (1924); and organized a distinguished research department in 1927 that concentrated on the study of schizophrenia. Funded investigations by the Memorial Foundation for Neuroendocrinology attracted Roy G. Hoskins (one of the country's foremost endrocrinologists) to be the Research Director, assisted by Francis H. Sleeper, Lewis B. Hill, and a host of investigators such as David Shakow, Elliot Rodnick, John Dollard, E.M. Jellinek, Paul Houston, Geza Roheim, Harry Freeman, D. Ewen, Cameron, and Jacques Gottlieb. Later association with the Worcester Foundation of Experimental Biology (Gregory Pincus and Hudson Hoagland, codirectors) would bring Harvard, Boston University, and Tufts into the research studies. The Great Depression of 1929 gave Worcester a brief opportunity to attract the best nurses and physicians and to demonstrate the possibilities of superior staffing. It was in this period that L. Cody Marsh introduced inspirational group therapy to mental patients.

After a brief period of rejuvenation brought on by the new somatic therapies of the 1930s, World War II depleted staffs and resources were diverted to the priority of the war effort, leaving the mental hospital system in a desperate condition. Without staff, the running of the institutions fell upon the patients. Patient leaders emerged who cared for other patients. Activities pertaining to food and shelter were largely carried out by patients, with but a few professionals left to supervise.

Albert Deutsch (26), who had chronicled the emergence of hospitals from asylums in 1937, shook public complacency when he described the level to which care of the mentally ill had fallen in his *The Shame of the States* (34). He was not the only critical voice, for the media blasted mental hospitals for the horrible neglect of patients. Public awareness of the extent of mental illness had increased as a consequence of the rejection rate for inductees, and as a result of the publicized psychiatric casualties of World War II. The shortage of mental health manpower to deal with mental problems had been stated many times. The climate was right for change.

The APA made a massive response to the plight of the mental hospitals. It called all superintendents together in 1949 at a Mental Hospital Institute. Their problems were identified and solutions developed. A section on mental hospitals was created at the APA annual meeting. A journal, *Mental Hospitals*, was developed to exchange information and to set forth improvements. Achievement Awards were established to give recognition to hospitals making significant improvement. The APA Medical Director visited institutions, and APA's Central Inspection Board surveyed hospitals* and made recommendations for improvement. These are but a few of the APA's activities instituted to improve mental hospitals. Later an APA unit, The Contract Survey Board, made consultation available by contract when an organization, a single hospital, or a state system wished to improve its program. A comprehensive planned program was developed by the field study team assigned.

Development of the Care of the Mentally Retarded

Care of the mentally retarded had a cycle of improvement (from the last decade of the 19th century to about 1912) and a slump into neglect following pessimism engendered by the studies on heredity, from 1912–1916 (26). A revival brought about by Walter E. Fernald's model institution improved the scene for a time, but the institutions succumbed to the depression, and conditions worsened during the World War, to improve again after exposures of shocking neglect.

---

* Two other surveys of note were made in the first half of the 20th century. Henry Hurd (head of an APA Committee on History) divided the country into regions (1911) making a committee member responsible for data collection on hospitals in the assigned region. As the purpose was to create a history of all existing mental hospitals, the data were usually supplied by the institution head and were not critical of performance. In 1937–1938 Samuel Hamilton was selected to conduct a survey of mental hospitals by the National Committee on Mental Hygiene with funds from the Rockefeller Foundation. Hamilton did promote APA standards and did make recommendations for improvement.

The period 1886–1912 was one of great growth in both the number of institutions and the number of residents in them. At the end of the 19th century there were 19 state and 9 private institutions for the feebleminded in 17 states. By 1924 there were 51 state and 89 private institutions in 43 states. In 25 years, the number of patients had grown from 6,000 to over 39,000 (36).

A significant advance in the mental retardation field was in extramural care. The first special class for the mentally retarded in the community was in Providence, Rhode Island, in 1896. The 1919 School Clinic Law in Massachusetts mandated special classes for the education of the mentally retarded. By 1923, there were special classes in 171 different cities around the United States (35).

Another significant advance in this field was the classification by mental age and the use of the Intelligence Quotient. Henry H. Goddard, Ph.D., at the Vineland Training School in New Jersey, visited Binet in 1905 and brought back his observations. With Lewis Terman, they developed a classification of the retarded by mental age into idiots, imbeciles, and morons (1910). The Intelligence Quotient made assessment of a child's potential for intellectual development easier than it had ever been before.

ADVANCES IN OTHER MEDICAL THERAPY

In the last decade of the 19th century, American Medico-Psychological Association members attending the annual meeting heard that physical training benefits the mental state (1890); B.W. Stone said that thyroid preparations were not helpful and could be dangerous (1892); S. Weir Mitchell encouraged the use of electrical equipment and hydrotherapy (1894); it was recommended that tuberculosis patients be isolated in separate quarters and their waste disinfected to protect others (1890); and Burke noted that the use of surgery in the mentally ill had remained steady since 1892 to demonstrated needs, as in gynecological conditions in women (1898) (20).

The first half of the 20th century brought refinements in some of the older therapies (such as moral treatment, occupational therapy, and hydriatics); continued use of restraint and seclusion for the control of violence; improved technique in psychotherapy; successful treatment of central nervous system syphilis, pellagra, and toxic-infectious psychoses; and new, effective treatments (such as insulin and electroconvulsive therapy) for functional psychoses.

Restraint and Seclusion

In 1839, John Connolly abolished restraint at Hanwell Asylum in England, but the APA founders rejected his stand and, in one of the earliest pronouncements of the Association, favored its limited use. For years the subject was debated. Gradually the use of restraint was diminished; strait jackets (camisole restraint), sheet restraint in a chair, cuffs, and isolation in a seamless locked room with only a bed or canvas-covered mattress remained. Chemical restraint with narcotics gave way to barbiturates. Led by New York and Massachusetts, states passed laws regulating the use of restraint and of seclusion (26).

Hydrotherapy

The use of water in treatment of the mentally disordered probably dates back to its use in Greek temples. In 1902 Emmett C. Dent, Superintendent of the Manhattan State Hospital in New York, read a paper at the APA annual meeting on the benefits to mental patients from hydriatic procedures. In 1912, Henry P. Frost, Superintendent of Boston State Hospital, cited John S. Butler's belief that shower baths benefited the mentally ill. Simon Baruch of New York planned a rational application of tub, spray, and douche in various medical conditions. The treatment became universal in mental hospitals over the next 30 years. Rebecca Wright's *Hydrotherapy in Hospitals for Mental Diseases* (published by Tudor Press, New York, in 1932) served as a textbook for correct application.

Each mental hospital's hydrotherapy unit had continuous baths in a quiet darkened room (ours at Worcester used a radio that piped in soft mood music). Patients were suspended for a half day or longer in a hammock in warm flowing water. The quieting effect was apparent. There were hot cabinets and steam cabinets in which the patient sat, and for more stimulating and invigorating treatment streams of hot water, cold water, or alternating hot and cold water were directed to the back of a standing patient, or a "needle" spray of water under pressure was applied. For the extremely disturbed and uncooperative patient, the wet sheet pack was used. Sheets wrung out in cold water were carefully wrapped about the patient's nude body, until trunk and extremities were encased and the "mummy" was then wrapped in blankets to retain body heat. The hazard of overheating was real, with fever sometimes reaching lethal heights. I was able to say in 1962 that the hydrotherapy suite and the modalities used were obsolete as therapy for the mentally ill (24).

Treatment of Focal Infection

The interest in surgery as a treatment for mental illness returned for a 20-year span with the belief in "autointoxication"—that foci of infection in the body either brought on or aggravated mental disorders (Sir Arbuthnot Lane in England believed that foci in the gastrointestinal tract were responsible). Henry A. Cotton was the advocate in the United States. In addition to the gastrointestinal tract (to be cleansed with colonic irrigations), the tonsils or teeth were believed to be the offenders (37, 38). The concern over infections of teeth led to the introduction of dentists into the mental hospitals.

Treatment of Central Nervous System Syphilis, Pellagra, and Toxic Infectious Psychoses

We have already noted the conquest of a disease—central nervous system syphilis—following Noguchi's identification in 1913 of the causative organism and the use of heat as therapy. St. Elizabeths led in the use of malaria in the United States in 1922, followed by similar work at the New York Psychiatric Institute and the Boston Psychopathic Hospital. Generation of heat by electricity (electropyrexia) was first demonstrated by Neymann and Osborne in 1929 (37, 39). It took until the end of World War II to make penicillin (discovered by Fleming in 1928) generally available. It eliminated 10 to 12 percent of all mental hospital admissions and made syphilis preventable.

Pellagra was the subject of a 1911 annual meeting presentation that assigned the cause to a toxin in spoiled corn. The work of Spies and others from 1928 to 1938 showed the disorder to be due to a deficiency of the vitamin nicotinic acid, and to be curable and preventable by a vitamin rich diet. Nutritional factors were discovered to be responsible for manifestations in severe alcoholism (such as delirium tremens, and Wernicke's and Korsakoff's syndromes), allowing therapy with vitamins to be made more specific (37).

Toxic infectious psychoses, once commonly presenting as delirium, became treatable and preventable with the introduction of sulfa drugs and penicillin.

The APA formulated standards for mental hospitals in 1925.* We shall note here only those standards that refer to therapy: hospitals must have qualified staff in connection with the following required units: a surgical operating room, hydrotherapy, occupational therapy, physical exercise, recreation, and social activities. Every patient, Adolf Meyer insisted, was to have a complete personality analysis with an attempt to understand physical, psychological, and social needs.

ADVANCES IN UNDERSTANDING OF THE
THERAPEUTIC INFLUENCES OF THE ENVIRONMENT

Concepts and practices underlying the potential therapeutic effects of the treatment setting have been in existence for a long time. They were expressed in moral treatment. When the belief that optimism would speed recovery gave way to pessimism in the latter part of the 19th century, trends were beginning to converge in a manner that would restore the conviction that the environment of the mental hospital could exert a positive therapeutic influence. Adolf Meyer helped to rekindle the spirit of inquiry through study of the whole patient, focusing on the development within the family, on the job, and in the community in an attempt to understand the stresses upon an individual. The Kraepelinian descriptive view of mental disorders as disease entities gave way, under Freudian influence, to acceptance of the concept that mental disease was a "unique reaction to life experiences in each patient" (40). The conviction slowly grew that attitudes of staff, relationships between staff and patients, and the relationships of patients to each other had an ameliorating effect. Bryan (30) noted that idleness and inactivity favored deterioration, whereas pressures to get patients to participate in work and social activities lessened the escape-from-reality phenomenon.

---

* Deutsch abstracts these in his book *The Mentally Ill in America* (26).

In 1939, Myerson (41) stated that the regression so commonly seen in schizophrenia was the result of hospitalization, not of the disease, and could be prevented if the hospital environment offered the right kind of stimulation. He called the marshalling of stimulating pressures the Total Push Therapy.

Further steps toward creating a therapeutic environment within the institution were taken by T.F. Main (42) and Stanton and Schwartz (43). The military experience in England of Wood (44) and Wilson and his co-workers (45), in which war neuroses were treated by an educational technique of open discussion and supportive staff relationships that altered attitudes toward symptoms, were basic to what would evolve in the 1950s into milieu therapy and the therapeutic community (46, 47).

ADVANCES IN PSYCHOTHERAPY

The psychotherapies, both individual and group (practiced for centuries with benefit when patients "talked through" problems with an understanding therapist) acquired new forms, greater depth, and improved results during the first half of the 20th century. Freud's psychoanalytic technique worked well in treating the neuroses. Early in the period, Adolf Meyer's analysis of the whole personality resulted in a better understanding of the psychobiological and environmental factors acting on the individual, and support and suggestion of the therapist improved behavior. Psychiatrists, by the 1930s, read books by Ives Hendricks (6) or Lawrence Kubie (48) as guides to Freud's technique.

In 1942, Levine, in his widely read book *Psychotherapy in Medical Practice* (49), advised that hypnosis was not very effective when performed in mental institutions, except in amnesia and in war neuroses. Psychotherapy was not indicated for mental retardation, for organic mental disorders, or for the major psychoses; however, it was useful after electroconvulsive therapy made patients more accessible. In 1944, Myerson (50) advised that psychoanalytic technique was of no value in treating schizophrenia, manic depressive psychoses, or any major mental disease.

However, Paul Federn, who began his studies of the structure of the ego in 1927, by the 1940s believed it was possible to modify psychoanalysis to benefit the psychotic individual. He avoided taking a history, for it aroused painful memories and sometimes caused a relapse; attention was focused upon current problems;

repression was encouraged; and no interpretations were made of positive transference (51). The frequency of treatment, its duration over time, and limited resources made general application of psychoanalysis impractical in all but a few specialized private mental hospitals.

However, understanding of psychodynamic forces did lead to a wider application of modified dynamic psychotherapy in the treatment of emotional and personality problems. The warmth, empathy, and understanding of the therapist interacting with the patient did foster improvement (52). The benefits from psychoanalytic and dynamic psychotherapy were an incentive toward the growth of extramural psychiatry and the movement toward private practice. Within institutions, focus on symptoms encouraged suppressive and supportive psychotherapy with a search for more effective short-term approaches. A variant of psychotherapy, narcosynthesis, developed out of World War II experience. Abreaction—the expression of a traumatic experience—was facilitated under intravenous barbiturates.

The utilization of group therapy, which started slowly in the first decade of the century, expanded rapidly after World War II. In 1907, an internist named J.H. Pratt employed the group process in patients with tuberculosis who felt ostracized from their communities, sharing their sense of rejection and their fears. The group met twice weekly for a lecture followed by discussion. In 1919 L. Cody Marsh used group therapy with institutionalized mental patients. He started out by giving lectures about mental illness, and by encouraging reading, attentiveness, and punctuality. By 1931, at Worcester State Hospital, he was gaining cooperative participation in an inspirational reality-testing session with a large group. The free expression of thoughts and feelings to others, in a small group, was encouraged by Triggant Burrows in 1925 (53). It was this latter model that was widely followed in the post-World War II period.

ADVANCES IN SOMATIC THERAPY

The somatic therapies started the revolution in the mental health service delivery system. The dramatic improvement that followed the use of electroconvulsive therapy in serious major mental illness made it possible to change the setting of treatment to one outside the state mental hospital system. It is interesting to note that all these new treatments were discovered in Europe. Confirmation of their effectiveness led to widespread application in the United States before World War II.

Insulin therapy was first used in mental patients in 1933 by Manfred Sakel in Vienna. After the discovery of insulin in the 1920s he and many others experimented with it in the treatment of major mental illnesses. Patients generally gained weight as their appetites improved. Insulin also had a desirable mild sedative effect. Induced insulin coma, carefully monitored and terminated with intravenous glucose, was carried out extensively in mental hospitals by a trained staff. Sakel noted that when some insulin-sensitive patients went into coma, they showed remarkable improvement when they came out (54, 55). Often 40 to 60 comas were induced in one patient to effect improvement. Results were best in schizophrenia. Remissions in schizophrenic patients who underwent induced comas were double the number of those remissions occurring spontaneously.

Von Meduna, in Hungary, believing that an antagonism existed between schizophrenia and epilepsy, began inducing convulsions in patients with camphor injections in 1924. In 1935 he switched to a soluble synthetic camphor preparation—Metrazole—which could be injected intravenously (56).

Shortly thereafter, a more effective and easier-to-administer method (which quickly replaced both Metrazole and insulin therapy) was discovered by two Italian investigators, Cerletti and Bini, in 1938 (57). They discovered that a controlled amount of alternating electric current, when passed through the brain, would produce convulsions (electroconvulsive therapy, or ECT). Introduced as a treatment for schizophrenia, this soon became the treatment of choice for agitated depressions. Depressive states were remarkably shortened and improvement was significant. Of all the somatic therapies, ECT made the most significant change in the treatment of major mental illness.

There has been considerable squabbling over who was the first to use ECT in the United States. My investigation shows that it was Douglas Goldman in 1939, with a machine patented by Franklin Offner (58, 59). Victor Gonda, one of the earliest to employ ECT, brought a machine to the United States from Europe and used it on patients in January 1940 (60). Other early investigators were Drs.

Impastato, Myerson (who published the first paper on ECT in the United States), Hughes, Smith, and Neymann (61).

Specialized facilities for giving ECT soon developed. It began to be used in office practice, in general hospital psychiatric units, and in private hospitals.

Another therapy, frontal lobe surgery, was first used in Portugal in 1936 by Monez (62) in the treatment of schizophrenia. It was popularized in United States by Freeman and Watts (63). After World War II extensive trials were instituted with favorable results reported in cases refractory to other forms of therapy (64). Its use was curtailed in the 1960s because it was thought to damage the brain, and the therapy still arouses controversy in the 1980s (65).

The advance in administrative psychiatry may not seem related to treatment, but the deployment of resources, the selection and retention of superior staff members, on-the-job training, and the organization of the total hospital environment exerts a vital force upon the therapeutic process. While the founding fathers of the Association were greatly concerned with administrative issues, and those members and leaders who followed continued to make advances in organizational standards and in management practice, it was not until 1936 that the concept of a total institution management system was set down in William A. Bryan's first U.S. textbook and now classic, *Administrative Psychiatry* (30). The changes in British administrative psychiatry are chronicled by Clark (66) beginning in 1942. Most of the significant developments in administration were to occur in the 1950s and 1960s and will be discussed later.

ADVANCES IN MEDICAL EDUCATION

The advances in psychiatric education during the 50 years from 1900–1949 were made predominantly by two men: Adolf Meyer and his pupil, Franklin Ebaugh. Meyer was the teacher and trainer of men who would become leaders in the field. Ebaugh was the catalyst to action. These two men, along with C. Macfie Campbell, William A. White, Titus Harris, and others, were to significantly improve the teaching of psychiatry. The period of change which had begun in the 1890s accelerated after the Flexner report in 1910 (67). The medical educational system improved and substandard medical schools were closed.

Before 1914, the teaching of psychiatry was didactic, descriptive, and focused upon the insanities. Teaching was limited to the clinical years and took place in isolation from the rest of medicine (68). As I have noted, Pliny Earle delivered a course of lectures in 1835 at the college of Physicians and Surgeons. In 1867 William A. Hammond was appointed professor of nervous and mental disease at Bellevue Hospital Medical College. In 1871 E.C. Sequin lectured on mental disease, as did Isaac Ray at Jefferson Medical College. It was in 1882 that the Association for the Protection of the Insane and the Prevention of Insanity sent a circular to the faculty of every medical school in the United States calling for the inclusion of the teaching of psychiatry, by lectures and demonstrations in clinics, to all medical students, as well as for the establishment of a chair in psychiatry and available clinical facilities. It was the establishment of psychopathic hospitals and psychiatric units in general hospitals and outpatient clinics that was to advance the teaching of psychiatry outside of the mental hospital (68).

In the period 1914 to 1931, the interest in mental hygiene, in prevention, in child guidance, and in community programs captured the attention of students. Teaching began in the preclinical years and was related to patients' deviation from normal. Psychotherapy was studied in relation to the theory of psychoanalysis (68).

After the survey of psychiatric teaching by the national Committee for Mental Hygiene in the 1930s, standards were formulated for instruction in psychiatry. Psychiatry was seen as an essential part of the general medical education. When the American Board of Psychiatry and Neurology was formed in 1934 (following Adolf Meyer's statement of the desirability of certification in his 1928 presidential address, and following an APA Committee on Medical Services [made up of A. Meyer, G.H. Kirby, and E.A. Strecker] report at the 1930 APA annual meeting), graduate and residency programs became structured (68).

The American Medical Association was to say in 1939, through its Council on Medical Education and Hospitals, "Psychiatry has not yet found itself in the medical curriculum," while noting that it was "one of the most underdeveloped areas in the medical curriculum" (68, 69).

Two events were to strengthen the teaching of psychiatry: Veterans Administration support, and the passage of the National

Mental Health Act in 1946, with the establishment of the National Institute of Mental Health in 1949. The VA, with the assistance of its Dean's Committees, established training programs such as the one at the Menninger Clinic for psychiatrists and mental health professionals. Under Robert Felix and Seymour Vestermark, the federal program (NIMH) would aid in the establishment of strong departments of psychiatry, provide stipends for residents, encourage career training in education and research, and fund training for much needed mental health professionals.

The 50-year span brought improvement in all of medical education, the rise of medical specialties (including psychiatry), the establishment of a certification process to ensure clinical competence, the creation of departments of psychiatry and neurology (first within departments of medicine and later free-standing), formalized residency training, the attraction of "90 day wonders" (military physicians trained in psychiatry for three months) into training in psychiatry, and the rapid expansion of the psychiatric professional pool.

Psychiatry had established itself as a medical specialty. A foundation for further advances had been laid. The period 1900–1949 was one also of growth in the number of psychiatrists, in change in the way they delivered services, and change in the organization that represented their strivings.

THE ESTABLISHMENT OF
A CENTRAL HEADQUARTERS FOR
THE AMERICAN PSYCHIATRIC ASSOCIATION

The American Medico-Psychological Association (the name that was adopted in 1894) had 400 members in 1900. Its membership activities and correspondence were the responsibility of the Secretary-Treasurer, and the Association address changed each time a new one was elected. The business and editorial functions of the *American Journal of Insanity* were conducted from the office of its Editors, Henry Hurd (1894–1904) and Edward N. Brush (1904–1931), at Johns Hopkins University. The journal's office moved to Toronto when Clarence B. Farrar became Editor (1931–1965).

By 1921 the organization had grown in size and now had 1,000 members. In that year the name of the organization was changed to the American Psychiatric Association. A seal bearing the likeness of Benjamin Rush was adopted in 1927 when the Association was incorporated. What was manageable when the organization was small became unmanageable as it grew. A more formalized structure was needed for communication and governance as well as for support of committee work.

Dr. Arthur Ruggles, Chairman of the Scientific Admission Committee, Clarence Hincks, Medical Director of the National Committee for Mental Hygiene, and members of the Association, appeared before the governing council to recommend the establishment of an office for the Association in the office of the National Committee for Mental Hygiene in New York City. On May 31, 1932, President Russell (70) introduced the matter for Council deliberation. The salary of a person who might be selected to be the Executive Secretary and Business Manager of the *American Journal of Psychiatry* was to be paid either in full or in part by the Association. After full discussion, action was deferred to the June 1 meeting of Council, with an invitation to Dr. Ruggles and Hincks to attend.

In June of 1932 the Council approved the employment of an Executive Assistant at the salary not to exceed $5,000, with an additional $1,000 for office expenses and travel. The offer of the National Committee on Mental Hygiene was accepted to finance an office and supply clerical service without charge. In the discussion of the actions taken, it was noted that the actual cost to the Association for the year beginning July 1, 1932, would not be $6,000 but $3,900 (advertising income increase was estimated at $1,000 and a saving of $1,100 in secretarial services for the *Journal* was effected).

After many years of expressed desire for a permanent headquarters, President Russell said with satisfaction that there would now be an address, telephone number, and name of a staff person on Association stationery. He expressed regret that the Association could not afford a Medical Director, but was pleased that it could finance a business agent.

On November 1, 1932, Austin M. Davies was appointed Executive Assistant and assumed his duties in the office of the National Committee of Mental Hygiene at 450 Seventh Avenue, New York City (71). The business office of the Association and headquarters was not as permanent in one location as had been expected, for the first of several moves was noted on April 1, 1934.*

Austin Davies (75) brought to his new post a knowledge of mental hygiene, teaching, sales, and business experience. He was a graduate of Brown University, with his graduate thesis on mental hygiene. For a time, he taught in the Kenilworth, New Jersey, public schools. Next he was a sales representative for a savings and loan company in Cleveland, and for the Babson Statistical Organization in Philadelphia. Just before coming to work for the APA, he worked in Philadelphia's Bureau of Unemployment Relief.

Davies was assigned three major duties: membership, business affairs, and expediting the President's and Council's actions. He processed membership applications, kept Association membership records, collected dues, published the directory, and assisted in the preparation of the Biographical Directory.

Business affairs, managed by Davies, included all those affairs of the *Journal,* running the annual meeting, and insurance. Advertising revenue for the *Journal* increased under a contract with the Stephen Herlitz Agency. Subscription accounts were kept, and all fiscal matters attended to, including printing. The scholarly editor was relieved to entrust all "the running of the Journal" to Davies, and praised his good work. As an insurance broker, he secured member and organization insurance policies.

It was Davies' responsibilities for the annual meeting that made him visible to members. He chose the site, selected the headquarters hotels, made all the arrangements for meetings and special events, operated the registration area, printed the program, arranged commercial exhibits, and attended to details such as corsages for wives of head table dignitaries at the annual banquet. A human dynamo, he dashed about to be present at the area of

---

* The office moved with the National Committee for Mental Hygiene to 50 West 50th Street, and then to other locations as follows:

July 1935: to 2 East 103rd Street (New York Academy of Medicine)
January 1940: to 50 West 50th Street
June 1948: to 1270 Avenue of the Americas
October 1949: to 9 Rockefeller Plaza
April 1964: to 500 Fifth Avenue
April 1965: to 17 East 82nd Street
October 1, 1965: New York office closed (72–74)

principal action or trouble. No obsessive record-keeper, he ran the annual meeting from a sheaf of onionskin papers he kept folded in an inside coat pocket.

Austin Davies' conservative approach, obsession with economy, and the efficient, prompt handling of orders from officers and Council won him strong support from the Association's leaders. He made it a point to greet new members and remembered their names. Relations with the National Association of Mental Hygiene were most cordial under Davies. In the discharge of his many duties, Davies had a small staff that never grew beyond 12. All but one of them, a competent bookkeeper, were clerical workers.

Davies was short in stature, affable, approachable, full of energy, and ingratiated himself with the "important people." His congeniality won him praise for devoted service to the Association. Noted also was his loving, protective, and solicitous attention to a shy and withdrawn wife. As a dedicated servant of the Association, he brought great strength to a loose organization, holding things together between meetings of Council. He was the right man for this stage of organizational development.

Times changed, but Austin Davies did not. He was certain that the new breed of leaders that emerged in the post-World War II era would bankrupt the organization. He resisted the movement toward a centralized headquarters in Washington. The dedicated servant became a controversial figure, surrounded by allegations of self-interest, ingratiation of VIPs, and the unforgivable booking into the wretched Chicago Morrison Hotel two years in a row.

Davies carried out prodigiously detailed tasks with limited resources, but by the 1940s, his position had become anachronistic; burgeoning membership and new, more liberal leadership pressed upon the Association to undertake a more active role in the affairs of medicine and in the world at large.

REORGANIZATION AND PROGRESS
TOWARD ASSUMPTION OF POWER

Several years before 1944, the Association started to plan an appropriate celebration of its 100th anniversary. The Centennial Annual Meeting was held in Philadelphia, the birthplace of the Association of Medical Superintendents. An editorial committee produced a magnificent commemorative volume: *One Hundred*

Years of American Psychiatry, 1844–1944; and the *American Journal of Psychiatry's* Editorial Board prepared a special centennial issue of the journal. The gala occasion featured, in drama, Benjamin Rush, as he lived in a perilous time. The APA President, Edward A. Strecker, a Philadelphian and a division psychiatrist in World War I, noted in his address member and Association service to the armed forces, as well as some of the major problems encountered during the war: the shortage of psychiatrists; the adaptation of treatment to return combat troops to battle; troop morale; prevention of breakdown; and the discharge of neuropsychiatric casualties from the armed forces (76). Dr. Strecker expressed a concern for a better world—a real democratic society expressed in the brotherhood of man—where dangers of national isolation would be overcome, and protection of minorities assured. He called on psychiatry to contribute to the search for an enduring peace (77).

At the end of the annual meeting in May of 1944, Karl M. Bowman assumed the presidency—a position he would hold until 1946, as no annual meeting was held in 1945 due to the primacy of the war. Dr. Bowman, in 1944, aware that the Association was approaching 4,000 members with stress upon the structure, asked, "Shall the American Psychiatric Association establish a permanent home with a library, museum, and general facilities for directing the work of the Association?" (78). It would take 14 years to acquire a permanent home, and 24 years to complete the facilities envisioned by Dr. Bowman.

At the Council meeting in December 1944, Dr. Bowman invited three distinguished leaders who asked to be heard: General William C. Menninger, Office of the Surgeon General of the Army; Captain Francis J. Braceland, Office of the Surgeon General of the Navy; and Robert H. Felix, Chief of the Mental Hygiene Division of the U.S. Public Health Service. The group appealed for greater Association participation in solving psychiatric problems in the armed forces, for leadership in public education, medical education, and training of psychiatrists, and in social planning for the post-war period. In the discussion of how these goals might be achieved, the appointment of a full-time leader who would be the Medical Director was suggested.

After the guests had been excused, the council (accepting the advice of Mr. Austin Davies, who urged avoidance of precipitous and possibly too costly action) formed a study group: a Committee on Reorganization under the chairmanship of Karl Menninger. The charge was to suggest how the APA might be altered to meet responsibilities for more effective action. This was to correct sluggish and cumbersome machinery for Association action, update the organization's structure, establish better channels of communication, and redefine organizational purpose.

At the January 31, 1945, meeting of Council, the Reorganization Committee suggested that instead of a Medical Director, the Association hire several persons to attend to public relations, psychiatric education, hospital standards, and research. The report was unanimously accepted. However, a suggestion to enlarge the committee to include advocates of change was rejected. Instead, the committee was instructed to get expert opinion from leaders, members, and other associations. It did request input from many individuals. A questionnaire and letter was sent to all members inviting their opinion. The response demonstrated a shocking lack of interest, for only eight percent of the membership responded, with about one-half of these expressing satisfaction with the organization as it then operated. The poor response led to acceptance of the Reorganization Committee's suggestion that a full discussion of issues over two days be provided at the 1946 annual meeting.

In his Presidential Address, Dr. Bowman (78) noted that public interest in psychiatry was aroused, making this the right time to expand the Association's role. He suggested the establishment of a Psychiatric Foundation to inform the public of the need for recognition of incipient mental disorder and its early treatment, raise money, train psychiatric researchers, and fund research projects. Next, he addressed organizational issues. "Should the Association," he asked, "be a small elite body or represent all of psychiatry? Should associate memberships be developed for clinical psychologists, social workers, nurses, occupational therapists and others?" (78, p. 21). He favored an organization that included only psychiatrists. He urged the appointment of a full-time psychiatrist in a central headquarters, the journal to become a monthly publication with added editorial support staff, and the development of four groups of minimum standards to cover: 1) the teaching of psychiatry in medical schools; 2) hospitals and clinics; 3) classification of mental disorders; and 4) a model commitment law.

Bowman found fault with the structure of sections at annual meetings (such as forensic, convulsive disorders, psychoanalyses, and psychopathology of childhood). As they had considerable autonomy and ill-defined functions, they often duplicated the work of standing committees, formed committees, and generated reports outside of the Association's channels for approval of statements made in the Association's name. "If sections exist only to generate an annual meeting program," Bowman said, "they should be abolished and the Program Committee take over this function. But if annual meeting sections are to continue as foci for special research, then many additional topics are important enough to be represented in a section such as military psychiatry, alcohol, psychosomatic medicine, shock and group therapy" (78, p. 23.)

The forum held at the 1946 annual meeting in Chicago was the first of several sessions devoted to policy that the Association was to hold in the years to follow. D. Ewen Cameron, speaking on the "Future of the Association," called for the Association to assume a leadership role in building social order of the future. To start action, he advocated staff support for certain standing committees such as Medical Education and Public Education. It was during the 1946 annual meeting that a group of "Young Turks" formed the Group for Advancement of Psychiatry (GAP) that was to become active in support of change in the APA (86).

In May of 1947, the affairs of the Association were still conducted by those members who attended the business session (300 in 1946, 700 in 1947) in town meeting fashion. The Nominating Committee's candidate for President-Elect was William Menninger, who was elected. However, the slate for councilors was challenged from the floor by a proposed slate of three different nominees. The alternate slate was elected with the strong support of GAP members present in numbers, with the intent of providing a governing body supportive of Dr. Menninger's policies for change. (William Menninger was also the current President of GAP.)

In a stormy session, the Reorganization Committee's plan for change in the Association was defeated. To make the organization more democratic, it proposed a House of Delegates and a Board of Trustees. However, constructive steps were taken with the vote of the membership to increase the dues, to become more active in leadership in psychiatry, and to establish a central office under a Medical Director with the assistance of a public relations officer. Conservative opposition stated that such moves were too costly and would bankrupt the organization. Opposition failed to persuade the members present, and the vote favored the actions noted.

Samuel Hamilton, President during this turbulent 1947 session, noted the following in his address:

1. An appropriation made over an 18-month period to the National Committee on Mental Hygiene to establish a Psychiatric Placement Service to help psychiatrists and other mental health professionals returning from the military service to find suitable jobs; some 900 persons had used this service
2. The first use of multiple nominations in the election of councilors
3. The ambitious plans of the Committee on Standards under the chairmanship of Mesrop Tarumianz since 1945; it proposed to survey and rate mental hospitals and to seek outside funding for the project
4. The problem of affiliate societies (the first had affiliated in 1934. The number increased to 11 by 1943. Five more were added and two awaited admission in 1947. These bodies sent nonvoting delegates to sit with the Council at the expense of the local society. The by-laws provided for the establishment of district branches by petition. Hamilton recommended riding the swirling current for awhile longer before enforcing districting. He noted that affiliate societies had as members some not eligible for APA membership.)
5. Establish a separate Treasurer and form a Budget Committee (79)

Steps toward establishment of a central headquarters moved swiftly after the eventful 1947 session. By February 1948, Daniel Blain was selected to be the Association's first Medical Director. Blain was, at the time of his appointment, Chief of the Division of Psychiatry in the Veterans Administration, a post he held for 2½ years with distinction. In a short time he had established 49 new mental hygiene clinics, created the policy that all VA general hospitals have psychiatric units, constructed well-planned new psychiatric hospitals, and instituted an extensive training program for psychiatric residents and clinical psychologists (see Appendix D and references 80, 81).

Dr. Blain reported for duty in April 1948 and opened a cubby-hole office on I (Eye) Street in Washington, D.C. In May 1948 he gave his first report as Medical Director, indicating that he would search for revenues outside the Association to support his ambitious plans. No better man could have been found than Daniel Blain to set in motion the revitalization of the Association.

Winfred Overholser, who had been the Secretary-Treasurer from 1941–1946, was elected APA President in 1948. In his address (82) he stated that the town meeting style of government was no longer feasible or democratic or representative for an association of 5,000 members, 24 standing committees, 5 sections, and 17 affiliated societies. Overholser also noted (82):

1. The continuing effort of the Committee on Reorganization to establish a more democratic structure
2. The appointment of Daniel Blain as Medical Director
3. The receipt of grants from the Rockefeller Foundation to support the inspection of nursing in all public mental hospitals and to improve the teaching of psychiatry in all medical schools
4. The Association's involvement through its Committee on International Relations in an International Congress on Mental Health in London (1948)
5. APA's participation in the war effort (outlined in defense of criticism of APA's role)
6. The need to establish principles for psychiatrists covering relationships to patients, families, community, and society; to elevate standards of interprofessional conduct; to cover reimbursement for services; to promote positive mental health, including a stand on sterilization and contraception; to take a stand on administrative policies affecting public and private care of the mentally ill; and to develop favorable attitudes toward research, etiology, prevention, and treatment of the mentally ill

The recital of gains and the aspirations for the future contrasted greatly with the bitter floor fight at the 1948 business session of the annual meeting in Washington, D.C. The Nominating Committee's candidate was the popular, gregarious Charles Burlingame, Psychiatrist-in-Chief of the Institute of Living in Hartford, Connecticut. Dexter Bullard, head of Chestnut Lodge (a private psychiatric hospital in Rockville, Maryland) nominated from the floor for President-Elect George S. Stevenson, the Medical Director of the National Committee for Mental Health, widely known for his work in prevention, community psychiatry, and the international mental health scene. Bullard's vilification of Burlingame (probably be-

cause of his advocacy of electroconvulsive therapy and psychosurgery, while Bullard's orientation favored a psychotherapeutic
approach) aroused passions. GAP was blamed for the discord but
was actually not involved in the floor nomination (83). Once again
the assembled members rejected the proposal to change the system
of governance to a House of Delegates and a Board of Trustees.

In the fall of 1948 the Association gained another outstanding
staff member when Blain appointed Robert L. Robinson as the
Association's public relations officer. Robinson was a graduate of
St. Lawrence University and the Fletcher School of Law and
Diplomacy at Tufts University. During his army service
(1941–1946) as a captain, he had been an information and education specialist with writing skills and editorial experience. Robinson's talents admirably complemented those of Blain. He was the
action arm of the idea man, developing the most promising of ideas
that streamed from Blain's innovative mind. It was a stimulus–response arrangement of superior level performance that
helped the Association gain recognition and power (84).

In November 1948 the Central Inspection Board was formed
with the mandate to survey and evaluate mental hospitals. By
December 1948 friction between the functions of the Executive
Secretary and the Medical Director led Blain to request a job
description to define areas of responsibility.

In April 1949 the first ongoing national continuing education
program was launched, with the first Mental Hospital Institute. It
set in motion an Association-wide effort that improved institutional
care of patients. Blain's idea became a reality when Robinson
wrote the grant application that secured $25,500 from the Com-
monwealth Fund to finance the project. Edited proceedings of the
institutes were prepared by Robinson (84). Communication was
improved by a journal—*Mental Hospitals*—and achievement
awards were established for innovative new programs.

At the annual meeting in 1949 in Montreal, a last ditch fight by
conservatives was launched to shut off the funds for the Medical
Director's office and stop what was seen as the radical move from
the primary concern of psychiatry—the clinical care of patients.
In April 1949 the Committee on Preservation of Psychiatric Standards was formed to lobby for their position. Known as "Robey's
Rangers" (its leader was Theodore Robey, M.D., of New Jersey),
they tried unsuccessfully to stem the reform movement.

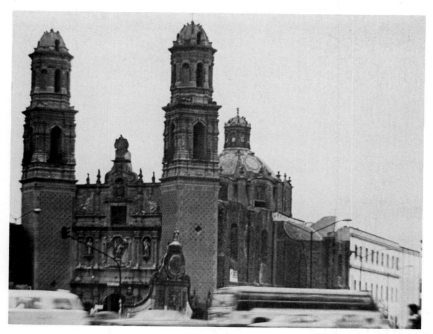

Church and Hospital de San Hipolito (the dome-topped building behind) in Mexico City, the first mental hospital in the New World (1566–1986). Photo by José Antonio Martinez. Courtesy of Ramón Parres.

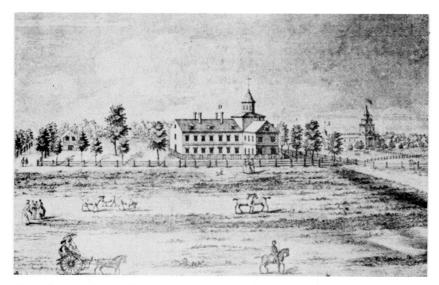

The old Pennsylvania Hospital, where the first hospital unit for care of the insane was provided in the colonies (1752). Courtesy of George S. Layne, M.D., of Bristol, Pennsylvania.

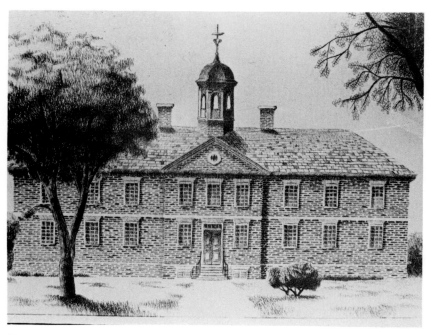

The first mental hospital in the United States, Williamsburg, Virginia, 1773 (from an original etching by John E. Costin).

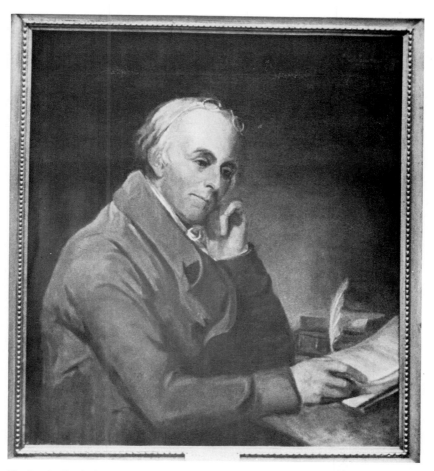

Benjamin Rush (1746–1813), father of American psychiatry. A copy of the Peale portrait (in Independence Hall) with hands from a portrait by Sully.

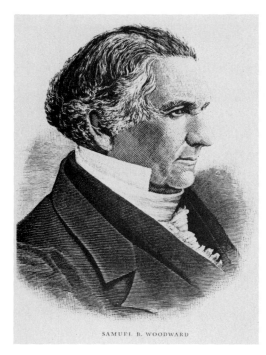

SAMUEL B. WOODWARD

Samuel B. Woodward (1787–1850), cofounder of the American Psychiatric Association and its first President. Courtesy of the National Library of Medicine.

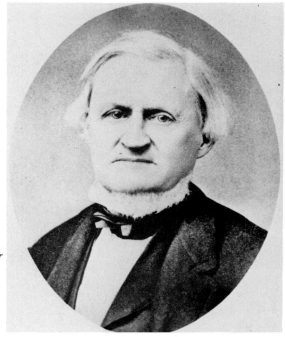

Francis T. Stribling (1810–1874), cofounder of the American Psychiatric Association. Courtesy of the National Library of Medicine.

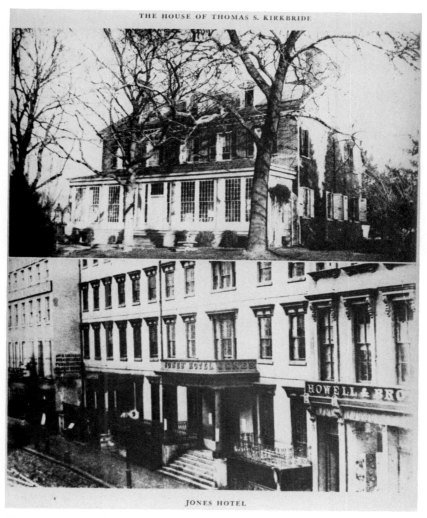

THE HOUSE OF THOMAS S. KIRKBRIDE

JONES HOTEL

The home of Thomas Kirkbride and the Jones Hotel. Courtesy of the National Library of Medicine.

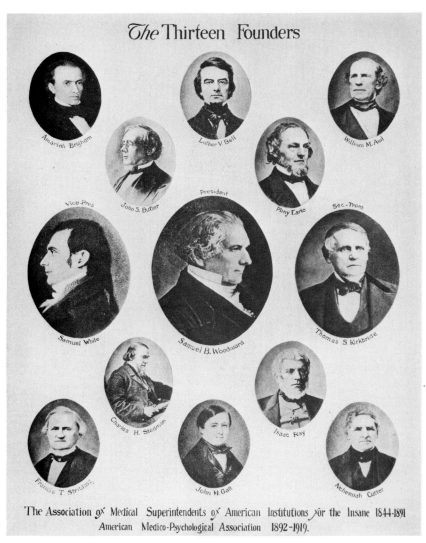

The Founding Fathers. Courtesy of the American Psychiatric Association Archives.

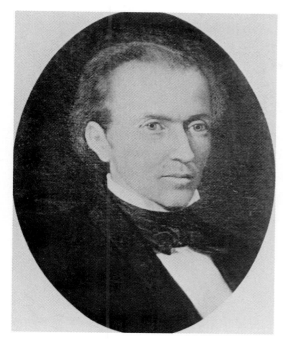

Amariah Brigham (1798–1849), founder and first Editor of the American Journal of Insanity *(July 1844)*.

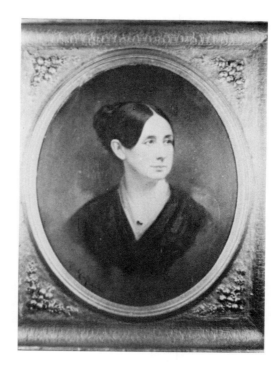

Dorothea Dix (1802–1887), social reformer, founder of 32 mental hospitals. Copy for the American Psychiatric Association of a portrait by Samuel Waugh (1865). Original in Dixmont Hospital.

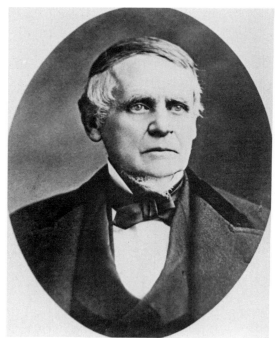

Thomas B. Kirkbride (1809–1883), founding father, first Secretary, and officer of the Association for 26 years.

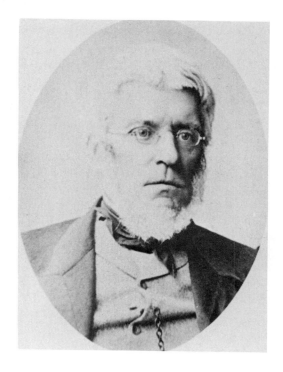

Isaac Ray (1807–1881), founding father and internationally renowned medico-legal expert.

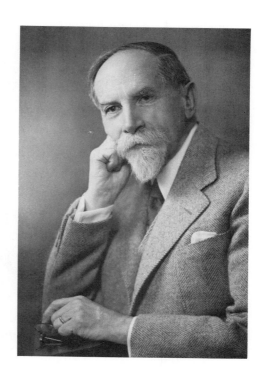

Adolph Meyer (1866–1950), dominant psychiatrist in the U.S. for 50 years. Author of the concepts "psychobiologic whole" and "common sense psychiatry." President of the American Psychiatric Association in 1927.

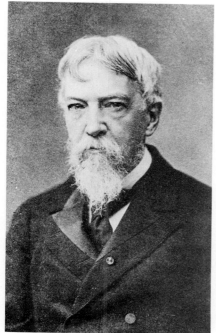

Silas Wier Mitchell (1829–1914), founder and first President of the American Neurological Association (1875). Poet, novelist, and catalyst to change the American Psychiatric Association.

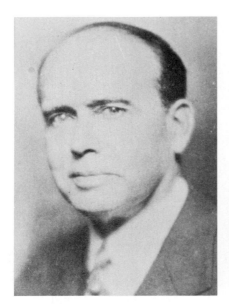
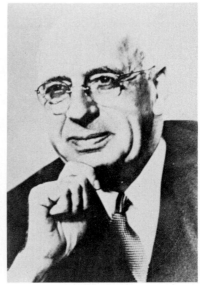

Clifford W. Beers (1876–1943), founder of the mental hygiene movement (1909) and of the national citizens organization (left).
Clarence M. Hincks (1885–1964), founder of the Canadian Mental Health Association (1918) and its head for 30 years. For eight years (1930–1938) he served as Director for the U.S. and Canadian Associations (right).

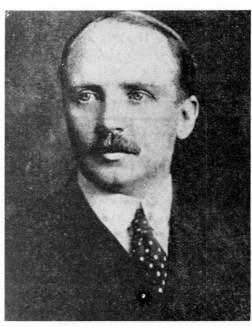

Thomas W. Salmon (1876–1927) played a key role in the development of military psychiatry in World War I. Director of the National Mental Health Association. He became the first non-superintendent President of the American Psychiatric Association, 1923–1924.

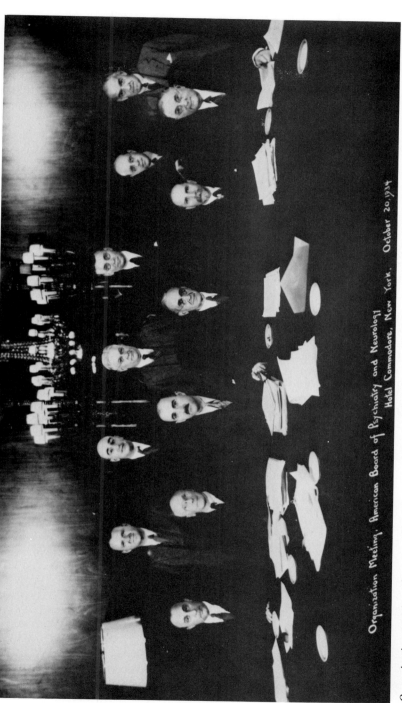

Organization meeting, American Board of Psychiatry and Neurology, October 1934. Front row: C. Cheney, C. Macfie Campbell, Walter Freeman, H. Douglas Singer, Adolf Meyer, and George Hall. Back row: F. Ebaugh, L. Casamajor, J.A. Jackson, L. Ziegler, L.J. Pollack, and E.G. Zabriskie.

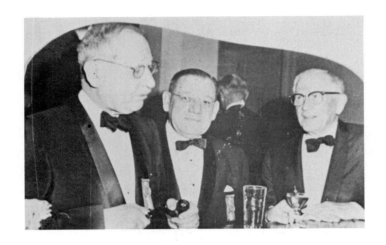

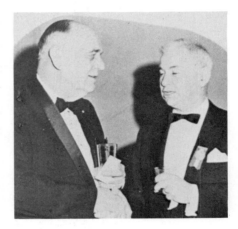

Top, left to right: Harry Solomon, Robert Felix, Karl Bowman
Middle: William Menninger, Francis Braceland
Bottom: John Whitehorn, Zigmund Lebensohn, Karl Menninger.

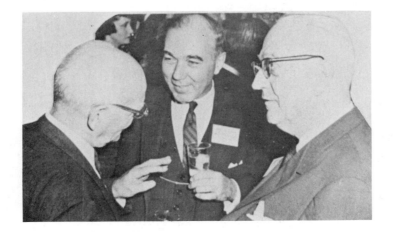

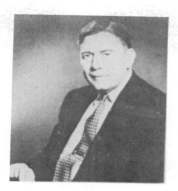

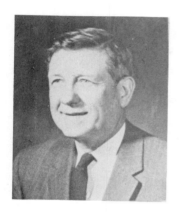
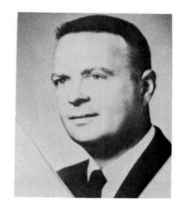

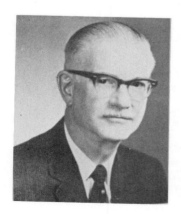
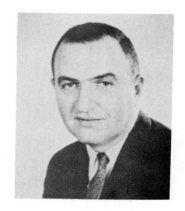

The Medical Directors and Executive Secretary.
Top: Austin Davies—Executive Secretary (1932–1964)
Middle: Daniel Blain (1948–1958), Matthew Ross (1959–1963)
Bottom: Walter E. Barton (1964–1974), Melvin Sabshin (1974–present)

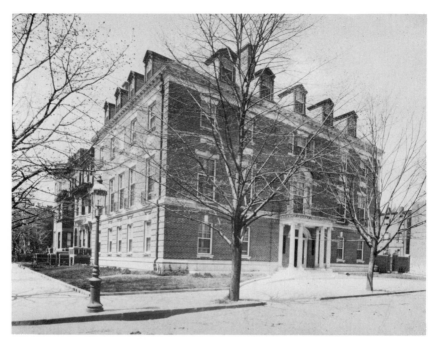

The Parsons Mansion (1910) . Note gas light, brick gate entrance to rear, absence of planting.

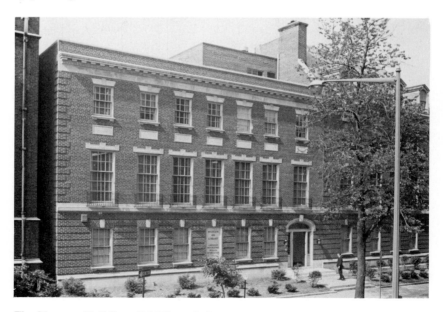

The Museum Building (1967) on R Street.

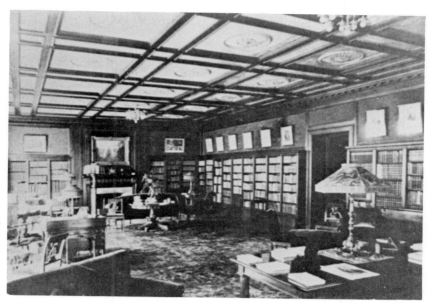

Parsons library at 1700 18th St. N.W., Washington, D.C.

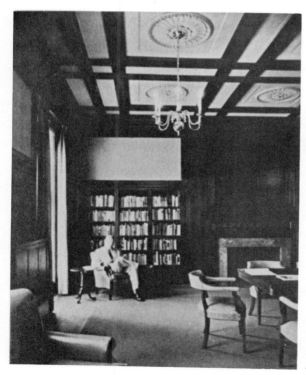

*The Modern
Founders Room,
American Psychiatric
Association, 1959.*

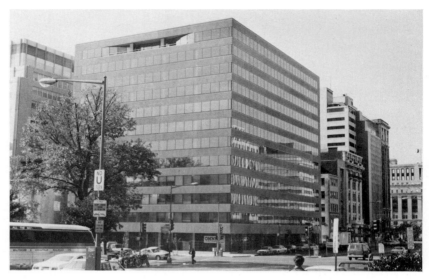

The American Psychiatric Association headquarters building, 1400 K St. N.W., Washington, D.C.

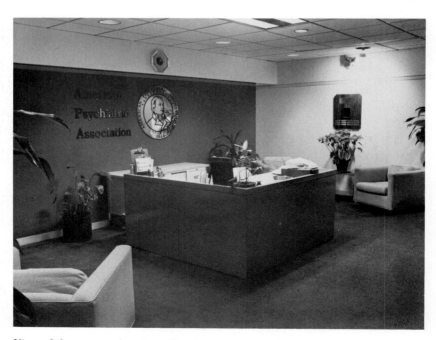

View of the present American Psychiatric Association lobby.

A Committee on a Permanent House was formed in December 1948, made up of five New York members and five Washington, D.C., members. This committee was asked to search for a building in either city and to investigate the suitability of the "Mansion" at Philadelphia in April 1949.

Job descriptions were approved to delineate the functions of the Medical Director and the Executive Assistant in May 1949. Essentially all business of the Association was to be handled in the New York office, and all professional affairs in the Washington office, with one exception: the Central Inspection Board would operate out of New York (November 1948).

The presidency of William Menninger in 1949 consolidated the movement of the Association toward reorganization, which made it more responsive to member needs and society's expectations. Menninger's Presidential Address noted the origin of the stimulus for change, assessed the current scene and remaining problems, and offered guidelines for the future of the Association (85). In the past there had been periods of turmoil such as that aroused by S. Weir Mitchell's criticism of psychiatrists' isolation, and by the appointment of Southard, the first nonhospital superintendent APA President (1919). There was also the "revolt" to form the Orthopsychiatric Association (1921) with its multidisciplinary membership. The dissatisfaction with the Association's participation in World War II in 1944 was the cause of the current press for the APA to exercise a leadership role in psychiatry. Menninger noted that conflict aroused member interest in Association affairs. There were common interests and divergent special needs of groups of psychiatrists that were only partially met by sections. For most members, the Association provided only an annual meeting and a journal. Only a few were involved in committees. Many of these committees never met, a few came together once a year for half a day, and many never developed a product. Menninger instituted a program to stimulate committee productivity. All met at one place and time to enhance information exchange and collaboration. Councilors were assigned to sit in on deliberations. Funding was provided to encourage more than one meeting, if needed, with emphasis upon productivity. Menninger noted (85):

- The work of reorganization was completed with many of the committee's recommendations adopted.

- Communication was improved largely by the enormous impact of the Medical Director, through personal contact, travels to local areas, with other groups, and by a newsletter.
- A start had been made on training needed manpower.
- Affiliate societies in time would become District Branches; local committees to relate to national ones were urged.
- A sound financial structure had been established.
- The need to integrate psychiatry into general medicine was recognized.
- The need to coordinate the efforts of mental health professions and mental health organizations in advancing shared goals was recognized.
- The need for psychiatry to play a greater role in governmental affairs, military planning, the VA, and various federal departments concerned with health policy was acknowledged.

Steps taken to bring together such groups as 12 professional journal editors and the superintendents of mental hospitals in a newly created section of the annual meeting, and leaders of all mental health professions at the Mental Health Institute and a conference of Mental Health Committees of State Medical Societies, were also noted by Menninger.

Menninger's leadership extended psychiatry's social role, increased its power and influence through collaboration, strengthened its internal structure, solidified its financial base, and made the organization more responsive to both members and societal needs. In the span of 50 years the APA had grown in size tenfold, from 400 to over 4,000 members.

MISSED OPPORTUNITIES

Although the achievements of the APA by 1949 were many, there were also some missed opportunities:

- The slow pace of the organization to face the problems of growth and change
- Complacency and inaction when the National Committee for Mental Hygiene filled the vacuum and assumed leadership in the war effort, in child psychiatry, in hospital surveys, and in mental hospital improvement

- Lack of monitoring psychiatric organization in the armed forces and in planning before World War II
- Minimal support of armed forces during World War II (individual APA members made major contributions, often with support from other organizations in which APA leaders were involved)
- Opposition of the APA membership to the formation of psychiatric units in general hospitals
- Absence of collaboration with the parent organization of developing mental health professions, especially clinical psychology, social work, occupational therapy, rehabilitation, and pastoral counseling (Individual APA members were involved; the organization was not. Psychiatric nursing was an exception—schools for training nurses were established in mental hospitals and affiliate training was provided for nurses enrolled. APA central staff included a nurse consultant.)
- No organizational involvement in the rapidly expanding Veterans Administration hospital system
- No advocacy for upgrading training for state hospital physicians (this came from outside the APA)
- Lack of a newsletter and monthly journal for more rapid dissemination of information to members until the end of the period

The foundation upon which the advancement of psychiatry as a medical specialty was laid was composed of the building blocks of theory, discoveries, standards, and a system of care similar to that of other medical specialties.

The concept of mind–body unity in a whole person integrating biological, psychologic, social, and cultural factors provided a broader base for research than had the preoccupations with the elusive search for organic causes of mental illness. The Freudian revolution provided new insights into psychological causative factors. Psychoanalytic theory stimulated analysts to study psychosomatic illnesses.

New discoveries drew psychiatry closer to all of medicine and led to specific therapies in certain illnesses such as pellagra, vitamin deficiency disorders associated with alcoholism, syphilis (discovery of spirochete, its sensitivity to heat, and control by penicillin), and some toxic infective disorders (successfully treated by sulfa drugs and penicillin). Tuberculosis units in mental hospitals were closed when effective treatment was developed.

The introduction of somatic therapies, especially electroconvulsive therapy (ECT), made it possible for the first time to
produce a rapid remission in a major mental illness.

New discoveries of chromosomes and inborn errors of metabolism brought new insight into the causation of some forms of
mental retardation. The introduction of the IQ test sharpened
diagnosis. School clinics brought psychiatrists out of their institutions and extramural programs sent residents of state schools into
the community.

Standard setting sought to improve mental hospitals. Surveys
produced recommendations, and when recommendations were followed and problems were corrected, hospitals were certified as
meeting standards. The creation of the American Board of Psychiatry and Neurology sought to assure the competence of the clinician by examination and certification as a diplomate. It also
stimulated medical education in psychiatry to meet national standards.

Changes in the system of care moved psychiatry out of its
isolation in mental hospitals into settings similar to those of other
medical specialties, but with unique features to cover patient need
for transitional facilities from hospital to community living. Child
guidance clinics, with their multidisciplinary teams, grew into the
specialty of child psychiatry and encouraged the emergence of
clinical psychology and psychiatric social work.

The development of the psychopathic hospital, the psychiatric
unit in the general hospital, the day hospital, the halfway house,
and ambulatory care in clinics and in doctors' offices moved
psychiatry further out of the mental hospital.

Psychiatry's assumption of power as a medical specialty and in
society did not take place without a struggle. The conflict between
conservatives who advocated that psychiatry be solely concerned
with clinical service to patients, and liberals who favored a wider
social responsibility, stimulated member interest in the Association.

Central to the advance of psychiatry was strong leadership
typified by the two great leaders of the APA at the end of this
period in 1948. General William C. Menninger, the APA President, moved to make the Association more responsive to patient
needs and society's expectations. Daniel Blain, the first Medical
Director, inaugurated new programs, raised funds to finance new

directions, and established a new power base within the Association in support of its objectives.

At the end of this period the American Psychiatric Association emerged reorganized and revitalized, ready to undertake the even greater challenges in the years ahead.

6

Medicine and Society:
Toward Shared Authority and Power
1950-1986

In an organizational society good leadership at the top is not enough . . . to function effectively interdependent teams at different levels need leaders; when everyone is prepared to manage self and job, leadership must become like Lao Tzu's best of all leaders, a valued resource that enhances individual power by consensus and education rather than a feared control mechanism that limits it by force.

—Michael Maccoby, *The Leader*, 1981*

The United States emerged, in the second half of the 20th century, as a superpower among nations. The other superpower, the USSR, tightened its hold on Eastern European countries within the communist bloc and expanded its influence into Afghanistan, Cuba, and Latin America. China's Peoples Republic spread communism beyond its borders into neighboring countries. The "free world" turned to the United States for help in the containment of communism.

The period from 1950–1986 has been a time of technological marvels such as nuclear power, lasers, computers, space exploration, and automated industry. The world has discovered, however,

* Reprinted from Maccoby M: The Leader. New York, Simon and Schuster, 1981. Copyright 1981 by The Project on Technology, Work and Character. Reprinted by permission of Simon & Schuster and the author.

that progress can be self-defeating: Nuclear missiles, for example, have the potential for destroying civilization.

An expanding population has demanded more energy and greater production of food. To grow more food, fertilizers and pesticides are used to increase the yield. The burning of fossil fuels produces acid rain, endangering vegetation and polluting lakes and rivers. Fertilizers have polluted the waters, while insecticides have killed birds and fish and contaminated the food chain (1).

The pressure for more food and more energy came in part from an expanding population. In 1950 the population of the United States was 150 million; by 1980, the population had increased to 220 million. The population of China was estimated to be 1 billion in 1985; the population of India and Pakistan, over 700,000; and the population of the USSR, 250 million.

POLITICAL DEVELOPMENTS

Communist Expansion: The Threat to National Security

The year 1949 was the year Mao Tse-Tung founded the Peoples Republic of China, bringing a large section of the globe into the communist system. In the same year, the USSR lifted the blockade of Berlin after testing the resolve of NATO (North Atlantic Treaty Organization, a defensive alliance against communism organized to protect any participant member from an attack). The alliance united the United States, Canada, and western European nations in the resolve to view an attack against any member nation as an attack against all. A massive airlift of food and supplies frustrated the Soviet attempt to isolate Berlin.

In 1950 Klaus Fuchs was found guilty of betraying British atomic secrets to the USSR, and in 1951 Julius and Ethel Rosenberg were convicted of giving vital information to the Russians and were sentenced to death for espionage against the United States. Senator Joseph McCarthy warned President Truman that the State Department was riddled with communists and communist sympathizers (2). The McCarthy Senate hearings (1950–1954), televised for the widest national publicity, implied that the government, media, theatre, and society were being undermined by the communists. One was presumed guilty if accused, or if one associated with a communist sympathizer.

A civil war, which the United Nations had predicted, began when communist North Korea invaded South Korea. The UN sent a multinational force to Korea under General Douglas MacArthur as Commander-in-Chief. The Korean Conflict was seen as a manifestation of the domino theory—when one nation was allowed to fall, all would topple.

UN troops gradually advanced, recaptured Seoul, and crossed the 38th parallel pushing into North Korea. The fear of another world war and a nuclear holocaust led the conflict to be designated a police action rather than a war, with combatants forced to accept a no-win policy. Some 2 million dead and wounded from 18 countries were sacrificed in a conflict that ended where it began, with no winners. American and UN intrusion into North Korean territory would encounter Chinese resistance, Chou En-lai warned the UN Assembly. Ignoring the warning, the UN authorized the invasion of North Korea to establish a unified democratic government. MacArthur was ordered not to use non-Korean forces north of the 38th parallel. He did so, beginning a feud with the administration on how to fight a war. When the combined forces reached the border with China, fighter planes crossed the border, with MacArthur advocating hot pursuit in order to bomb bases of operation. He was forbidden to do so because of fear of a war with Communist China. MacArthur disagreed, believing the rest of Asia would fall. Confident of victory, the 8th Army and South Koreans launched an attack for the Yalu River. Aerial reconnaissance had failed to detect a huge Chinese force moving into Korea by night. The Chinese communist army attacked in waves, decimating the opposition and forcing retreat. When an intransigent MacArthur lashed out at the administration for limiting use of options to crush the enemy, he was removed from command. The action was not popular. Senator Nixon demanded reinstatement, Senator McCarthy called President Truman "an s.o.b." who removed General MacArthur when drunk. A Gallup poll of public opinion favored MacArthur against Truman 69 to 19 (1).

Some 78 captured American airmen were subjected to psychological and physical torture in order to get them to confess that UN forces used germ warfare. Thirty-eight confessed (1). Brainwashing—coercive persuasion—was accomplished by placing prisoners in a hot box so small that standing was not possible; filth, degradation, isolation, starvation, sleep deprivation, and incessant interrogation by trained investigators who promised to stop the torture, led to confession.

A shocking disclosure after the armistice was signed was the extent of collaboration with the enemy among the 3,597 American prisoners who were released. Fifteen percent were active collaborators, 5 percent were not, and 80 percent signed peace petitions or something similar. Seventy-five Americans had agreed to become communist spies on returning home, and 25 refused to return to the U.S. Coercive persuasion proved to be an effective tool to change minds. In addition, there was a shockingly high death rate—38 percent—among prisoners. Many of these had starved themselves to death. The disturbing lack of discipline and absence of a sense of unity among prisoners led to a new code of conduct and raised doubt in the public mind that American troops were equal to the stress of an ideological battle for the mind.

Dwight Eisenhower, a popular hero of World War II, was overwhelmingly elected President in 1952. He continued the Truman policy of negotiation and secured a ceasefire agreement in Korea to end the bloody conflict. The war had claimed 33,529 American lives (1). The resolve to contain communist expansion was undiminished. Arms and assistance were given to the French in their struggle to keep Vietnam from falling to communism. The Southeast Asia Treaty Organization (SEATO) was formed in 1954 to maintain the uneasy peace that lasted until 1963 (2).

In 1958 Fidel Castro launched a total war in Cuba that culminated in a communist nation at America's doorstep. In 1961 an attempt by Cuban exiles in America (trained and supplied by the U.S.) to invade Cuba failed at the Bay of Pigs. President Kennedy assumed responsibility for the fiasco (2). When the USSR sent arms to Cuba and began construction of a missile base, President Kennedy demanded the base be dismantled. In the tense period of threats—the Cuban missile crisis—the two superpowers tested each other's resolve to stand firm. Khrushchev backed down, the base was dismantled, and the U.S. blockade of Cuba was lifted.

The Strategic Arms Limitation Talks (SALT) of 1970 led to a treaty to ban nuclear testing in the atmosphere in 1976.

From arms supply to the French in Vietnam followed financial aid and a military mission, with escalation of U.S. involvement in 1964 when the destroyer USS Maddox was allegedly attacked off the coast of North Vietnam. U.S. aircraft bombed bases in retaliation. Heavy fighting during the period 1965–1973 led to 45,948 American combat deaths, 303,640 wounded, and 10,298 noncombat deaths. Nine hundred thirty-five thousand American troops are estimated to have been involved in the Vietnam war, with U.S. expenditures of $109.5 billion. The intervention was unsuccessful and Saigon fell in 1975, with North Vietnam scoring a decisive communist victory. Later communist influence spread into Laos and Cambodia.

The prolonged war was unpopular in the United States, leading some eligible draftees to flee the country. Protests and demonstrations against the war were extensive. Returning veterans felt deserted and confused by public reaction to their sacrifice. As a byproduct, many of the military personnel abused drugs, which were plentiful in Vietnam. Once again doubts arose as to the ability of the U.S. to sustain its resolve in an ideological war.

The threat of communist expansion became very real in the coup in Czechoslovakia, the use of troops in Hungary, the "Cold War" in Europe, the attempt to take over South Korea, the conquest of Vietnam and Indochina, Cuba, China, and in the supply of arms to Middle Eastern nations and to insurgents in Latin America. The ideological struggle became even more troublesome as the communists took the side of the oppressed and powerless, with their support of the "collective good" in a controlled society.

What has evolved has been a movement toward compromise by communist and noncommunist governments. Each now has elements of the other. To motivate individuals to produce more food, "capitalistic free enterprise" was allowed by communist governments. Alternatively, nations opposing communism under the free enterprise system gave high priority to individual autonomy but found it necessary to move cautiously toward government-sponsored social programs to insure equity and the public good.

SCIENTIFIC DEVELOPMENTS

Nuclear Proliferation

In 1952, Great Britain and the U.S. developed the hydrogen bomb, as did the USSR in 1953. Atomic fission was succeeded by fusion and the potential for destruction multiplied. By 1967,

China and other countries possessed nuclear capability. As several nations held the power to destroy others, and as the superpowers counted missiles with nuclear warheads in the thousands with the potential to destroy civilization, the concern for control of nuclear proliferation became dominant.

Electrical energy, generated by nuclear reactors in this country and abroad, was at first seen as the answer to the energy crisis. However, after one nuclear reactor accident in 1979 at Three Mile Island, near Harrisburg, Pennsylvania spewed radioactive matter into the air, fears of disaster mounted. Every cracked pipe, stoppage for repair, and problem of disposal of nuclear waste was widely publicized in the media. In 1986, the reactor at Three Mile Island remains closed. "No nukes" has become a slogan of organized protestors who have tried in every way possible to stop further building of nuclear reactors and the closing of all. On April 28, 1986, another accident at a nuclear reactor occurred—this one in Chernobyl, U.S.S.R. It has prompted much fear and anger around the world. What will happen as a result of this accident remains to be seen.

The press for abolition of missiles and all nuclear armaments grew so strong that some were willing to support unilateral disarmament without a treaty or surveillance in order to insure that other nations would eliminate all nuclear armaments. Efforts at formal limitations of nuclear armaments have failed after repeated efforts. In this climate, the superpowers have stockpiled nuclear devices and have raced to build up military strength. Both the U.S. and the U.S.S.R. have become arms merchants, equipping nations perceived as their friends with military hardware.

Space Exploration: The New Frontier

At World War II's end both superpowers, knowing that German scientists had the capability of building mightier rockets than those used in the attack on London, persuaded the scientists involved to work in their countries.

In 1957 the Soviets launched a space rocket—Sputnik—the first Earth satellite, before a startled world-wide audience. This was the event that started the space race for technological supremacy between the superpowers.

The woeful lack of emphasis on the teaching of science in U.S. schools led to the passage of the National Defense Education Act in 1958. In the same year, The National Aeronautics and Space Administration (NASA) was established and richly funded to coordinate the development of space exploration. In 1958 the U.S. launched Explorer I with a 32-pound satellite, while the U.S.S.R.'s Sputnick III carried a 3,000-pound satellite. Progress was swift. Soon both countries were orbiting astronauts in satellites and conducting experiments in space. The Soviets were first to perfect a landing, while the Americans splashed down at sea. In 1969 the U.S. was first to land two men on the surface of the moon, and to return them safely in a lunar module that joined an orbiting space satellite. Next followed space probes (1969) and planetary exploration (1974). Marvelous pictures of Earth and of planets captured world attention. By 1970, spy satellites and commercial communication satellites were in use.

By 1980, technology had advanced to permit frequent space shuttle flights and orbiting sophisticated space laboratories. With a presence in space comes the threat of attack and a scramble to defend against it. The hope for treaties to insure the peaceful use of space, and collaboration of scientists in the pursuit of knowledge about the universe, now appears to have been only a cherished dream.

SOCIAL DEVELOPMENTS

The Civil Rights Movement

The race for advantage in space between the superpowers stimulated the leap in technology. Social progress in the same period, 1950 to the present, was energized by the model of protest used by the civil rights movement. From individual protests by courageous blacks who rebelled against where they were expected to sit—in the back of the bus, on a toilet designated for blacks only, or in a separate section of a restaurant—grew organized protests such as the city-wide boycott on the use of buses in Montgomery, Alabama, in 1955. In that year, the U.S. Supreme Court ruled that school segregation was unconstitutional, and declared in 1955 that segregation in parks, playgrounds, in tax supported colleges and universities (1957), and federal housing (1961) must end. When there was noncompliance, as was the case in Little Rock, Arkansas, in 1957, federal troops were called to enforce desegregation in the schools.

In the 1960s whites joined blacks in freedom marches, protesting peacefully and demonstrating support for elimination of discriminatory practices. Voting rights were secured in 1965. Not all followed the peaceful course charted by Martin Luther King, Jr., the charismatic black leader of the Southern Christian Leadership Conference. The year 1967 was marked by rioting, burning, and looting by blacks who were impatient at the slow pace of change.

The civil rights protest model has been employed by students seeking a voice in policy in college and university, by a broader cross-section of society against the U.S. war in Vietnam, by women seeking equal rights, by advocates of abortion and those opposed to it, and by those opposed to investments in racist South Africa.

The protest model has been employed by supporters of a variety of causes or perceived injustices. The protest against all authority extended from the 1960s into the 1970s. It was so general as to be caricatured by the challenge to the professor's "Good morning" with the class' "How do you know it's good?"

Some protesters dropped out of society and developed a counter-culture. However, in the 1970s to 1980s more traditional patterns have returned in the use of the democratic process.

Violence as a Political Statement

Assassination of political leaders who are seen as oppressors has been a social blight in the United States since the 19th century. Lincoln, McKinley, Garfield, and Kennedy were assassinated while President, and many more leaders (including Presidents Truman and Reagan) were the targets of unsuccessful attempts. Violence as a political statement reached a peak in 1968, when Robert Kennedy and Martin Luther King, Jr., were murdered, and violent protests rocked American cities and college campuses.

Catholics and Protestants killed each other in Ireland during years of violent protest, and this violence still continues. The Irish Republic Army (IRA) has used bombs to protest England's presence in Ireland. The Arabs and Israelis have battled each other for centuries. Acts of terrorism in the name of homeless Palestinians have threatened Israelis since 1948. Now, in 1986, Libya is staging terrorist attacks around the world, and the threat of violence is a common concern.

Selecting the Olympic Games of 1972—with the world watching on television—11 Israeli hostages (most of whom were athletes participating in the games) were seized and murdered. In 1979, the religious leader of Iran, Ayatollah Khomeni, ordered Americans working in the American Embassy to be seized as hostages. The intent was to punish and humble a superpower for its aid to the deposed Shah of Iran, and for its support of Israel, "occupiers of Palestine." Full worldwide media coverage was given to the event, which lasted for more than a year. The slaughter of 90 French and 200 American members of the "peacekeeping force" in Beirut in 1983 by suicide bombing of dormitory buildings was intended to demonstrate that a "foreign" presence was unwanted.

The taking of hostages to be used as bargaining chips for political ends, if possible, before the television cameras, has become common practice, but not the only technique employed. Foreign officers and leaders of governmental affairs have been killed and bombs have been thrown into crowds to make a political point.

Conservation

While 20th century America has witnessed violent upheaval, we have also made important attempts to preserve what is best and most beautiful in our country. The idea to preserve for future generations a part of the astounding wilderness with which the United States is blessed emerged before the country celebrated its centennial. On September 19, 1870, three men sat around a campfire in Yellowstone (Gen. H.D. Washburn, a surveyor; 2nd Lt. G.C. Doane, a vigilante law officer; and C. Hedges, a judge in the Montana territory) discussing what should be done with the amazing area they had been exploring for five weeks. It was Cornelius Hedges who said it should not be owned by individuals but should become a national park. All pledged to achieve that goal. They succeeded two years later when Congress created Yellowstone National Park, the first national park in the world. From that beginning grew the Park Service (a bureau in the U.S. Department of Interior founded in 1916), administering 24 million acres of land in 181 units scattered throughout the land. The Antiquities Act (1906) preserved, by proclamation, places of historical interest (3).

The desire to preserve the natural beauty of wilderness areas and places of historical interest extended in the 20th century to constrain individuals and industries from polluting land, water, and air. A stimulus to the conservation movement came from such eloquent champions as Rachel Carson in *Silent Spring* (1962), who brought to public attention the harmful effects of DDT and pesticides on birds and in the food chain. Barry Commoner, who wrote *The Closing Circle: Nature, Man and Technology* (1971), explained the nature of ecology and the ecosphere—poisoned air in Los Angeles, poisoned water in Lake Erie, poisoned land in Illinois, and genetic damage from atomic fallout. Barbara Ward and Rene Dubois wrote *Only One Earth* (1972), a report commissioned by the Secretary General of the United Nations Conference on the Human Environment, which summed up the importance of conservation for the world.

Progress has been made in the conservation of our natural resources. The Atlantic salmon returned to the Connecticut River in 1975. Rivers and streams, once sewers of human and industrial waste, are now cleaner, and many have become fit to swim in again. Serious efforts have been made to search out and clean up dumps of toxic waste. The insatiable demand for energy to fuel expansion has become critical. Every industrial expansion is now more closely scrutinized for its environmental impact.

Human Resources

The generation of the baby boom—born 1946 to 1964—are the workers destined to support an increasing number of aging Americans. The elderly are healthier than ever before, with more living beyond the age of 80 years when chronic illnesses take their toll. The aging group uses a greater number of health care and welfare resources in proportion to its percentage of the population than any other group. The birth rate has been shrinking to near zero growth, foretelling a smaller work force to support the increasing number of aged in the future (4). Japan has achieved a zero population growth. China, in the 1970s, made population control a major priority. India and third world countries are faced with population growth pressures that have strained their capacity to feed their populace.

The Economy

The state of the economy of the U.S. has been a major concern in the 1980s. In 1965 inflation troubled the government; a wage–price freeze was invoked but failed to control inflation. During President Carter's term in office (1977–1981), double digit inflation and a severe recession closed down factories, swelling unemployment rolls and threatening cities with bankruptcy.

In 1981, President Reagan succeeded in controlling inflation. The strategies involved were reducing the size of the federal government; severe cuts in federal programs; deregulation to permit a free market; reduced taxes; and a control of the money supply. Greater management efficiency to control costs, increased worker productivity, and renegotiation of union contracts at lower wages to hold on to jobs and to make American industry more competitive in the foreign markets have become widespread practices in the 1980s.

In spite of these efforts the national debt reached one trillion dollars, with the consequence of a disproportionate number of resources consumed in debt financing. The goal of a balanced federal budget has proved elusive due to our increased military spending to achieve parity with the U.S.S.R. Efforts to reduce the national debt have become a bipartisan goal of the 1980s.

Health care costs have soared out of sight. Expenditures in 1960 were $27 billion, and in 1983, $356 billion (5). As the proportion of the gross national product spent for health care increased from 3 to 11 percent in 23 years (5), the government and industry have sought ways to control costs. The health care system's voluntary efforts have made everyone aware of the problems. Under the threat of caps on spending and the potential for rationing health care, various strategies have been tried in the 1980s such as:

- Utilization review to determine necessity of hospitalization
- Peer review and professional service review organizations (to assess the appropriateness of intervention, length of stay, etc.)
- Prospective reimbursement schemes
- Health Maintenance Organizations (HMOs)
- Preferred Provider Organizations (PPOs), with contracts to lowest bidder to supply health care

- Payment on the basis of Diagnosis Related Groups (DRGs): a system with a fixed rate of payment for a given diagnosis

One of the most promising avenues for reducing costs has been encouraging the individual to be responsible for his or her own health through proper diet, exercise, and changes in lifestyle (no smoking, avoidance of alcohol and drugs, limitation of carcinogenic food additives, low salt intake, and so forth).

The United States, the superpower in the 1950s able to assist the world in maintaining stability, lost its position of preeminence. In the 1980s power has been shared with other nations. Once invented and technology for production worked out, a product could be marketed at lower cost with cheaper labor costs in other countries than in the U.S. This has affected the U.S. economy.

After the 1950s, investor owned for-profit corporations began to enter the health care field, buying or leasing general and psychiatric hospitals. They also operate chains of nursing homes, outpatient surgical and medical clinics, and, under contract, run hospital emergency rooms, offer management consultation, and provide other services.

The first step toward a revolution in information processing was taken in 1942 when the computer was invented in the United States. The huge cumbersome machines became smaller with the invention in 1964 of the silicon transistor microchip. Automated industrial adaptations employed computer-directed robots to perform repetitive tasks. Soon computers guided everything from missiles and space vehicles to the family motor car.

The computer's impact upon the health field since 1974 has been tremendous. The burgeoning literature of science could be stored in the memory of the computer, which could search and retrieve what was needed at terrific speeds. Hospital information systems, as a management tool, began in 1954 with automation of the payroll. Soon the computer was applied to personal records, bed and appointment scheduling, determination of patient characteristics, analysis of length of stay, allocation of resources, inventory control, food management, and outcomes of treatment.

In clinical practice, in addition to the above institutional uses, the computer could record patient information, provide information on drugs, analyze tests, produce data for insurance forms, and be applied in countless other ways (6, 7).

The electron microscope, perfected after World War II, had its beginning in the 1920s and 1930s. Its ability to magnify the hidden structure of the body changed anatomical foundations. The laser, invented in 1960, was a marvel. Laser photons produced tremendous light energy, could "see" into space or under the sea, visualize the human body, take meteorological readings, monitor engine performance, cut through steel or weld, destroy cells of cancer, coagulate a gastric ulcer, or repair a retinal tear in the eye. Laser beams could be a weapon of war or a versatile tool of medicine (8).

DEVELOPMENTS IN HEALTH SCIENCES

Infections and Communicable Diseases

The conquest of infections and of many communicable diseases was achieved in the 30-year period beginning in 1950. Sulfa drugs, although discovered in 1917, came into general use in the post-war period. Penicillin, discovered in 1928, proved valuable in World War II and became commercially available in the 1950s, with streptomycin appearing in 1952.

One of the truly remarkable advances in the health sciences was in the treatment of tuberculosis. The highly vulnerable American Indians and African black slaves had not encountered the disease before meeting the white man. In 1890, an astounding death rate of 9,000 per 100,000 population was reached among Indians; by 1940, the mortality under conservative management had fallen in the general population to 50 per 100,000, but the rate in blacks was about five times higher than in whites. Approximately 100,000 beds were devoted to tuberculosis patients, many of these in mental hospitals (9).

Streptomycin (1943), isoniazid (1912, though it was not used until the 1950s), and para-amino salicylic acid (PAS) proved to be powerful antituberculosis agents so effective that tuberculosis hospitals and tuberculosis wards in mental hospitals were closed.

Vaccines for smallpox, rabies (1885), diphtheria (1895), and tetanus were used in the conquest of communicable and infectious diseases. Added in the years after 1950 were other vaccines, such as those for yellow fever (1951), poliomyelitis (1954–1957), and rubella (1969). Smallpox was eradicated in the entire world as a result of the vaccine. Cases of measles in the U.S. dropped from 500,000 in 1962 to 1,500 in 1983 (9, 10).

Heart, Stroke, and Cancer

The clinical diagnoses of heart disorders improved markedly with the refinement of the electrocardiograph, which was introduced into clinical practice in 1920. When I was called in an emergency in the 1950s to see a patient whose heart had suddenly stopped beating, I sharply thumped the chest. This primitive method has been replaced by cardiopulmonary resuscitation (CPR) that saves many lives when followed by rapid transport to an intensive care unit in a nearby hospital. Two Russians, Gurvick and Yuniev in 1946, reported that a strong electric shock applied externally to the chest would restore cardiac activity. By 1952, Boston's Beth Israel Hospital used the method on a patient in cardiac arrest. The emergency use of the cardiac defibrulator (1956) and the development of a pacemaker (1960–1970) kept hearts beating. Heart-lung machines evolved from 1935 to 1955. Valve surgery, developed in 1952, and by-pass surgery, developed in 1967, became common operations in the 1970s. By 1976, surgical treatment could alleviate coronary heart disease, remedy damaged heart valves, remove aneurysms and replace obstructed areas with plastic tubes, and ream out or bypass occluded blood vessels, thereby reducing deaths by 25 percent (5).

Hypertension, too, could be treated and blood pressure lowered. Hydralazine (1946), reserpine (1952), alpha-methyldopa (1960), and chlorothiazide (1957) aided the control of hypertension. Within a decade, effective diuretic agents combined with low salt intake greatly improved the management of high blood pressure.

The improved control of hypertension and of diseases such as diabetes, along with the discovery of anticoagulant drugs, reduced the number of deaths from strokes by nearly 40 percent since 1970 (5). Federal concern for these leading killer disorders was recognized in 1965 in PL 89–239, the Regional Medical Programs Act, to aid in the struggle against heart disease, stroke, and cancer.

Deaths from cancer have steadily increased over a 50-year period (10). The era of chemotherapy for cancer began when Goodman and colleagues published a landmark article in 1946

(11) on nitrogen mustard therapy for Hodgkins Disease, lymphosarcoma, leukemia, and other disorders. In terminal cases resistant to radiation, 26 out of 67 were alive after nitrogen mustard therapy was instituted.

When recognized early, surgical removal, radiation, chemotherapy or some combination of these, resulted in some 48 percent of all cancer patients living at least five years after treatment. Other chemical agents, such as methotrexate (1947), mercaptopurine (1951), and many others have become weapons to fight cancer.

Research

The massive influx of federal dollars ($100 million) to support cancer research, granted by The Cancer Act of 1971, leads me to comment on the role of Mary Lasker in moving the federal government to support research activity in a manner that also made possible greater funding of mental health research. Mrs. Albert D. Lasker, a wealthy citizen concerned for the poor state of health of the people in the United States, had worked as a volunteer to help streamline the American Cancer Society. Mary Lasker teamed up with a friend, Florence Mahoney, who was an experienced campaigner for the improvement of health programs. In December 1944, the two supported Senator Claude Pepper and asked him to emphasize the need for medical research. Lasker money financed the National Committee Against Mental Illness with Mike Gorman, a crusading journalist who strove to improve care of the mentally ill, as its Executive Director (10).

The stimulus of government involvement led, in 1945, to the establishment of a Mental Health Division in the Public Health Service, and, in 1946, to the National Mental Health Act and the National Institute of Mental Health.

The National Institutes of Health budget by 1967 was over one billion dollars. In 1950 the National Science Foundation created a division of Biological and Medical Science to support basic research (not clinical research, which was NIH's role). The major support in Congress during this period of massive infusion of federal funds for research came from the leadership of Representative John Fogarty and Senator Lister Hill. Also during this same period, the VA system was given funds to develop its research capability in the health sciences.

In 1950 Margaret Sanger persuaded Gregory Pincus of the Worcester Foundation for Biological Sciences to develop an effective method for birth control. In collaboration with John Rock (a gynecologist and expert in endocrine therapy of infertility), Pincus used progesterone in 1952. Commercial preparation became available in 1957. Birth control by the "pill" spread rapidly worldwide. Later, intrauterine devices were introduced along with progesterone compounds to prevent fertilization.

Successful transplantation of organs awaited the solution of the body's natural tendency to reject a foreign tissue, the discovery of an effective anticoagulant of blood, and mechanical devices that would sustain life during the transfer procedure (8). Immunosuppressive agents were developed; heparin, one of the more effective anticoagulants, was discovered; and the renal dialysis machine, first applied in animal experiments at Johns Hopkins in 1913, was further developed as a prototype in 1945 and perfected in the following decade. As early as 1908 Alexis Carrel transplanted kidneys in dogs and cats, but it was not until 1951–1953 that the procedure was successful in humans in work done at Boston's Peter Bent Brigham Hospital (10).

By the 1980s kidney, liver, and corneal transplants were done successfully. With the use of living organs for transplant, and also because machines could sustain life, it became essential to define brain death (1972), and, when appropriate, to cease heroic efforts to keep a patient alive (1976) (12).

After World War II, artificial limbs were developed to restore function with refinement under electric power. Artificial hip joints replaced damaged joints. Hearing aids helped the deaf, as did microsurgery.

The Cost of Health Care

Health insurance, started in the 1940s, expanded to cover most U.S. citizens who were employed. Federal programs such as Medicare (1965) covered those over 65, and Medicaid (1965) covered the needy with state participation. Third parties became involved in nearly every physician–patient relationship, with a need to have access to a patient's records in order to pay benefits. This seriously strained traditional confidentiality.

Hill-Burton legislation (1965) provided funds to improve hospitals, with $2 billion added to the $4 billion already appropriated, to benefit some 1,880 facilities (8). The Comprehensive Health Planning Act (PL–749) passed in 1965 established planning programs for health care facilities in all states.

Two issues came to the forefront of concern in the 1970s, with a profound impact upon the health field: ethics and liability. The advance of science and new technologies raised all manner of ethical questions, such as, "When does human life begin?" In 1975, K.C. Edlin was found guilty of manslaughter for performing a "legal" abortion. A "test tube" baby was born in England in 1970. Artificial insemination, surrogate mothers, fetal surgery, genetic engineering, and the "right to die" raised ethical questions.

A liability crisis arose in the 1970s that caused near-panic among physicians when insurance companies cancelled malpractice insurance. Variability in individual response to drugs with toxic side effects, slight risks of injury with patients not forewarned, and the patient's perception of less than successful treatment led to patient lawsuits against doctors. The cost of defensive medicine and high liability premiums were added to already soaring health care costs.

The 1980s has ushered in a period of general concern over escalating hospital and physician costs for health services. The response has been to fashion controls varying from caps on fees, prospective payment schemes, extension of contracts to the lowest bidder to provide services, and many other schemes to keep costs contained.

Concern with the Effects of Drugs, Alcohol, and Tobacco

Since 1960, the introduction of more potent drugs targeted to specific symptoms carried a greater likelihood of serious side effects. Drugs can produce blindness, hearing loss, neurological damage, and even death. The 1962 tragedy of the drug thalidomide causing serious birth defects illustrates this point.

Once again, people were made aware that the ingestion of excessive alcohol during the early months of pregnancy could increase the risk of birth defects. Although fetal syndrome due to alcoholism had been known to occur for many years, it became a real concern after 1960. The abuse of alcohol, driving while drunk, and damage to health by drug abuse have been issues of major concern since the 1970s. The relationship of cigarette smoking to heart disease and cancer led to the removal of cigarette advertisements from television, and to warnings of its danger to health printed in all cigarette advertisements and on all cigarette packages.

Since 1960 it has become popular to exercise, jog, ingest less salt, eat low cholesterol foods, include fiber in the diet, be concerned about carcinogens in food additives, and be concerned with the potential for harm of many chemicals in common use.

Federal Policy and Medical Manpower

Federal policy, under the G.I. Bill, entitled veterans of World War II to educational benefits. Many sought admission to medical schools. In 1950, 25,000 individuals applied for 7,000 openings in the first-year class (10).

Under federal immigration legislation and because of the shortage of physicians in the post-World War II period, it was easy for a foreign medical school graduate to enter the U.S. under the status of temporary visitor and convert to permanent resident (10).

In the 12-year period from 1960 to 1972 the number of foreign medical graduates increased by 43,000. By 1972, 46 percent of the physician licenses issued were to foreign medical graduates. It had been hoped that they might become family physicians and settle in underserved areas. They did not, preferring to practice in the same densely populated areas as U.S. medical school graduates. Foreign medical graduates did not include only citizens from foreign countries; in 1974, some 5,000 Americans who had been denied admission to U.S. schools were enrolled in foreign schools (13).

Fewer physicians became general family doctors and more became specialists; the shortage of family doctors that resulted was most apparent in inner cities, in rural areas, and in family practice. More physicians remained in academic centers, as full-time faculties expanded tenfold in the 30 years beginning in 1930 (10).

A controversial federal policy determined that a physician shortage existed, and the 1968 Health Manpower Act broadened support for medical education and allied health personnel. The number of medical schools increased from 82 to 116, with double the number of graduates (10). The quality of medical education improved during the period, as did the competence of faculties; continuing medical education became a highly specialized and costly business. In the 1980s the concern has become the oversupply of physicians, with a call to reduce the size and numbers of medical schools, and to end the influx of graduates from schools outside of the United States.

ADVANCES IN PSYCHIATRY

More advances in the field of psychiatry have been made in the 35 years from 1950 to 1985 than were made in all of the 18th and 19th centuries. Perhaps the most significant events were:

1. The discovery of effective drug therapy, exploration of how drugs worked, and new knowledge about the role of chemical transmitters in the nervous system
2. The development of the National Institute of Mental Health with a massive infusion of funds into training, research, and clinical service
3. The action that followed the Joint Commission on Mental Illness and Health recommendations derived, from a survey of the field, a determination of needs and the support of President Kennedy (The Community Mental Health Movement was a spin-off of the Commission's study)
4. The development of a widely accepted classification of mental diseases (The American Psychiatric Association's *Diagnostic and Statistical Manual of Mental Disorders*), which has facilitated research, diagnosis and treatment, and the establishment of standards and accreditation of psychiatric facilities
5. The extension of legal involvement in the mental health field, expanding self-determinism into the right of the mentally ill to treatment and to refuse it; to the adoption of the legal principle of informed consent; to the court established standard that admission be to the least restrictive alternative to hospitalization; and to the redefinition of liability beyond the standard of negligence to include outcomes of medical treatment that were less favorable than expected
6. The advances in the field of medicine that had a profound effect upon the practice of psychiatry: the conquest of tuberculosis and infectious diseases, cardiac surgery, heroic measures to sustain life (with its stimulus to the growth of consultation-liaison psychiatry), computer applications, and new

diagnostic aids such as computerized axial tomography (CAT), positron emission tomography (PET), and nuclear magnetic resonance (NMR); the APA, as an organization, was directly involved in many of these developments

Advances in Research and Theory

Drug Research

The discovery of drugs that would alter feeling, thinking, and behavior (drugs that had psychotropic effects) began in 1949, when Cade, in Australia, tested the use of lithium in patients with mania (14). Rauwolfia alkaloids were used in India in psychotic patients for a very long time. Reserpine, introduced in the U.S. between 1952 and 1953, had but limited usage, quickly being replaced by more effective antipsychotic agents (15).

Made from a synthesis of aniline dyes, phenothiazine was shown to have antihistaminic and sedative properties (16). Phenothiazine was first used in 1951 by the surgeon Laborit, who described its peculiar effect upon consciousness (16). It was Delay and Denniker who first used the drug between 1952 and 1953 in psychiatric patients (17). While searching for an analegesic drug, P.A. Jensen in Belgium (1959) developed butyrophenones, later widely used in the U.S. as haloperidol (16). Iproniazid was discovered in 1952 to inhibit monoamine oxidase (MAO), and a few years later tricyclic antidepressants were discovered, with imipramine used in clinical trials in Switzerland by Kuhn (1957–1958) (16). The first clinically effective antianxiety agent was meprobamate (1957), followed in 1960 by the benzodiazepines—chlordiazepoxide and diazepam.

The discovery of drugs effective in the treatment of mental disorders stimulated further research into their mechanisms of action. The antipsychotic drugs, Carlson suggested in 1963, blocked dopamine receptors in the brain (18); and Kety (19) believed that dopamine blockade was only part of the biological process in schizophrenia, and that other neurotransmitters may be involved—an abnormality of dopamine beta-hydroxylase could be important in the causation of schizophrenia. The theory states there is a defect (an expression of the genetic component in schizophrenia) in the enzyme DBH, which converts dopamine to

norepinephrine, and the underactivity of norepinephrine is corrected by a blockade of the specific dopamine receptors in the
brain (19).

The antidepressant drugs potentiate the action of cate-
cholamines and, in particular, norepinephrine and serotonin.
There are demonstrable changes in catecholamine metabolism in
states of elation or depression. Since 1968, it has been found that
levels of a major metabolite of norepinephrine—3-methoxy 4-
hydroxyphenyl glycol (MHPG)—are lower in periods of depression
and higher in periods of elation in persons suffering from affective
disorders. It has been postulated that a genetic–familial defect in
the neuroregulatory mechanisms is a cause of affective disorder.

The benzodiazepines widely used in anxiety disorders exert a
sedative, widespread inhibitory effect in the central nervous system: anticonvulsant and muscle relaxant activity and depression of
the limbic system of the brain. Their diffuse inhibitory effect is
accompanied by anticonvulsant and muscle relaxant properties.

Neuropsychiatric Research

In the same period of exciting advances in neurochemistry,
another old strand of interest was revived—that of the study of the
brain with theories advanced to explain emotional and behavioral
disorders on the basis of defects in the structure and function of
the nervous system.

In 1973, MacLean (20) established that the striatal cortex is
concerned with movement and the storage of learned behavior, that
the limbic system* functioned to integrate emotionally determined
behavior related to self-preservation, and that the neocortex controlled cognitive functioning, information processing, and decision
making, leading either to action or to its inhibition (20, 21).
Experimental verification with lesions or stimulation of the limbic
system confirmed its influence on emotions and behavior. Arnold
(22) stated that emotions derive from the appraisal of input from

---

* Papex, in 1937, proposed a theory that emotional expression and emotional
experience are separate phenomena and identified the locus of emotional
integration in the brain in structures to which MacLean, in 1952, gave the name
the limbic system.

the sensory system, mediated by the limbic system, and are related to affective recall with action controlled by circuits connected to the frontal lobe.

Arousal, alertness, or altered consciousness were discovered to be located in what was termed the reticular activating system (23).

Memory and learning functions were theorized to be performed in many areas of the cortex, with impairment of memory being correlated with the destruction of cortical tissue. RNA is involved in long-term memory and interference with its synthesis impedes learning, while increased availability results in more rapid learning (23).

Between 1950 and 1960, both chemical and electrical transmission was demonstrated to be characteristic in nerve function. Stereotypic, rapid, and inflexible behavior was found to be the action of electrical transmission, while slower, more complex behavior utilized chemical activity. Neurotransmitters and neuroreceptors were identified with receptor specificity for the transmitters they bound. All chemical neurotransmitters were found to act on the surface of cell membranes (24). Axelrod (25) made this concept more understandable when he said that when nerve impulses reach the end of an axon, certain events occur to transfer the impulse to the second neuron. An electrical depolarization of the presynaptic membrane permits the release of the chemical neurotransmitter (such as acetycholine or dopamine) stored in presynaptic vesicles.

Research into the Affective Disorders

Brodie and Sabshin (26) have stated that the most significant breakthrough in the psychiatric field has been in the biology of affective disorders. The biogenic amine hypothesis declared depression to be associated with a deficiency in catecholeamines, particularly norepinephrine.

After a more rigorous method of twin study was instituted to establish zygosity (to adhere to diagnostic criteria and to study monozygotic twins separated from their biological parents), Kety and Rosenthal (27, 28) demonstrated "a genetically determined vulnerability to schizophrenia that interacts with the environment in the development of the illness" (26, p. 1315).

Genetic studies conducted in 1957 identified the 22 pairs of chromosomes, how they are transmitted, and, in 1959, the sex-determining chromosomes XX and XY (29). Some 50 gene-determined metabolic abnormalities were identified. The hereditary message in DNA was transferred to RNA and then to microsomes in the cell cytoplasm. Down's syndrome was found to occur when a disjunction occurred at chromosome 21 with an extra chromosome. Inborn errors of metabolism (such as phenylketonuria or PKU) that were associated with mental retardation, if detected early, could be successfully treated with dietary control. It would now be in the realm of possibility for tissue and organ transplants to correct congenital enzymatic defects (23).

Beginning in the 1950s, the stages of sleep were identified, along with physiological and metabolic changes that occur during each of these stages, especially during the REM cycle (1967)—EEG patterns and the recall of dreams. Behavior changes, often incapacitating, were discovered to follow sleep deprivation. Sleep disturbances began to be studied in relation to mental disorders. More precise diagnoses of sleep disorders have led to treatment clinics and to better management of those affected (23).

Psychoanalytic Theory

The popularity of psychoanalysis reached its zenith in the 1950s and 1960s. Psychoanalysts headed medical school departments of psychiatry. It was a time of consolidation and refinement, but not of new theory building.

Frieda Fromm-Reichmann, utilizing as a foundation Harry Stack Sullivan's 1947 formulation, said, "emotional difficulties in living are difficulties in interpersonal relationships" (30). She applied Sullivan's concept to serious mental illness. Using the art of interpersonal relationship and the science of psychotherapy, mutual trust and respect and a more open transference were her goals. She interpreted the dynamics of content. She discovered that the mutual understanding of the patient's overt and covert (inner thoughts and reveries) mental processes could lead to insight and behavior change. She avoided free association and the use of the couch.

Existential analysis originated from Kierkegaard's philosophy in the mid-19th century. Martin Heidegger (1949), Albert Camus

(1955), Jean Paul Sartre (1956), Ludwig Binswanger (1963), and others contributed to the expansion of the philosophical concept of existentialism (31, 32). Existentialism is a "viewpoint on man that recognizes the unique place and presence of individual human existence and the centrality of human action and freedom with human existence" (32, p. 927). It promotes human freedom of action based upon choice and gives primacy to ethical commitment.

While the psychoanalytic method emphasized that the doctor should be out of sight, neutral, objective, and rational in analysis of verbal data, the existential method emphasized the countertransference to reduce the distance between doctor and patient, feelings (at the expense of verbal formulations), and the here-and-now, as opposed to the past (33).

At the 1956 APA annual meeting in Chicago, the morning session of the joint meeting with the American Psychoanalytic Association was devoted to the biographical account of Freud given by Ernest Jones. The next day, the Academic Lecturer was Percival Bailey and his topic was "The Great Psychiatric Revolution." Bailey led an attack on psychoanalytic theory and upon analytic practice. The address evoked the expected controversy (34–36). In 1952 Leon Eisenberg had predicted "the historian of psychiatry, fifty years from now, will regard Freudianism as a curious cultural phenomenon that constituted a conceptual barrier to progress" (37).

In 1962 Barton (38) commended psychoanalysis for its contributions to understanding human behavior, but criticized it for the diversion of so many hours of the psychiatrist's time from the many who needed help to the few, and criticized its cost and failure to prove its superiority over other methods of treatment.

The factors of time and cost led many to revive the earlier explorations of Franz Alexander on *brief psychotherapy*. Castelnuovo-Tedesco (1965) advocated 10, 20-minute sessions (39), and Mann began a prolonged trial of 12 hour-long sessions of time limited psychotherapy (40).

Transactional analysis, made popular by Eric Berne in 1964 (41), utilized Sullivan's interpersonal theory and communications theory. The concept is that transactions (communications exchanges) take place between individual ego states (parent, adult, or child) and evoke a complementary reply, or a reply addressed to an ego state other than the one addressed. Intrinsic to transactions are rewards, or "payoffs" (41). *Games People Play* (40) and Harris' *I'm OK, You're OK* (43) were enormously popular during the brief and soon discarded period of popularity of transactional analysis. In an assessment of psychoanalysis, John Romano (44) states, "There has emerged a more sober view of the efficacy of analytic psychotherapy, disenchantment with its earlier claims of success, and perhaps more important, the feeling that it seems to be stuck on a conceptual basis with very few germinal ideas emerging" (44, p. 39).

Psychosomatic medicine, which began in the 1920s with adherence to psychoanalytical theory under the dominance of Franz Alexander until about 1955, turned into an attempt to correlate emotions and other psychological variables with measurable physiological variables (45). Lipowski and his associates (45) provided an overview of advances in the field in 1977. He proposed a tripartite definition of psychosomatic medicine: 1) the scientific study of the relations among biological, psychological, and social factors in determining health and disease; 2) a holistic approach to the practice of medicine; and 3) consultation-liaison psychiatry. Contributions to theory and to clinical practice have been made by many investigators. Some of the areas of study are: relation of psychosocial stress and physiological responses; coping mechanisms; relation of life change to illness; the role of separation and loss on bodily functions; and the measuring of psychological variables as they modify bodily function and contribute to illness (45).

Behavior modification and biofeedback developed as a result of animal experimentation by Beckhterev in 1912 (46), as a result of the formulation of the conditioned reflex theory by Pavlov in 1927 (47), as well as a result of the work of Thorndike in animal learning (1898) (48) and that of B.F. Skinner in learning theory and operant conditioning (49–52).

Behavior modification is "founded on the premise that all social behavioral expressions, healthy or maladaptive, are learned or represent distortions or deficits in the learning processes of the growing human" (21, p. 788). Modification of behavior is possible by extinguishing original learning experiences. New learning experiences are associated with the arousal of emotion through gratification (pleasure) or aversion (pain). Desensitization and reinforcement, either positive or negative, are tools for the process.

Biofeedback employs bioelectric instrumentation, either visual or tonal, to indicate a change in the action potential when the subject makes a conscious effort to modify a physical state such as muscle tension or a tension headache.

The behavior therapies emphasize the shaping and controlling of behavior through cognitive methods or through laboratory principles of learning (42). In the 1970s, although widely utilized, the behavior therapies remained controversial. There has been evidence of behavior therapy's lasting benefit in the treatment of phobias, in a variety of neurotic conditions, in sexual dysfunction, and in stuttering. Token economies—operant conditioning—can change the behavior of patients while in hospital. Control of variables, comparisons with other accepted strategies over time, and sound research design have only begun in the 1980s (53).

Social Psychiatry

Social factors in the causation of mental illness have been known to be intertwined with the broader issues of indigency and welfare for a very long time. Edward Jarvis (1855), in his report *Insanity and Idiocy in Massachusetts*, showed the poor to be disproportionately represented in the number of cases identified as insane or idiots. Earlier I noted Faris and Dunham's finding that the highest rate of mental disability occurred in inner city slums. This led to the hypothesis that social disorganization might cause mental disability, or that a downward drift of the mentally handicapped might be responsible for the higher rate of disability.

Social causation of psychiatric disorders has been explored by many investigators. Perhaps the most influential studies were conducted by August B. Hollingshead and Frederick C. Redlich in 1938—the New Haven Study (54); by Srole and colleagues in 1962—the Midtown Manhattan Study (55); and by Leighton in 1959—the Sterling County Study (56). From these studies emerged the following theories:

• Untreated rates of psychiatric disorders in an urban setting demonstrate an inverse relationship between the overall rates and social class. The highest rate was in the lowest class (57).

- Sociocultural conditions have measurable consequences, reflected in the differences in mental health observed in the population (57).
- Different types of psychiatric disorders show markedly different relationships to social class and to urban versus rural settings (57). Neuroses and manic depressive disorders do not show an inverse relationship to social class (57).
- Sociocultural disintegration in a poorly functioning social system manifests its ineffective functioning in deficiencies in communication, weakness of leadership, breakdown of shared values, and in-group hostility and violence (21).

Violence as a manifestation of aggression and hostility has been extensively studied in animals and in man both as an individual and as a group. As I have already stated, the use of terrorism and violence to make a political statement has increased in the 1970s and 1980s. Rape as an instrument of vengeance, power, and violence is a concept that has been advanced by Susan Brownmiller (58).

Another form of violence that has captured public attention since the 1970s has been family violence—abuse of the aged, spouses (particularly wives), and children. "Studies of the syndrome of child battery have found a defect in the mothering or fathering of the abusing parent. The defect is one of attitude, not ability or willingness to care for the child. The defective attitude views the child as existing for the parents' pleasure and satisfaction, and repeats what the parents themselves experienced when they were children" (12, p. 258). Child abuse has most often been held as a manifestation of narcissistic rage.

It was the research investigations of Kinsey (59) and Masters and Johnson (60) that provided a framework for the examination of theories of sexual behavior. For example, the appetitional theory holds that sexual expression is rooted in a diffuse or unfocused biological drive that can be organized, amplified, or diminished in terms of the available social definitions of the sexual. According to Stoller (61), among the elements of social scripts in the sexual realm are conceptions of self, gender role identity, and conditional social and cultural learning.

An attempt was made by Grinker in the 1950s to develop a unified theory of human behavior (62). Developments in many sciences, including the biological, psychological, and social, provided a foundation for the effort. Of all the attempts, the one made by Bertalanffy—general systems theory—was the most successful (63). The system was a set of interrelated units that could be closed (with impenetrable boundaries) or open as in living systems. The system received input of energy, matter, or information. Inputs are processed consuming energy as patients enter a hospital ward (a system) along with staff and other resources (input). In the process of treatment the patient is changed and now can cope with stress. The outputs from the system can be expressed in action, with feedback to correct system function. It is possible to embrace within the system multiple variables, multiple levels of the biopsychosocial process, integrate them (relate parts to the whole) and relate the system as in the example of the hospital ward to other systems such as the support system (food, housekeeping). The concept of boundaries limiting input or semipermeable (admitting some inputs and excluding others) and of energy exchange provide a means of dealing with complexity (64).

THE FEDERAL ROLE IN THE ADVANCEMENT OF PSYCHIATRY

The National Institute of Mental Health, the Joint Commission on Mental Illness and Health, and Other Organizations

The establishment of the National Institute of Mental Health in 1946 inaugurated substantial federal support of the mental health system (63). It was the most significant event in the growth of the field of psychiatry in the 35 years from 1946 to 1981.

An earlier 19th-century effort to broadly involve the federal government in the care of the mentally ill failed. The culmination of Dorothea Dix's crusade was her attempt to convince Congress (which she did), only to fail when the President vetoed her plan to finance improved care of the mentally ill with land grants.

The passage of the Harrison Narcotic Act in 1914 set in motion a chain of events that would expand the federal role from simply the control of narcotic addiction to include care of the mentally ill. In 1929 Public Law 70–672 established two farms for confinement and treatment of those addicted to narcotics and authorized two hospitals to be built to investigate addiction, its treatment, and rehabilitation. The hospital at Lexington, Kentucky, opened in 1936 with Lawrence Kolb, Sr., M.D., as its Medical Director. There Kolb pioneered research in drug addiction. (The second hospital for the treatment of narcotic addiction was opened in Fort Worth, Texas, in 1938.)

The Narcotic Division became the Division of Mental Hygiene in the U.S. Public Health Service under the direction of Walter L. Treadway, M.D., in 1930. He had been a proponent of the creation of such a division, along with Toliaferro Clark and Thomas Salmon (who was APA President from 1923–1924). The Division was responsible for administration of the narcotics farms and hospitals, and for investigative studies of both narcotic addiction and mental illness. The Division also assisted states in providing services for addicts, developed medical and psychiatric services in federal prisons, and studied and gathered statistics on mental disease.

Treadway was succeeded by Dr. Kolb as Director of the Division in 1938. It was Kolb who pressed for the building of a National Psychiatric Institute. The concept was supported by the APA, the AMA (Section on Nervous and Mental Diseases), the American Neurological Association, and the National Committee for Mental Hygiene.

World War II interrupted planning for a national institute, but it did shockingly demonstrate the need for an institute of applied research. A million men were rejected as unfit for military duty by reason of mental disorders. Psychiatric casualties in combat were all too frequent, and there were staggering shortages in professional manpower.

With the end of World War II, agitation among the public to refurbish deteriorated state mental hospitals and to remedy the neglect and abominable treatment of the mentally ill, the perceived need for research in the field that lagged far behind the rest of medicine, and the severe labor shortages resulting in understaffing of facilities put pressure upon Congress to provide federal support. Strong voices advocated legislative action. APA leaders and Thomas Parran (Surgeon General, U.S. Public Health Service) supported bills in Congress introduced by Representative J. Percy Priest (Tennessee) and Senators George Aiken (Vermont), Lister Hill (Alabama), Robert LaFollett, Jr. (Wisconsin), Claude Pepper

(Florida), and Robert Taft (Ohio). In July 1946, the National Mental Health Act was passed by Congress and signed into law by President Harry Truman. The historic, milestone Act provided "for research relating to psychiatric disorders and to aid in the development of more effective methods of prevention, diagnosis and treatment of such disorders, and for other purposes." The other purposes specified research, investigations, experiments, demonstrations, application of results, training of personnel, and assisting states to improve the system in the areas of prevention and treatment of mental illness.

Robert H. Felix, M.D. (President of APA from 1960–1961) was fortunately chosen to be the first Director of the federal enterprise in the mental health field within a month after passage of the Act; before federal funds were available, with a grant of $15,000 from the Greentree Foundation, he convened the appointees (made by the Surgeon General, Parran) authorized under the Act. The National Advisory Mental Health Council had six leaders in psychiatry and six outstanding lay leaders. (The psychiatrists appointed were David Levy, William Menninger, John Romano, George S. Stevenson, Edward Strecker, and Frank Tallman.) Felix demonstrated his genius as an administrator by selecting a top-flight staff of experts; by wise policy decisions; by swift incisive action to put a comprehensive program in place in the areas of training, research, and clinical service; and by innovative action to move away from traditional practices. By 1947, Congress appropriated funds to inaugurate stipends for postgraduate training of psychiatrists and mental health professionals, and for research (65).

In April, 1949 the National Institute of Mental Health was established with Robert Felix as its Director. From a Quonset hut on the grounds of the National Institutes of Health, the federal program had already been underway for three years. As NIMH expanded, it would soon be too large for the space it was able to squeeze out on the NIH campus, and too big for the rented quarters in Bethesda. In the 1970s spacious quarters assembled NIMH's many programs in a new campus in Rockville, Maryland. As this is not a history of NIMH, we shall only cite a few of the steps taken along the road to formation of the Alcohol, Drug Abuse and Mental Health Administration (ADAMHA).

In the 1950s basic research in genetics, neuroendocrinology, and sociology was underway. Training grants expanded the labor pool. Medical school departments of psychiatry and expanded faculties were funded. APA's conferences on medical education (to provide direction in education) received financial support. The 1955 Mental Health Study Act supported the Joint Commission on Mental Illness and Health. The 1956 Health Amendments Act provided alternatives to hospitalization and to development of paraprofessionals.

In the 1960s the Community Mental Health Center Act (1963) and the Mental Health Center Staffing Amendments (1965) launched the community mental health center movement. The 1966 Narcotic Addict Rehabilitation Act (and the addition of alcohol in the 1968 Amendments) led to the establishment within NIMH of a center for the study of alcoholism and drug abuse and a national program to apply research findings to clinical practice. The National Clearing House for Mental Health Information was also founded in the 1960s to make the burgeoning literature in the field readily retrievable.

Shortly after Felix retired (1964) and Stanley Yolles was appointed to succeed him, NIMH, with its many centers supporting various programs, became a unit of what was called the Health Services and Mental Health Administration. Later, when the alcoholism and drug abuse program grew at an amazing rate, they were split off—this reorganization became ADAMHA.

It is difficult to imagine the growth of the field of psychiatry without the help of NIMH. Its leadership kept it on target toward building a strong mental health system. It was not only the catalyst to development, but also the means of support to achieve objectives. NIMH's strength came from its readiness to accept expert opinion (specialist panels assisted its internal operations) and it was receptive to ideas arising outside the organization's structure.

One such call for an assessment of the status of the field, its projected needs, and a master plan to guide growth came from Kenneth Appel, President of the American Psychiatric Association in 1954, in an address to a conference of state governors. As a consequence of his suggestions, a planning body was created that brought together the APA and the AMA.

Political activism by some of the most influential leaders (including Kenneth Appel, Leo Bartemier, and William C. Menninger) succeeded in convincing Congress to establish a funded commission (PL–182, the 1955 Mental Health Study Act) to survey the resources in the United States and to make recommendations for combating mental illness. ($1,250,000 was appropriated, and grants from foundations and participating organizations raised the total funding to about $1.5 million.)

The APA was joined by the AMA, whose Chairman of its Council on Mental Health was Leo H. Bartemier. With APA and AMA spearheading the effort, some 36 organizations became the Joint Commission on Mental Illness and Health. The employed staff worked under the Director, Jack R. Ewalt (President of the APA from 1963–1964). (I was a member of the APA group to plan the Commission, APA's representative member on the Joint Commission, and served on the Committee on Studies and on the unit that produced *Current Concepts of Positive Mental Health.*)

The final report, *Action for Mental Health* (66) (written by Greer William, distinguished science writer on the Joint Commission staff) was widely read, as were the eight other monographs and two books that appeared on the work of the Commission. *

Action for Mental Health was built on the theme of society's rejection of the mentally ill, and stressed the importance of a change in attitude as a precondition to the solution of three major problems: labor, facilities, and cost. Among its many recommendations were the following:

---

* The monograph series, all published by Basic Books, included:

Jahoda M: Current Concepts of Mental Health, 1958
Fein R: Economics of Mental Health, 1958
Albee GW: Mental Health Manpower Trends, 1959
Gurvin G, Veroff J, Feld S: Americans View Their Mental Health, 1960
Robinson R, deMarche DF, Wagle MK: Community Resources in Mental Health, 1960
Plunket RJ, Gordon JE: Epidemiology and Mental Illness, 1960
Allinsmith W, Goethals GW: The Role of Schools in Mental Health, 1962
McCann RV: The Churches and Mental Health, 1962

Related to the work of the Joint Commission were:

Pugh TF, MacMahon B: Epidemiologic Findings in U.S. Mental Hospital Data. Boston, Little Brown, 1962
Schwartz MD, Schwartz CG: New Perspectives on Mental Patient Care. New York, Basic Books, 1962

- Support of a balanced research portfolio in the search for new knowledge
- Manpower recruitment with use of extenders
- Support of education and training of psychiatrists and mental health professionals
- Establishment of psychiatric units in general hospitals
- Development of small public mental hospitals with fewer than 1,000 beds
- Conversion of large mental hospitals into rehabilitation centers for all chronic diseases, including mental disorders
- Development of a system for community care, including children and adults with aftercare, day and night treatment, and alternate facilities to reduce the need for full hospitalization
- Public information to assist the public in acquiring an accurate perception of mental illness and the caretaking professions.

Equally as important as the recommendations for change and the books of facts and opinions published to support them, was the highly successful social action taken to implement the findings of the Commission.

NIMH staff and advisory groups such as the Braceland Committee developed programmatic details. The National Association of Mental Health held a national conference of its leaders followed by regional and state conferences to acquaint all social policy makers with the Joint Commission's objectives.

The President of the APA (Walter Barton, 1961–1962) made implementation of the Joint Commission's recommendations his principal objective, urging district branch action and "stumping the country" urging corrective action.

It was fortunate that at this critical time the country had a President in the White House who read extensively. He digested the report, called for support of the recommended change in the Executive Branch, and delivered the first-ever message to Congress on Mental Health and Mental Retardation.*

---

* John F. Kennedy, Speech to Congress, U.S. Congressional Record, 88th Congress, 1st Session, 1963, CIX part 2 1744–49, and as H.R. Document 58

See also Am J Psychiatry 120:739-830, Feb 1964

President Kennedy proposed a "wholly new emphasis and approach to care for the mentally ill," promising "If we launch a broad new mental health program, it will be possible to reduce the number of patients now under custodial care by 50 percent or more." The "bold new approach" to mental illness and mental retardation was to use federal resources to stimulate state, local, and private action. Congress authorized grants to states for construction of comprehensive community mental health centers and for planning grants. The latter, relatively small sums, were to initiate a most important planning process, which brought into focus deficiencies in the system and established priorities for remedial action.

The discussion of the proposed action that followed revealed that both the American Medical Association and the American Hospital Association were opposed to the entrance of the federal government into the delivery of health services. Following negotiations that were focused on withdrawal of active lobbying against the special needs of the mentally ill (with a long history of government support of the public system of care), an important conference was sponsored by the APA. Its objective was to bring together representatives of the 50 states, major health and professional organizations including AMA and the American Hospital Association (AHA), and members of key congressional committees to explore the advantages and disadvantages of the proposed "bold new approach." A nearly unanimous vote in Congress supported the Community Mental Health Center Act of 1965.

At about this time a similar effort on behalf of children was organized under congressional authorization (PL 89–97 Social Security Amendments of 1965). Authorized was a "study of resources relating to children's emotional illnesses," funded in the amount of $1 million.

The Joint Commission on the Mental Health of Children (JCMHC) was formed (after a joint planning effort between the APA and the Academy of Child Psychiatry) by 46 participating organizations with liaison representatives from such federal agencies as: Children's Bureau; Division of Indian Health; National Institute of Neurologic Diseases' Social Rehabilitation Services; National Institute of Child Health; HEW; and NIMH. The Commission organized itself into six task forces and five committees, each with members and consultants. Altogether some 500 leading authorities in the field of childhood and adolescence contributed to

Commission work. Reginald S. Lourie was the President and Chairman of the Commission, and Joseph M. Bobbitt the Executive Director. As in the earlier Joint Commission, contracts were made for field studies.*

Crises in Child Mental Health revealed that only one-third of children who needed care for mental and emotional disorders received it. Over one million received no care at all. After providing an overview of society's attitude toward children, the report described special problems of minorities and the nature of emotional disturbances in children and adolescents. The report's recommendations included:

- A child advocacy system, with a National Advisory Council on Children, State Child Development Agency, Local Child Development Authority, and Neighborhood Development Councils
- Pilot demonstration of case finding and outreach by evaluating 100 child development councils
- Manpower development
- Family planning
- Prenatal care and comprehensive pediatric services
- School health and mental health programs, including college mental health services
- Mental health service by clergy
- Remedial mental health services to include:
  information and referral
  developmental and psychoeducational assessment
  treatment of child and family
  special education programs
  rehabilitation
  residential care

---

* The final report of the Commission, *Crises in Child Mental Health: Challenge for the 1970s* (1970), along with five other related volumes, was published by Harper and Row:

Robinson HB, Robinson N (Eds): Mental Health: From Infancy Through Adolescence, 1973
Josselyn IM: Adolescence, 1973
Lustman SL (Ed): The Mental Health of Children: Services, Research, and Manpower, 1973
Social Change and Mental Health of Children, 1973
David HP (Ed): Child Mental Health in International Perspective, 1972

Unlike the Joint Commission on Mental Illness, there was no general consensus that recommendations be adopted, and no dramatic change in the service delivery system for children occurred. The advocacy system did not catch on and the pilot demonstrations were not funded. However, the NAMH did hold a series of conferences on clinical issues. While all were agreed on the need for a commitment to children and adolescents, there was opposition to a government operated advocacy system, and amazement at the neglect of clinical issues in the Commission's report.* In spite of the adverse reception of the advocacy proposals, significant gains did follow with the efforts of the Academy of Child Psychiatry, APA, NAMH, and NIMH. More child psychiatrists were recruited and trained. Community mental health centers required the addition of services to children and adolescents. Services to children improved slowly.

Still another assessment of need occurred during the presidency of Jimmy Carter. An urgent demand for an update in the care of the mentally ill led President Carter to appoint a President's Commission on Mental Health (Executive Order #11973, February 17, 1977). Twenty commissioners were appointed by the President. Rosalynn Carter, the First Lady, was an active participant, with the title of Honorary Chairperson. Thomas A. Bryant was Chairperson, with a staff of 32. There were three psychiatrists among the commissioners—Allen Beigel, Mildred Mitchell-Bateman, and George Tarjan—and many more on the task forces. The Commis-

---

* For a critical assessment, see the Group for Advancement of Psychiatry's Report #82 (1972). The interdisciplinary debate in the Commission between the behavioral scientists in the majority, and clinicians in the minority, resulted in the low priority given in the report to a system of treatment for children with emotional illness. Criticized was the concept of an advocate other than parents, and the omission of a plan for financing the advocacy system.

(I was the Assistant Secretary on the Board of Directors on the Executive Committee, and APA representative on the Commission. Signs of disaster went unheeded, the science writer failed to complete his project, the money ran out, and the Commission came to an abrupt end before its reports were completed. The APA came to the rescue and provided assistance and space, while Reginald Lourie scurried about to gather contributions to pay a recruited staff research associate, Barbara J. Souder. She performed a minor miracle by ensuring that all books were written, edited, and published, coordinating efforts of Task Force and Committee members.)

sion was charged "to conduct public hearings, inquiries, and studies as may be necessary to identify the mental health needs of the nation" (P.L. 89–97, 1968). The specifics included an assessment of how the mentally ill were being served or underserved. The one-year study by task forces and 35 panels of experts produced a four-volume report.* Its major findings were:

- Substantial numbers do not have access to mental health care of high quality at reasonable cost.
- Rural and inner city areas are underserved.
- Racial minorities are inadequately served.
- Children and adolescents are underserved.
- More human and fiscal resources are needed.
- Coordination with the general health system should be developed.
- A community network should be developed as a support system.

Congress passed, and the President signed, the Mental Health Systems Act in 1980. The economic recession and fiscal crises due to unemployment and inflation nullified the good intentions, as the Act was not funded.

There were other organizations that contributed to the advancement of psychiatry during this period: The National Association of Private Psychiatric Hospitals (1933) vigorously campaigned to have all of its member hospitals accredited.** The Academy of

---

* Report of the President's Commission on Mental Health, Superintendent of Documents, U.S. Government Printing Office, Washington, DC (040–000–00390 to 00393). Three of the volumes are appendices containing task force findings.

** Accreditation was granted by the Joint Commission on Accreditation of Hospitals (1952). The American College of Surgeons had moved in 1916 to upgrade hospitals by establishing standards and by surveying hospitals to assure that standards were met. In 1952 this activity became a joint responsibility of a commission composed of representatives from the AMA, Canadian Medical Association, American Hospital Association, American College of Physicians, and the American College of Surgeons. It was not until 1970 that the Accreditation Council for Psychiatric Facilities was formed, applying a modification of APA standards. The Psychiatric Council did not survive a decade, but a mechanism for input from organized psychiatry into commission standards was provided by the employment of consultants.

Child Psychiatry (1959) promoted the advancement of services to children.

ADVANCES IN DELIVERY OF SERVICES

A dramatic shift in the delivery of services to the mentally ill came to pass in the decade of the 1950s. It was almost as revolutionary as what had transpired in the care of tuberculosis. In spite of rising hospital admission rates for mental illness, the population in public mental hospitals declined sharply. Ambulatory care became the dominant pattern of service delivery.

The practice of psychiatry in the office expanded. Psychoanalysts who had dominated the private practice field were joined by psychiatrists, then by clinical psychologists and social workers as psychotherapists. With the advent of psychoactive drugs, over 20,000 psychiatrists in 1980 provided direct service to patients in the office. In the 1980s it has become common for psychiatrists to practice in multiple settings, serving in the office, in the general hospital, teaching in the medical school, and serving as a consultant to other agencies and facilities.

The change in the focus of service delivery from inpatient care to ambulatory care is illustrated by the following figures:

1955   1.7 million patient care episodes
              inpatient, 77 percent; outpatient, 23 percent; daycare, 0 percent

1977   6.9 million patient care episodes
              inpatient, 27 percent; outpatient, 70 percent; daycare, 3 percent (67)

1955   outpatient care episodes accounted for 200 episodes per 100,000 population

1977   outpatient care episodes accounted for 2,000 per 100,000 population

1955   daily average census in U.S. mental hospitals was 539,681 (36)

1979   daily average census in U.S. mental hospitals was 233,384

Census was still declining in the 1980s, reaching below 130,000

In the 1980s, more than 1,000 of the nearly 7,000 general hospitals had psychiatric units. Another 2,000 had some psychiatric services. By 1970, the general hospital was the primary element in the inpatient care system for acute mental illness requiring inpatient service. Approximately one in five ambulatory doctor–patient encounters took place in the general hospital, and one-half of those took place in the emergency room (67). A notable achievement in the shift of locus of care to the general hospital was the reduction of the time of stay in the hospital for an episode of care (approximately 11 days, with one-half of these remaining in the hospital for 7 days or less) (68). One-half of the public mental hospitals had average stays of 29 days or more, indicating the use of the public system for the more serious chronic mental disorders.

The dramatic drop in the census of 304 state and county mental hospitals and 24 VA psychiatric hospitals in the United States (1975) was due to three major factors: new treatments, administrative reform (informal admission, greater patient responsibility for self-management, work programs, and open hospitals), and a conceptual shift to a belief that long hospitalization was unnecessary and undesirable, and could even be harmful (67). In the 1840s separation from family and community stress was seen as essential to recovery. It was believed that as long as the patient remained amidst the objects and scenes which precipitated and aggravated the disease, the patient could not recover. The mental hospital gave the patient, in this view, the enjoyment of more liberty than did any other place (69).

Social policy from 1970 to 1980 was expressed in the concepts *deinstitutionalization* and *the least restrictive alternative to hospitalization*. The former concept expressed the belief that through preparation of patients for release and support after release, long-term chronic patients were better cared for in the community. The concept of the least restrictive alternative to hospitalization was formulated by the courts, and expressed the assumption that the mental hospital was to be used as the last resort after all other possible placement had been exhausted.

The mentally retarded as well as the mentally ill were best cared for in the community, in the accepted social view. In the case of the

mentally ill, deprivation of liberty (confinement in the mental
hospital) was to take place only if the individual was dangerous to
self or to others.

Consultation-liaison psychiatry became an accepted mode of
practice in the 1970s. It had been hoped that internists might
become the primary specialists in psychosomatic medicine. They
did not. Internists found greater discernible benefits to patients
when they pursued more precise diagnosis made possible by
laboratory technology. Psychoanalysts, the pioneers in the psychosomatic field, withdrew when they found that their interventions
produced limited results. While "the predisposing and precipitat-
ing role of emotional factors had been convincingly demonstrated," physical and social factors complicated the process (70).

Life-threatening arousal of fear and anxiety in cardiovascular
surgery, the emotional tension of vascular hypertension, the stress
upon individuals with peptic ulcer, and the emotional concomi-
tants of irritable bowel syndrome, asthma, and eating disorders,
were prevalent reactions to illness in the general hospital. Therefore, the growth of hospital psychiatric services and the presence
of psychiatrists led to increasing referral for all forms of psychosomatic problems.

As noted earlier, the Community Mental Health Center Act
(1963) and the Mental Health Center Staffing Amendments (1965)
launched the Community Mental Health Center Movement. The
1960s featured federal Great Society programs, with the government playing the role of initiator and supporter of national social
welfare programs. The public "attitude toward social service and
political process rejected Social Darwinism for a more
compassionate belief that the crucial elements in the individual
maladjustment was the social and legal matrix in which the illness
or instability occurred" (70). Failure to overcome social disadvan-
tage due to minority status, slum housing, unemployment,
wretched childhood, and incorrect attitudes was seen as the cause
of mental illness. In this optimistic (and unrealistic) view, better
mental health could change society. Providing public education,
psychotherapy, a new place to live, and a job were seen as the
tasks of the mental health professional.

The NIMH goal was to establish 2,000 community mental
health centers (CMHCs). Each center was to provide comprehensive mental health care for a defined population (catchment area)
of 75,000 to 200,000. Consumers (citizens) were to have a control-

ling voice on Boards of Control (71). The basic services to be provided included inpatient, outpatient, emergency, partial hospitalization, and consultation (prevention) to other service systems. The Health Services Act of 1975 (P.L. 94–63) would add new services to the original five: screening, follow-up, transitional living arrangements, complete treatment services for children and the elderly, plus alcohol and drug abuse programs.

The high hopes of the 1960s were reduced to doubts in the 1970s and to hostility of the nonmedical mental health care system toward psychiatrists in the 1980s. In the 1970s, social activism was encouraged to influence the political system; housing, jobs, and education were viewed as more important than medical care; the health care dollar, used for recreation and relief of stress, was justified as prevention; treatment was given to the worried well, neglecting the sick; severe, chronic mental illnesses could be avoided; and there was a lack of coordination with state mental and local general hospitals.

There is hostility toward psychiatrists in the 1980s. Discontinuities (failure to relate to state mental hospitals and psychiatric units in general hospitals) in treatment subverted the goal of continuity in patient services. The emergence of a nonmedical mental health care system has resulted in the rejection of the medical model in favor of a social–psychological one, downplaying the role of biological factors in the causation of mental illness. The nonmedical mental health care system is reducing the role of the psychiatrist to prescribing psychoactive drugs. Through diagnosis, treatment, planning, and management, nonmedical mental health professionals seek to override psychiatrists' opinions. Psychiatrists who had originally participated fully in the development of the Mental Health Center movement withdrew, leaving clinical psychologists, social workers, and paraprofessionals as the dominant staff members.

By 1975, 26 percent of admissions for mental and emotional problems were to federally funded CMHCs. Thirty-nine percent were to outpatient psychiatric services, and 35 percent to all inpatient hospital services (VA, state, general, etc.). There were 196 CMHCs in 1970, and 691 in 1980 (19 percent of all mental health facilities) (72).

The medical system has become a formidable rival to the CMHC system in the 1980s. The growth of general hospital psychiatric units to over 1,000 have made inpatient, outpatient, emergency, and daycare services under psychiatrists' supervision available in the local community. Furthermore, approximately 60 percent of all males and 40 percent of all females with a principal diagnosis of mental disorder were treated by physicians in their offices (psychiatrists see 40 percent of males and 59 percent of females) (68).

In 1970 there were 310 state and county public mental hospitals. In 1980 this number had declined to 280 (70). There was also a shift in age groups treated in state hospitals. The proportion of young adults increased; most of this increase was due to additions of patients aged 18 to 44 being treated for alcoholism, drug abuse, or schizophrenia. While still a major treatment resource for severe and chronic mental disorders, the central role of the state hospital has given way to the outpatient psychiatric clinic and the psychiatric unit in general hospitals. More ambulatory psychiatric disorders are treated by physicians other than psychiatrists, and more patients with mental disorders are cared for in the welfare system than in the mental health system.

The 1980s has witnessed a backlash in response to the policy of deinstitutionalization. The civil rights protests of the 1960s viewed commitment of individuals as depriving them of certain inalienable rights. Community-based treatment was seen as more humane and more therapeutic. The law expressed this ideological concept in restricting commitment to those who are dangerous to themselves or others, specifying the rights of patients, and requiring placement in the least restrictive environment. Mentally ill individuals are now free to be homeless and live in the streets, to reside in jails and prisons, and to be confined in nursing homes in the community without treatment. Welfare costs have soared and efforts have been made to reduce them. The expected cost savings did not occur with the shift in the focus of care. Expenditures by all mental health facilities rose from $3.3 billion in 1969 to $8.8 billion in 1979, with much of this due to inflation (72).

ADVANCES IN THERAPY

The most significant advances in therapy since 1950 have been changes in the locus of treatment, in the types of patients treated, in the emergence of effective drug therapy, in the increasing specificity of pharmacologic agents, in the introduction of behavioral therapy, in deinstitutionalization, and the renewed interest in responsibility for one's own health.

Change in Locus of Treatment

While community mental health centers were evolving and general hospital psychiatric units expanding, public mental hospitals developed strategies to prepare patients for community placement and to smooth the transition while providing continuity of care. Factory-in-hospital programs and industrial therapy with paid employment prepared patients to work. They were modeled after similar programs in England and Holland of the 1950s and 1960s (73, 74). Veterans Administration Psychiatric Hospitals established comprehensive physical medicine and rehabilitation programs adding (to occupational therapy, physical therapy, and industrial therapy) corrective, recreational, and educational therapies (75). Job placements, halfway houses, sheltered workshops, social clubs, and aftercare assisted patients in making the transition to community living (76–78). Another program to provide continuity of care was the *unit plan*, originated in Clarinda, Iowa, in 1961. It divided the mental hospital into units related to the community in which the patient originally resided, to provide a connection between patients and therapists in community agencies following release to insure the monitoring of treatment.

The seminal study conducted in 1954 by Stanton and Schwartz (79) revealed that many patient symptoms were directly related to the informal organization of the mental hospital. Stress on employees, conflicts, personal problems carried into the work place, or disagreements among staff exerted an influence upon patients and their symptoms, and influenced their response to treatment. Many studies followed the impact of the social setting on treatment.

Changes in the Types of Patients Treated

Changes in the types of patients treated were related to the disappearance of tuberculosis wards in the mental hospital, and to the successful treatment of syphilis and toxic-infectious diseases. When funding shifts occurred in the late 1960s and accelerated in the 1970s, the aged patient was seldom admitted to the mental hospital, and mental hospital admission became limited to the dangerous.

There was a marked rise in the number of admissions for drug abuse and alcoholism in the 1960s. Young adults with personality disorders became a dominant group among patients in public mental hospitals. As a result of deinstitutionalization, chronic mental patients were released into the community in large numbers, and have become, in the 1980s, the focus of concern as a result of neglect, absence of treatment, and lack of supportive networks for these people.

The Emergence of Effective Drug Therapy

The ferment in psychopharmacology of the 1950s produced meprobamate (known widely by the trade names Miltown or Equinil). Meprobamate was developed by Ludwig and Perch in 1951, who noted its muscle relaxant and sedative properties. Meprobamate was the first widely used antianxiety drug (Dixon demonstrated its beneficial effects in 1957). Sternback (1960) introduced chlordiazepoxide (Librium), a drug that also has anticonvulsant action, in 1960. Diazepam (Valium) was discovered shortly thereafter. Valium and Librium became two of the most widely prescribed of all drugs. Their addictive quality would be discovered later (80).

The introduction of antidepressants in the 1950s largely replaced ECT, amphetamines (for patients with psychomotor retardation), and barbiturates (for the agitated). Iproniazid, introduced in 1951 for the treatment of tuberculosis, was seen to produce elevation of mood. In 1952 Selikoff and Delay confirmed ipromiazid's beneficial effects in treating depression. Other monoamine oxidase (MAO) inhibitors also demonstrated antidepressant qualities. A root compound of the next class of antidepressants had been synthesized as early as 1891 by Thiel and Holzinger. It was not until 1959, however, that tricyclic antidepressants came into clinical use in the U.S. Clinical trials a few years earlier were begun, first in schizophrenia when the similarity in structure to chlorpromazine was noted, and then with great success in depression (80, 81).

One of the first comparative studies of the effectiveness of five forms of treatment in schizophrenia—drugs alone, drugs plus psychotherapy, ECT, psychotherapy, and milieu therapy—was that of May (82) in 1969. He found antipsychotic drug therapy the most effective and least expensive of the treatment modalities used.

The introduction of effective pharmacologic agents was associated with a host of awesome toxic side effects. Some antianxiety drugs have addictive properties; lithium can cause neurological symptoms, gastric upsets, renal damage, coma, and death; antidepressant drugs can be used for suicide and cause anticholinergic effects, sexual difficulties, delirium, and urinary retention; antipsychotic drugs may induce glaucoma, skin reactions, aplastic anemia, cardiovascular changes, dystonias, parkinsonism, akathesia, and tardive dyskinesia. Toxicity of potent drugs that alleviate symptoms have led to increased vulnerability of psychiatrists to liability suits in the 1970s and 1980s.

The efficacy of antipsychotic and antidepressant drugs in the treatment of psychosis has been proven in many controlled studies. In the 1980s, one area of research was the use of neuroendocrine tests as a predictor of response to treatment. For example, the dexamethasone suppression test (DST) and the thyrotropin releasing hormone test (TRHT) were found useful in helping the clinician to decide which class of drugs should be used in therapy. An increasing number of the new drugs introduced had fewer side effects and greater specificity toward target symptoms.

ADVANCES IN PSYCHOTHERAPY

Classical psychoanalysis was at its peak in the United States in the 1950s. Its purity was being threatened by application to character disorders, borderline syndromes, and schizophrenia. New knowledge of ego and its function, of developmental psychology, and of the importance of social and cultural factors contributed to change in technique. Psychotherapeutic techniques range from uncovering or insight approach to a variety of supportive therapies. The former has as its objective the "achievement of psychological changes through emotional insight into the unconscious aspects" of mental life (81). The supportive approach uses the patient–therapist relationship to reveal one's problems to a concerned, stable, and supportive therapist. The usefulness of this approach has been demonstrated in situations of crises, in situations in which uncovering techniques have been too threatening for the patient to handle. Adolescents, children, and the elderly fare better with treatment other than classical psychoanalysis. The high cost of classical psychoanalysis has led to the less expensive brief psychotherapy. A variety of modifications now are practiced.

Milieu Therapy

Milieu therapy, in an earlier era called "moral treatment," is defined as "the process directed to the patient's emotional and interpersonal needs that marshals all environmental resources, including attitudes and behavior of staff to meet determined needs" (83). Just as moral treatment had been regarded in the past, milieu therapy, in the period after 1950, was regarded as an essential element in every inpatient treatment program. Smith and King (84), in a study of organizational effectiveness, demonstrated that more than a humanistic concern for patients was essential to successful treatment. A reactive and supportive environment, coordination, and decision-making have a pervasive influence upon patient care. The Cummings (85, 86) developed a set of milieu principles for application on the inpatient ward, and Maxwell Jones (87, 88) applied the concepts of milieu therapy in a novel way, giving rise to staff and patient participation in a therapeutic community. Jones set forth principles of distribution of power to patients, blurring of mental health professional roles, and elimination of hierarchies that influenced social and community psychiatry. The therapeutic community movement developed in the 1950s and flourished in the 1960s (81).

Behavior Therapy

Behavior therapy became an accepted treatment technique in the second half of the 20th century. Examples of the application of behavioral techniques had been cited for centuries. The classical conditioning experiments of Pavlov (1927) and the laboratory studies of Skinner (1938) on operant conditioning were the roots from which the principles underlying behavior therapy emerged (89–91).* Many others made major studies that aided formulation of principles of behavior modification both before and after 1950 (81). Skinner (1953) reported studies on the application of operant conditioning on the observable behavior of severely disturbed mental patients (91). Wolpe (1958) described many of the techniques used in behavior therapy (92). By the 1960s behavior

---

* A brief history of behavior therapy can be found in reference (79). A comprehensive source can be found in Kazdin AE: History of Behavior Modification. Baltimore, University Park Press, 1978.

therapy outgrew its learning theory origins and its model of stimulus–response. In 1973 an APA Task Force Report, "Behavior Therapy in Psychiatry," endorsed the clinical use of behavior therapy; and in 1981 an APA Task Force Report, "Biofeedback," described clinical applications and an assessment of results. Clinical usage expanded markedly and medical schools established departments of behavioral medicine with the development of specialty practice (79).

Interpersonal Therapy

Interpersonal therapy stems from the work of Adolf Meyer and Harry Stack Sullivan. The treatment period is short (12–16 weeks) and is oriented toward symptom relief and the resolution of immediate interpersonal difficulties. It focuses on here-and-now problems.

Cognitive Therapy

Cognitive therapy, introduced in the 1970s, appears to benefit some types of depression. This approach utilizes short-term therapy directed toward symptom relief. Symptoms offer clues to verbal thoughts or pictorial images and beliefs. Negative cognition plays a pivotal role in the development and maintenance of a psychopathological state (81). Modification of beliefs and attitudes is the therapist's goal, secured through clarifying the ways in which the patient conceptualizes events, and his or her basis for assumptions. Patients are given homework assignments to develop objectivity by recording stereotypic responses to events, identifying assumptions underlying their responses to events, and testing alternative approaches and assumptions (81).

Family Therapy

While Nathan Ackerman (1937) pioneered the concept (borrowing from early practice in child guidance) it was not until the 1970s that a remarkable growth in family therapy took place. At first, the whole family worked with the same therapist at the same time. As the number of nonmarried couples living together has increased, however, and as separation, divorce, and remarriage have become common events, the scope of application of family therapy has changed.

Sex Therapy

Sex therapy became more widely applied after several events: the Kinsey survey of sexual habits of men (1948) and women (1953); the widespread use of oral contraceptives introduced in the 1950s; and the "laboratory" study of Masters and Johnson, *Human Sexual Inadequacy* (1970). The more effective treatment of sexual disorders has increased the demand for help with such dysfunctions as impotence, premature ejaculation, orgasm inhibition, pain due to muscle spasm, and sexual phobias.

Hypnosis

Hypnosis, popular in the 19th century, was utilized in World War II; by the year 1970 it became selectively used in medical, psychiatric, dental, and psychological practice. Research has aided in developing clinical scales useful in the determination of responsivity to hypnosis.

Group Therapy

Group therapy increased markedly in clinical practice after World War II. Stemming from Pratt's (1907) groups of tuberculosis patients, Cody Marsh's inspirational sessions with mental hospital patients in the 1930s, and Moreno's (1957) role playing (psychodrama), the practice has extended to therapist-led groups, self-help groups (such as Alcoholics Anonymous and Recovery, Inc.), consciousness-raising and encounter groups, and sensitivity training groups. The focus of these groups is often upon interpersonal exchanges among group members and with the therapist.

There are many variants of group therapy which have had limited applications as variants of psychotherapy: Janov's primal therapy (which addresses the basic need for love and gratification); Rolfing (developed by Ida Rolf in the 1960s, and based on the assumption that misalignments of the body structure can be restored to balance by such direct interventions as massage and transcendental meditation); reality therapy (introduced by William Gasser in 1965 to counter the ethical neutrality of psychoanalysis, it seeks to teach the patient to face reality and be responsible for his or her actions; love and discipline are important tools of a responsible, tough, human, sensitive therapist); and many others.

Quality Control of Psychotherapy

Since 1950 concern for the quality of care and the efficacy of treatment has increased. Organizations have developed quality control units to insure proper application of treatment for a given diagnostic entity. Measurement has improved and corrective steps have been taken when studied profiles have shown deviation from expectations. Stimulus to expansion of quality control has come from several sources. Control of costs demands proper utilization of resources. Class action legal suits have challenged the adequacy of treatment given to hospitalized patients. For-profit enterprises—the emergence of corporate hospital and nursing home chains, the expansion of contractual service for emergencies, for outpatients, and clinical and laboratory services, have required monitoring to insure that the quality of care is not sacrificed to make a profit for a corporation.

Outcome studies of treatment results and comparisons of different therapeutic modalities have also expanded in the 1970s and 1980s. Accountability for money and resources expanded, as public policy has stimulated scientists to demonstrate that their interventions did, in fact, make a difference.

A unique and notable organizational activity was originated in 1977 under the stimulus of Jules Masserman, the President of the American Psychiatric Association. Masserman appointed a Commission on Psychiatric Therapies (with APA Board of Trustees approval) to assess therapies in current usage, to critically examine the literature, and to analyze findings to differentiate between effective and noneffective therapies. Such an enterprise was not without hazard; the organization had set out to bless one therapy and damn another. The individual who followed his or her medical judgment would run the risk of liability when he or she deviated from the standard of *the authority.* Many consultant experts assisted APA's Commission in the discharge of its task. The quite remarkable product of the Commission's findings was published in two volumes. *Psychotherapy Research: Methodological and Efficacy Issues* (93) and *The Psychiatric Therapies* (81). The former volume was published in 1982; the latter volume, published in

1984, is a valuable resource on the state of the art in psychiatric therapy.

THE EMERGENCE OF ADMINISTRATIVE PSYCHIATRY

Just as the environment shapes the processes that take place within it, positive or negative environmental factors influence the treatment process. "Management is the process by which a group of people are united to achieve an agreed upon purpose. It is getting things done with the cooperation of individuals who have been assigned responsibility for specific tasks" (94, p. 11). "Mental health (or psychiatric) administration is the management process formed from the interaction among general health administration, clinical psychiatric care of patients, program elements, and the organization itself, as well as the environment in which the structure exists including the attitudes, values, and belief systems" (94, p. 790). Success in treatment is greatly influenced by the interactional processes among patients, among patients and staff, and among members of the staff.

The extraordinary importance of joining the elements of health administration and clinical psychiatric care—with its dependence upon social, psychological, and biological factors—with sensitivity to the interactional process in a total environment, has created a major problem. Is administration in psychiatry a specialty area? Should psychiatrists and mental health professionals be trained as clinician–executives to join the diverse elements in mental health administration? Should mental health organizations follow the general hospital model, with lay administrators responsible for business affairs, and a medical director in charge of medical and psychiatric clinical care?

These questions express the major problems in administrative psychiatry. In an earlier period, the psychiatrist was the administrator of the hospital for the mentally ill and for the mentally retarded without question. In the 1970s and 1980s, as administration has increased in complexity, as resources have dwindled, and as the delivery system has changed, psychiatrists have become a minority among administrators of mental health organizations at all levels. As the private system has expanded, the public system has lost its ability to attract and to hold the best psychiatrists. As a consequence, psychiatry has diminished in influence upon social policy, sacrificed its power to effect change, and tarnished its public image. In the 1980s the APA has launched a major effort in an attempt to reverse events by demonstrating concern for the chronic patient, concern for improvement in psychiatric patient care, and development of psychiatric leadership in the public system.

There are arguments for generic training in administration: there is a common theory and knowledge base; skills used are the same in any setting; human behavior is not very different from one organization to another; retraining clinicians is too expensive; and psychiatrists have priced themselves out of the market as administrators. These arguments are less cogent when one realizes that insufficient training in the unique requirements of mental health administration is common in the educational system of general health administration.

Some of the unique elements of the mental health system are:

- Heavy dependence upon public funding and regulation for accountability (knowledge of the political process and public relations is required)
- More legislative and judicial action than other branches of medicine, which affects every aspect of psychiatric practice
- Service delivery changes that require extensive planning effort to support deinstitutionalized patients
- A troublesome population with unique needs, for whom care continues into community placement, with support required after the episode of acute treatment ends
- The fostering of a climate of understanding in which interpersonal relations, attitudes, and values support behavior change in patients with sensitivity to the reactive environment (94)

The developing knowledge base in regard to mental health administration stems from two main sources:

- The field of generic administration, with its massive literature
- The accumulated theory and practice from the fields of psychiatry, psychology, sociology, and anthropology

The Founding Fathers of the APA banded together in 1844 to share in the solution of administrative problems. At the start they were more interested in the administrative than the clinical aspects of their work, as illustrated by the committees they formed in 1844. Woodward pioneered the model organization; Kirkbride developed standards and design for mental hospitals; Ray was the expert on the law; and Earle corrected the outcome statistics. Bell understood the political process and probably assisted Dorothea Dix in becoming the expert politician she was.

Through the years, small groups of members of the APA have developed moral treatment, experimented with organizational structures, and established programs such as outreach clinics, aftercare, family care, and many more.

It was not until 1936 that Bryan published the accumulated experience. *Administrative Psychiatry* (95) became a classic; it aided in the establishment of a subspecialty field in psychiatry under that name. Bryan's model of clinical care, teaching, and research was adopted by NIMH as its organizational structure. The book was the first to stress the importance of public relations and public education to gain community support, to obtain the essential resources for goal attainment, and to stress accountability for the use of public money.

One important stimulus to the development of administrative psychiatry was the APA's organizational response to the public exposés of the decay in the public mental hospital system during World War II. Testimony on the need for reform came from an assemblage of nearly all U.S. public mental hospital administrators called by Blain in 1949—the Mental Hospital Institute—chaired by the charismatic Mesrop Tarumianz, M.D. From this organization (which became the oldest continuing educational effort in administration, attracting close to 1,000 persons annually) sprang the Central Inspection Board (CIB), the Architectural Project, the Mental Hospital Service Program (distributing books, articles, and films to participating organizations), and a forum for the various groups to meet together to discuss common problems. Librarians, nurses, social workers, occupational therapists, psychiatrists in general hospitals or the public system, and business administrators met at the time of the Institute. A direct spin-off of these meetings was the founding of such organizations as the Association of Mental Health Librarians, the American Association of Psychiatric Administrators, and the Association of Mental Health Administrators.

In 1953, the APA established a certification process for psychiatrists in mental hospital administration, with a qualifying examination under the direction of a Committee on Administrative Psychiatry, later under the Council on Medical Education and Career Development. Opportunities for specialized training were limited, so most applicants for certificates qualified through apprentice training and self-study. Although many—if not most—public mental health system psychiatrists were certified, there was scant evidence that diplomate status was useful or was even a criterion in the selection of an administrator.

Greenblatt and his associates (77) captured the explorations in social treatment and efforts to improve patient care through organized programs in 1955, in the book *From Custodial to Therapeutic Care in Mental Hospitals*. In 1956, Ewalt's *Mental Health Administration* (97) outlined a community mental health program, described the functions of a mental health center, instructed in the obtaining of support through the political process, and stressed the utilization of volunteers. In 1960, the Group for Advancement of Psychiatry's Committee on Hospitals produced a monograph entitled *Administration of the Public Psychiatric Hospital* (98). This short volume emphasized the importance of the environment for psychiatric care, the role of the administrator, and influences of the informal organization upon the psychiatric hospital. An annotated bibliography accompanied the text on selected administrative topics.

The presence of Duncan Macmillan of Mapperly Hospital in England at GAP committee meetings, a visit to America by T.P. Rees (who described the "open door" policy widely endorsed in England), and a brief note on Querido's home-visiting teams to prevent hospitalizations stimulated Americans to study progress of administrative methods in Europe. In 1961 an APA publication (written by Barton, Farrell, Lenehan, and McLaughlin) summarized the significant findings of these European methods. A direct consequence of the visit of various groups of American psychiatrists to Europe was application of changed attitudes toward patients: a greater respect for the dignity of individuals and a greater emphasis on self-care; factory-in-hospital programs; home visiting; and extension of rehabilitation programs.

The stimulus of working under two great administrators, Bryan and William Menninger, the several years of work on conceptualizing aspects of administration in the GAP Hospital Committee, and the broadening horizon provided by many visits to European and North American mental hospitals provided the background for the writing of Barton's comprehensive textbook, *Administration in Psychiatry* (38). From its publication in 1962, it was the sole definitive source for guides to mental hospital management for over a decade.

In 1970, APA published a position paper on confidentiality (99) and established a Task Force on Confidentiality, whose work in Task Force Report #9 summarizes their work in *Confidentiality and Third Parties* (100). A broader view emerged from an APA Conference held in 1974. The report of the conference *Confidentiality* (101) stands as a significant landmark to maintenance of the confidentiality of health records.

In the 1970s the APA, after producing a revision of its standards, played a key role in organizing the Accreditation Council for Psychiatric Facilities within the Joint Commission for Accreditation of Hospitals. The APA also joined with two other organizations—the Association of Mental Health Administrators and the Association of University Programs in Health Administration (AUPHA)—in forming a National Task Force on Mental Health and Mental Retardation Administration. Some of the more important products of this joint effort were *A Guidebook to Curricula in Mental Health Administration* (102), which was the first listing of training opportunities in mental health administration; *Continuing Education For the Health Profession* (103); three annual national conferences on the subject of education for mental health administration, the first of which was held in 1973; and the Task Force's final report (104), covering development of the field of mental health administration, the knowledge base, and a suggested curriculum in mental health administration.

In the 1980s the APA has included courses in administrative psychiatry as part of its continuing education offerings at its annual meetings. The departure of psychiatrists from all executive level posts in the public mental health system has reached crisis proportions. The APA responded by forming a committee on Psychiatric Leadership in Public Systems to assess the situation and to make recommendations. Panel and paper presentations on administrative topics are included in the annual meeting program, and the APA has established an achievement award in administrative psychiatry to enhance the prestige of the field and to make members aware of the profession's responsibility to maintain quality care for patients in the public sector. The election of two presidents of the APA with credentials in Administration—George

Tarjan in 1983 and John Talbott in 1984—were important steps toward the recognition of the field.

The awareness of the need for training in administration was slow to develop. As the pace of change accelerated and uncertainties multiplied, it became evident that more than common sense and clinical skills were needed to manage organizational complexity. The knowledge base continued to expand. Talbott and Kaplan produced a comprehensive textbook, *Psychiatric Administration* (105); Barton and Barton produced *Mental Health Administration: Principles and Practice* (94) in two volumes, and a third volume, *Ethics and Law in Mental Health Administration* (12), provided a complete reference source for the field. *What's New in Administration* (106) provided quantitative methods to help manage uncertainty; reported technological advances in treatment requiring new administrative arrangements and programs and the development of computer assisted management information systems. Other new additions to mental health administration were problems in role definition; scarcity of resources; more regulation and external controls; with a greater need to understand ethics, law, politics, public relations, and marketing. As a consequence, administrators became more responsive to society and to the internal needs of the public mental health care delivery system.

As is so often the case in the United States when a problem area is identified, an organization was founded (1979): the American College of Mental Health Administration. It brought together an elite group of clinician–executives, joining psychiatry with psychology, social work, and nursing to cope with the common problems of expanding educational opportunities in mental health and mental retardation administration, developing status and prestige to clinician–executives, and encouraging research in administration.

ADVANCES IN MEDICAL EDUCATION

It was the shortage of psychiatrists in meeting military needs during World War II, and the lack of knowledge about psychiatric disabilities by the physicians in the military services, that provided the major incentive for change that expanded the psychiatric professional pool and the teaching of psychiatry in medical schools. The APA had fewer than 3,000 members in 1942, too few to fill Military requirements. To supplement the demand, general physicians were assigned as neuropsychiatrists. To teach them the essentials of psychiatry, the army established the School of Military Neuropsychiatry (1943–1945), from which 1,000 physicians graduated in a three-month course to serve as neuropsychiatrists (107).

Other factors that induced changes in the teaching of psychiatry were:

- Increasing specialization in educational systems that were isolated from one another
- Evident deficiency of research by psychiatrists and the lack of training in research methodology
- The need for a greater number of minority psychiatrists and women in the service delivery system
- Technological and other scientific advances in diagnosis, in social and behavioral sciences, in neuroscience, and in psychopharmacology
- The initial predominance of psychoanalytic psychotherapy, followed by disenchantment with this method as a practical therapeutic modality (essential to understanding, but too costly in time and money for general application)
- Broadening of psychotherapies to include crisis intervention, family, marital, and sex therapies
- New roles in the community and as consultants to medical and surgical services

The expansion of the federal role from 1950–1970 provided the funds to greatly expand departments of psychiatry in the medical schools, to develop career teachers and research investigators, to support the training of extenders (clinical psychologists and psychiatric social workers and nurses), to offer incentives to general practitioners to train as psychiatrists, to train paraprofessionals (mental health workers and emergency medical technicians), and to fund surveys, demonstrations, and conferences. Federal funding, wisely administered by NIMH, was the primary agent in providing the means to effect change.

Prior to 1950, the American Board of Psychiatry and Neurology outlined (in 1946) the basic subjects and clinical training in three full years of residency training in psychiatry. Also required in the teaching centers were competent teachers, collaborative work with mental health professionals, and social agencies. In 1972, the Residency Review Committee for Psychiatry and Neurology and the AMA Council on Medical Education detailed recommendations in a *Guide For Residency Training Programs.*

The Group for the Advancement of Psychiatry report, *Medical Education* (1948), recommended that undergraduate medical students see and study patients from the first year on, concentrating on growth and development in the first year of training, on psychopathological conditions in the second, and on supervised clinical training in the third year of residency. Within the three-year period, six months were to be spent in neurology and six months with the psychoses; in addition, some time was to be spent with children, with the mentally retarded, and in the study of the neuroses. A later GAP report, *The Pre-Clinical Teaching of Psychiatry* (1962), provided an overview of the experience up to that time, with a recommended educational sequence.

The American Psychiatric Association and the Association of American Medical Colleges, with NIMH grants, held two conferences that shaped the pattern of the teaching of psychiatry for the following decade. The product of the 1951 conference was *Psychiatry and Medical Education* (108), and that of the 1952 conference was *The Psychiatrist, His Training and Development* (109). The demand for greater detail was answered in 1956 by the APA's Committee on Medical Education in *An Outline for a Curriculum for Teaching Psychiatry in Medical Schools* (110).

The Cornell Conferences, held in Ithaca, New York, in 1951 and 1952, reflected the ambiance of the time: confident expectancy of a bright future and the belief that goals articulated would be achieved. Psychiatry was to expand its role in the medical school; to develop integrated teaching with other departments; to experiment with new curricula; and to offer courses in each of the four years utilizing seminars, group field visits, movies, audiotapes, and one-way windowed rooms. Included was to be the teaching of interviewing techniques, doctor–patient relationships, disorders of children, and psychosomatic and social psychiatric medicine. The 1952 conference stressed the fundamental position of the teaching of psychodynamics and the great urgency of expanding the psychiatric profession.

It is not surprising that the hope and promise of expanding psychiatry in medical education, and of the dominance of psychodynamics, came at a time when there were great leaders in American psychiatry who had a special interest in educational issues, as well as the ability to achieve goals. John Whitehorn was the APA President from 1950–1951. He was a superb teacher, administrator, and student of emotional function. He espoused the development of social-psychodynamics and held that psychoanalysis contributed to the understanding of personal relationships and social roles. From 1951–1952, the APA president was Leo H. Bartemier, one of the world's leading psychoanalysts. He stressed the doctor–patient relationship and sought to improve psychotherapy and enhance its effectiveness. At NIMH, two great champions with similar viewpoints, Robert H. Felix and Seymour D. Vestermark, turned concepts and ideas into reality with policies favoring medical education, support of faculty, and development of the professional pool in psychiatry.

In the tumultuous and revolutionary climate of the 1960s, actions designed to strengthen medical education and continuing education were taken by the AMA, the World Health Organization (WHO), and the APA.

Gradually, over a period of two decades, an awareness developed that the elaborate plans to distribute and pay for medical care and the increase in the number of physicians and specialists would not assure the application of the new knowledge for the benefit of the sick patient. The pace of change was so rapid that what one learned quickly became obsolete. The valiant effort to keep abreast of the literature by reading journals was not enough, nor did attending lectures remedy the problem of keeping up with the latest developments in the field.

In 1961, the AMA set in motion a cooperative study (by AMA, AAMC, AHA, APA, and other medical specialty organizations) that resulted in the formalization of required continuing medical education. The Joint Study Commission produced a highly readable and informative report, *Lifetime Learning for Physicians* (111). While the recommended cooperative nationwide "university without walls" for continuing medical education, estimated to cost $25 million, was·not implemented, the concepts and ideas were put into general use. In 1972, the APA published *Prospects and Proposals: Lifetime Learning For Psychiatrists* (112).

What did transpire from the program was a voluntary system under AMA sponsorship with a certificate issued to physicians who, in a three-year period, completed the required number of credit hours of continuing medical education (CME). After conducting a survey, the AMA extended to state medical societies, universities, and organizations such as the APA, the right to approve CME presentations for credit. States, for renewal of medical license, frequently required evidence of an AMA CME certificate or its equivalent; and organizations—such as APA—required completion of CME credits for continued membership.

Other notable efforts to enhance medical education in the 1960s were: the World Health Organization's *Teaching of Psychiatry and Mental Health* (113); GAP's *The Preclinical Teaching of Psychiatry* (114); and two surveys—AMA's, *The Graduate Education of Physicians* (The Millis Report) (115), and AAMC's *Planning For Medical Progress Through Education* (the Coggleshall Report) (116). The Millis Report of 1966 was notable for its call for teaching centers to accept responsibility for control of the graduate medical education process, eliminating the internship (with its fragmentation of educational process, discontinuities, exploitation of interns, and integration of clinical experience within the university setting) and coordinating residency. The Coggleshall Report advocated that medical education be planned as a life-long continuum.

To keep abreast of changes in medical education, the APA held two conferences, as it had done in the 1950s: one on graduate psychiatric education in 1962, and the other on psychiatry in general medical education in 1967. A new generation of psychiatric leaders had achieved a strong position for psychiatry in the medical school. The emphasis was less on the struggle for power and time in the curriculum, and more on specific learning objectives with appraisal of results.

The respective products of these conferences—*Training the Psychiatrist to Meet Changing Needs* (117) and *Psychiatry and Medical Education II* (118)—provided expert opinion on new developments (in social psychology, ecology, biological science, behavioral methods, and psychopharmacology), but eschewed definitive guidelines during a time of social upheaval.

Student protest in the 1960s made faculty more accountable, and gave students a voice in planning and decision-making and a seat on important committees. Women and minorities pressed for elimination of discrimination for admission to medical school, for residency appointments, and for appointments to faculty positions.

In 1952 there were 7,500 psychiatrists; in 1962, 13,000. In 1952 there were 2,456 psychiatric residencies, with 1,784 posts filled. In 1962, of 4,231 residencies offered in psychiatry, 3,245 were filled. Perhaps the most significant results of the APA medical education conferences of the 1960s were the emphasis upon outcome and evaluation of the quality of care; the assessment of clinical performance; the focus on attitudes of residents in training, and the impact of training on the resident; and the endorsement of new methodologies in education (videotapes, patient management techniques, and computer simulations). The swing away from a primary psychoanalytic focus became evident, with a move toward a biological and sociological orientation. The shift to the biologically oriented chairpersons of departments of psychiatry was manifested in the 1970s.

As the cost of medical care continued to increase, and as governmental expenditures for health rose to over 39 percent of the national total expenditures (118), the clamor for accountability and control of soaring costs became insistent. Recognizing the criticism of psychiatry and facing drastic modification in the support of medical education, the American College of Psychiatrists addressed the issues in 1973, in *Psychiatry: Education and Image* (119). Individualization, diversity, and training in multiple settings were key elements in the preparation of psychiatrists, with proof of competence obtained by examination.

The establishment of 28 new medical schools offered a rare opportunity to develop innovative mental health teaching programs. With an NIMH grant, the American Association of Chairmen of Departments of Psychiatry explored the prospects in a 1972 conference. There had been freely expressed dissatisfaction with the health care system in the 1960s. The outcry was for more consumer input and control, and for a greater number of human services. The recurrent theme of interdepartmental integrated teaching was stressed with examples of educational programs in new settings (120).

As the organization had done in the past, the American Psychiatric Association made a major contribution to the advancement of psychiatric education in the 1970s. An APA Task Force on the evaluation of Community Mental Health Centers, with NIMH grant support, provided the stimulus for a conference held at the University of Illinois Medical School in Chicago (1972) on *Evaluative Methods in Psychiatric Education* (121). Multiple choice testing was examined, as were other measures of competence (such as patient management problems, computer aided simulations, film and videotape, recordings, clinical performance, attitudes of residents in training, etc.). In sum, evaluation was seen as essential to learning, with appropriate measures to be applied for the assessment of clinical skills, and knowledge represented by the cardinal aspects of the learning experience (121).

A conference sponsored by the APA, the American Association of Chairmen of Departments of Psychiatry, the Academy of Child Psychiatry, and the American Association of Directors of Psychiatric Residency Training, with NIMH grant support, was held at Lake of the Ozarks, Missouri, in June 1975. The report of the conference appeared in two volumes: *Psychiatric Education: Prologue to the 1980s* (122) and *The Working Papers of the 1975 Conference on Education of Psychiatrists* (123). Marked changes had altered the delivery system for mental health services, affected the role of psychiatrists, eliminated the internship, restricted the accepted authority of leaders, caused consumers to demand accountability and regulation to control costs, altered the funding base, and challenged the image of psychiatry. It should be noted that the request for funding the conference was rejected until the representatives of consumers and residents in training were added, the proposed research curtailed, and the budget for the conference drastically reduced. Perhaps the most significant findings of the conference were:

- A shift from emphasis upon process to the product of psychiatric education
- A need for better data for long-range planning
- A need for greater flexibility and individualization in the design of educational curricula
- Demonstrated competence of psychiatric residents measured before completion of training
- Research in education
- Study of the economics of training
- An outline of the essentials for residency education, with a clear statement of goals and objectives

Roy Grinker, Sr. (124) stressed the importance for the good psychiatrist to be first a good physician, able to diagnose and treat disease; to be sensitive to hidden feelings, able to communicate with an awareness of the effect of personal values; and to have a capacity to integrate the totality. John Romano (44) emphasized the importance of the introduction of psychology and the social sciences into medical school teaching; the expansion of educational programs in psychiatry to nurses and social workers who had new roles in therapy; the greater precision now possible in diagnosis; and the need to study the nature of delivery systems.

With a demonstrated commitment to continuing medical education, the APA (following immediately on the successful pioneering experience of the American College of Physicians) instituted a comprehensive self-assessment evaluation program. The first test was given in 1969, the second in 1972, and test programs have been repeated at intervals in the 1980s. Each successive self-assessment test attracted more APA members. Although the test is costly, it has proven to be a profitable and self-sustaining venture.

Herbert Pardes, former head of NIMH, has articulated clearly the *Challenge to Academic Psychiatry* (125) in the 1980s. The loss of capitation funding for medical schools, cuts in Medicare and Medicaid programs, and retrenchment in all federal support, have made financing psychiatric education a central issue. The marketing of services of academic centers has come to public attention. The need for sound public relations and active involvement of psychiatry in the political arena has become evident in the fierce competition for limited resources.

CHANGES IN NATIONAL POLICY AFFECTING PSYCHIATRY

National policy was to develop manpower to combat shortages in the post-World War II period. The shortages of psychiatrists and in particular child psychiatrists, mental health professionals, and mental health workers led to federal support of education, expansion of full-time faculties, and residency or trainee stipends. Physicians in general lacked good instruction in psychiatric disabilities and in sensitivity to the emotional accompaniment of medical illnesses. This deficit had to be corrected by competent teachers of psychiatry. Career teachers were therefore supported by the government, as were career research investigators. A projected shortage of physicians had to be corrected by capitation funding for expanding the medical school student body and for building new medical schools. Foreign medical students and

Americans studying abroad were given the opportunity to train in the United States. In the 1980s the physician pool has expanded to the point where an oversupply is predicted.

Problems, however, have remained. Some specialty areas such as child psychiatry are still underserved. There are still shortages in inner city and rural areas. Psychiatrists in urban practice face increasing competition from other mental health professionals in solo practice. The prediction of an oversupply of physicians in the 1990s foreshadows further competition for psychiatrists, for it seems likely that primary care physicians will treat more mental disorders without referral.

Equal rights and nondiscrimination as national policy have given favored treatment to minorities. Blacks and Hispanics have been supported in order to meet qualifying standards, and medical schools have been encouraged, through incentives, to recruit more minority group students and to seek qualified minority faculty members. Women in psychiatry residencies have increased from 17 percent to 30 percent, with further gains evident. Efforts have been made to eliminate discriminatory practices.

Patient rights have been guaranteed by judicial action and legislation. Standards of care have been enforced by class action suits. Deprivation of liberty (by commitment) is now allowed only when the individual is dangerous to self or others. The right to refuse treatment has been upheld. The least restrictive alternative to hospitalization must now be found. Work by patients is to be a voluntary option and is to be paid.

Research on human subjects must now be approved by an Institution Review Board, patients must be allowed to refuse to participate and to withdraw at any time, and to be subject to rigid safeguards. Psychosurgery has been drastically restricted, and fetal research and genetic research are now strictly controlled.

Cost control has become a national priority in the 1980s after utilization and peer review failed in the 1970s era of accountability for government funds. A fee schedule for Diagnostic Related Groups (DRGs) has been used under Medicare to control costs for medical procedures and treatments. The special problems posed by dependence on proper outside supports after a patient's release from hospital, and on fixing a period of time for treatment and a fee for a diagnostic entity in psychiatry, led the APA (in 1983) to institute a study of feasibility of the DRG system in psychiatry.

Restrictions on lobbying by tax exempt organizations has led the APA to establish a separate Political Action Corporation (PAC) to lobby on behalf of mental patient interests in the 1980s.

The heyday of federal support of psychiatry in the 1950s and 1960s ceased when the recession of the late 1970s caused federal belt tightening. Congress wanted to support the public mental health system, but the strong conservative, President Reagan, prevailed in enforcing retrenchment in most federal entitlement programs.

7

Building a Stronger
American Psychiatric Association
After 1950

It takes all the running you can do to keep in the same place.

—Lewis Carroll (1)

A stronger and more influential American Psychiatric Association came into being after 1950. The structure of governance changed; an Assembly of District Branches was formed, and the Association became more democratic. Benefits to members increased. There was greater involvement in the legislative policymaking process, in the courts, and in collaborative action with other medical and mental health organizations. The Association assumed a more responsible role in society and extended its influence to the medical profession.

The structure of the APA in 1950 had changed but little in the more than 100 years since the organization was founded. The annual meetings, held each year for a week in mid-May, continued to provide a forum for the members to meet in committees, to learn of scientific advances, to conduct the Association's business, to hear reports, and to elect its officers in the town-meeting style. Business between meetings continued to be conducted by an elected council. The council was composed of elected officers (President, President-Elect, Secretary, Treasurer, and nine elected Fellows as counselors—three elected each year for a three-year term). The council continued to meet at the time of the annual meeting and at three other times during the year.

As I have noted in Chapter 5, the ferment within the organization led President Karl Bowman (1944–1946) to appoint a Reorganization Committee to study the organizational structure and to develop a comprehensive plan. The APA had a headquarters under an executive officer, Austin Davies, for more than a decade; but structural change, growth in programs, and an increase in the organization's power did not take place until the advent of strong medical leadership.

Daniel Blain, M.D. (1898–1981), was the innovative leader; Matthew Ross, M.D., in the four years from 1958 to 1962 fostered growth of the assembly and selected several key staff persons; Walter Barton, M.D., Medical Director for 11 years (1963–1974), built a strong organization; while Melvin Sabshin, M.D., Medical Director from 1974 to the present, has extended and strengthened educational programs, liaison relationships, and international participation, has developed new programs, and has made the APA a force in the political arena.

Because of their influence upon the organization and its growth, I shall sketch the background of the Medical Directors and focus on their contributions.

THE MEDICAL DIRECTORS

Daniel Blain, the first Medical Director, served from 1948 to 1958. He came to the APA from a post he had filled with great distinction—Chief of the Department of Psychiatry at the Veterans Administration headquarters in Washington, D.C.*

Some of Blain's major achievements were:

- Establishment of the Washington headquarters in its elegant building at 1700 18th Street
- Recruitment of such key staff members as Robert Robinson, Pat Vosburgh, Ann Whinnie, Ralph Champers, Lucy Ozarin, Charles Goshen, Charles Bush, and many others

---

* In addition to the brief biographical sketch describing the background of each Medical Director found in Appendix D, the following published information will supply those interested with further details: for Dr. Blain (2–4); for Dr. Ross (5, 6); for Dr. Barton (7). For Dr. Sabshin (8) see *Psychiatric News* 9:1–34, Sept. 18, 1974.

- Organization of the Mental Hospital Institute in 1949 (the oldest continuing education program)
- Publishing of the magazine *Mental Hospitals* and the *Mail Pouch*
- Organization of the joint enterprise on hospital architecture with the American Institute of Architects (1957)
- Establishment of the General Practitioners Education Project in 1957 with funding from the Lasker Foundation (later funding was provided by NIMH). Blain selected Charles E. Goshen to head the project
- Development of the Central Inspection Board with state surveys of psychiatric hospitals and a Consultation Program for system improvement (1950) with Ralph Chambers as Director
- Promotion of professional development, with more women in medicine, and organized a National Commission on Mental Health Manpower
- Working aggressively to develop insurance benefits for the mentally ill (Group Health Insurance and United Automobile Workers)
- Traveling extensively, visiting some 500 mental hospitals to express APA concern and interest in the public and private systems of care

Blain inspired trust and loyalty in APA staff members. Although not an administrator, he was a great leader. He provided the flow of creative thought, while Robbie Robinson translated the ideas into actions as, for example, in the case of the first Mental Hospital Institute or the first Conference on Medical Education. Robbie wrote the grant applications, arranged the meetings in detail, and produced reports. Once an activity was proven effective, Robinson turned it over to others, and began the development of another of Dan's ideas.

Blain was kind and energetic, impatient with administrative aspects of the job, letting others define the task and solve the problem. His was the broader vision of relieving suffering of the mentally ill and building a more caring society.

Some years after Blain's retirement from the post of Medical Director, when he was APA's President (1964–1965), his call for a policy retreat led to a major overhaul of the organizational structure. The Airlie House Conference was convened at Blain's request to make the APA more responsive to the changing times and capable of prompt action. Blain also had a marker put on Benjamin Rush's grave acknowledging his many contributions, and his recognition as the Father of American Psychiatry.

Matthew Ross was handicapped from the start, for it was his bad luck to follow a great leader. Ross had been highly visible as Speaker of the Assembly (1956–1957). His social skills and personal charm projected the image of a young potential leader when the Council selected him to succeed Blain. But Ross had been in solo private practice. He had never had administrative responsibility for an organization and so was miscast as Medical Director. Lacking managerial expertise, he was, in the author's opinion, an ineffective administrator.

Ross made two outstanding appointments to the APA staff: *Bartholomew V. Hogan,* Rear Admiral of the Navy and its recent Surgeon General (1955–1961), who had extensive credentials in administration (9); and *Donald W. Hammersley, M.D.,* who had been a unit chief at Madigan General Army Hospital and then Director of Professional Services and Education at the Topeka VA Hospital, when he came to the APA in 1961.

Ross requested the Council to clarify his responsibilities and in March of 1960 a job description was approved. The intent was to improve management and to clarify relationships with Council and APA components. The job description statement, excerpted below, was approved in March 1960.

The Medical Director must be a Fellow of APA, appointed by the Council and responsible to that body under the immediate supervision of the President. The principal functions of the Medical Director are to:

- Administer the activities of the Association in accordance with APA objectives
- Coordinate, staff, and stimulate liaison with other professional organizations, and develop a budget (with the help of the Treasurer and Executive Assistant)
- Provide staff assistance to APA components
- Prepare agenda for Council and its Executive Committee
- Direct the Mental Hospital Service and its journal, *Mental Hospitals*
- Express concern for the information services, the library (document collection, permanent records of association, press clippings, photographs), publications, membership activities, and

Council approved projects (such as the Architectural Study Project, General Practitioner Education, and State Surveys)

The New York office under Austin Davies as Executive Assistant continued to be responsible for membership records, dues collection, and the business affairs of the *American Journal of Psychiatry.* The publication office of the *American Journal of Psychiatry* continued in Toronto under the editorship of C.B. Farrar.

Ross contributed to the maturation of the Assembly, advocated public policy that favored the mentally disabled, and fostered community psychiatry. He was responsive to the diverse elements within the Association, but when promises were unfulfilled, allegations of unreliability were heard.

In January of 1963, the Council accepted the resignation of Matt Ross, who went to Holland as a Fulbright Research Scholar. Dr. Hogan was named Acting Director until April 1, when the new Medical Director selected by the Council was to take office.

*Walter E. Barton** became the third Medical Director and served for 11 years (1963–1974). Unlike his predecessors, Barton had an intimate knowledge of the APA. He had served on Committees, on the Governing Council, and on its Executive Committee (1952–1955). In addition, he had held many important posts as APA's representative to other organizations, such as the AMA and the Joint Commission on Mental Illness and Health. Immediately preceding his appointment, Barton had been President-Elect and President of APA from 1960–1962. He was most reluctant to accept the post of Medical Director because he had been active in the investigation of the troubled affairs of the staff in the central office. The insistence of the Council that he was admirably suited for the job overcame his objections.

Barton began his duties as Medical Director by clarifying authority and responsibility through the development, jointly with an executive staff cabinet, of policy and procedure manuals, personnel manuals, and operational manuals.

---

* Because the author cannot be objective about his own performance, assessment was requested from former and present APA staff and past Presidents of the Association. The same opinion statements were obtained on Matthew Ross. Medical Directors were asked for self-assessment, but only Dr. Sabshin submitted one.

The long talked about central headquarters became a reality. The delicate negotiations to retire the much loved Editor of the *American Journal of Psychiatry*, C.B. Farrar, was completed, and the Toronto office closed. Similarly, Austin Davies was retired and the New York office closed.

The consolidation of all APA administrative offices was followed by reorganization of the staff into discrete divisions. Hogan as Deputy Medical Director was assigned the responsibility for personnel management, support of the Assembly (with Ann Whinnie), relations with governmental agencies, and foreign affairs. He was superb in the conduct of his activities, as well as a master physician-politician, and contributed much to the creation of a smooth-running and efficient organization.

Donald Hammersley served as Chief of Professional Services representing the APA in all substantive committee activities requiring psychiatric clinical input, both in house and outside the organization. He was also in charge of the Mental Hospital Service and consultant to staff on medical problems.

Pat Vosburgh was named Editor of *Mental Hospitals* (which, in 1965, was to become *Journal of Hospital and Community Psychiatry*), and built a fine support staff (Betty Keenan, Teddye Clayton, Betty Cochran, and Ed Pace as Business Manager).

Evelyn Meyers was appointed Managing Editor of the *American Journal of Psychiatry* under the new Editor, Francis Braceland. She surrounded herself with a highly competent staff of assistant editors.

Robert Robinson (10) was designated head of Public Affairs. Robbie (1915–1980) was the staff member with the longest service—31 years. He was an action-oriented, convivial man who made outstanding contributions to the APA. Among them were:

- Development of Dan Blain's ideas into the Mental Hospital Institute, and became Editor of its Proceedings
- Arrangement of the 1950s conferences on medical education at Ithaca and produced their two reports
- Improvement of communication with members, first through the *Mail Pouch*, and then through the highly successful *Psychiatric News*, serving as its first Editor
- Establishment of APA's open press policy and organized a national conference with the National Association of Science Writ-

ers as cosponsor (with grant support from the Ittleson Family Fund, Albert and Mary Lasker, Division Funds, and the Harris Foundation). The conference defined public relations issues predicted to become more urgent. Robinson wrote about these issues in a monograph entitled *Psychiatry, the Press, and the Public* (1956)

- Initiation of the *Psychiatric Glossary* and *Scientific Proceedings in Summary Form* of the annual meeting
- Organization of a fund drive (1954–1955) to finance the purchase of the headquarters building at 1700 18th Street
- Assisting in the development of the Joint Information Service under the brilliant author of its 15 successful books, Raymond Glasscote
- Development of APA's first best-selling publication, *DSM-II*, in collaboration with Paul Wilson
- Initiation of the formation of a government relations department under Caesar Giolito to orchestrate legislative lobbying.

Other departments were developed under strong leadership: Business Management, Manpower and Personnel, and Meetings Management. Barton secured grants for studies of insurance (Louis Reed), information processing (Paul Wilson), manpower development (Lee Gurel), and physician continuing education (Hugh Carmichael).

Other achievements under the Barton tenure were:

- Growth of staff from 48 to 116 persons, with greatly expanded programs and staff support of APA activities
- Construction of the Museum Building and renovation of the 1700 18th Street headquarters to accommodate the expanding activities (1966)
- Development of international meetings with Alfred Auerbach
- Attendance at meetings in Japan, Mexico, Scotland, Scandinavia, Spain, the U.S.S.R., the Caribbean, and the Netherlands, varied from 250 to 600, with an average of 200 APA travelers. APA often presented gifts to host organizations. Many of the countries visited responded to APA invitation to meet in the U.S. at APA annual meetings
- Origination of the reorganization model for APA introduced at President Daniel Blain's Airlie House Conference

- Development of strong ties with AMA and other medical specialty organizations. Formed the Coalition for Mental Health to develop unified support for mental health legislation
- Organization of the conferences on community mental health (1963) that led to passage of the Mental Health Act in Congress
- Successfully fighting to include psychiatric benefits in Medicare legislation, and continued the cooperation with UAW on mental health insurance begun by Blain and Harvey Tompkins
- Identification of promising young psychiatrists and involved them in APA work
- Salvaging (with Reginald Lourie) the work of the Joint Commission on Mental Health of Children, making publication of its volumes possible
- Promotion of training in administration for mental health professionals

Barton was the benevolent authoritative leader who fostered staff growth, pursued a prudent fiscal policy setting aside reserves for future building, and possessed the skills to coordinate disparate elements in the APA into a smooth and efficient organization. He restored integrity in leadership and brought the organization into the big league of medical specialty organizations.

At the height of his success, while enjoying immense prestige (it was said "he was the role model of what a psychiatrist should be"), and with the knowledge of more power accumulating around the Medical Director than it should, Barton followed his own textbook dictum encouraging administrators to retire after 10 years, and asked to be relieved. The APA had become a strong organization with an excellent staff and high morale, respected in the community of medical specialty organizations.

Melvin Sabshin, the fourth Medical Director, was appointed by the Board of Trustees in October 1973 and assumed his duties at APA on September 1, 1974. The long lead time permitted an orderly transition. The staff was prepared for change and anticipated the coming of a leader with a proven track record of administrative achievement and a thorough knowledge of APA as an organization.

Sabshin came to the post from the Abraham Lincoln School of Medicine of the University of Illinois in Chicago, where he was acting Dean and professor of psychiatry, and former Chairman of the Department of Psychiatry. His scholarly interests in research methodology, psychiatric concepts, administration, social and community psychiatry, and depression resulted in many publications in the literature.

Under Sabshin's directorship, membership has grown from 20,000 in the 1970s to more than 31,000 in 1986. The Association's budget climbed from $3 million annually to $15 million. Programs have diversified; new APA components have multiplied; rising costs of patient care and cost containment problems have contributed to the erosion of the psychiatrists' image; and budget cuts, as well as legislation and judicial actions, have made it essential for the APA to aggressively struggle to preserve quality patient care and to protect psychiatry's turf.

The most significant new developments under the Sabshin regime have been:

- Establishment of the Corporation for the Advancement of Psychiatry (CAP), a political action committee to lobby for psychiatric interests, with Robert J. Campbell, President, and a Board of Trustees representing the seven APA areas
- Expansion of Members Benefits and Services Program and Directory to include professional liability coverage; life, accident, health, and disability insurance; retirement plan; legal consultation; and Avis car rental discount
- Founding of the American Psychiatric Press, Inc., with Ron McMillen as General Manager and Shervert Frazier, M.D., as Editor-in-Chief; this corporation publishes, in addition to APA publications (Directories, *DSM-III*, and the *Psychiatric Glossary*), a Psychiatry Update series, Clinical Insights monographs, Private Practice monographs, Progress in Psychiatry monographs, reference books, textbooks, professional books, tapes, and books for the general public
- Organization of an Office of Economics, under Deputy Medical Director Steven S. Sharfstein, M.D., to keep members informed and up-to-date on insurance coverage for mental illness and the financing of service delivery. The American Psychiatric Press has published books that summarize the Office of Economics group studies
- Planning, fund raising, and developing a new headquarters building at 1400 K Street, N.W., with sale of properties at 1700 18th Street

The *governance* of the Association was changed, as recommended by the Key Conference (to be discussed later), to give greater power to the Assembly. The Board of Trustees continues to be the ultimate authority, with responsibility for constitutional committees, ad hoc committees, and liaison representatives. The Assembly derives its power through member-elected representatives from the District Branches, its minority and resident-in-training members, and through the seven Area Councils. Jointly, the Board and Assembly operate Commissions (such as Government Relations, Public Affairs, Medical Education, Psychiatric Services, Standards and Economics of Care, and Research, together with related Committees, Task Forces, and Boards.

The headquarters office has been reorganized to create divisions under Deputy Medical Directors such as Education (Carolyn B. Robinowitz, M.D.), Professional Services (Donald Hammersley, M.D.), Business Administration (Jack White), Economics (Steven Sharfstein, M.D.), and Minority Affairs (Jeanne Spurlock, M.D.). Expanded have been legislative functions in the Government Relations department under Jay Cutler; legal consultation under Joel Klein; and Public Affairs under John Blamphin.

To the strong legislative network, with its District Branch representatives, has been added a similar network concerned with public relations, with the support of a Commission on Public Affairs and a staff department. A new Office of Research has been added to relate to foundations and to coordinate research constituencies.

Fellowship programs and resident and medical student involvement have expanded. The Association has increased its interest in professional accountability with a new Office of Peer Review (responsible for review programs of CHAMPUS and other health insurance plans). The ethics process has been refined and elaborated under the direction of Ms. Carol Davis and Mr. Joel Klein. The Council on Professions and Associations has been terminated, and its activity has become a staff function. There has been increased liaison activity of the APA, particularly with AMA, the Council of Medical Specialty Societies, the Joint Commission on Accreditation of Hospitals, the American Association of Medical Colleges, the American Board of Psychiatry, and especially with federal agencies.

Sabshin has directed in the teleocratic leadership style—oriented to process more than structure, to interaction more than procedure. He is incredibly intelligent, a superb communicator, and has the ability to avoid conflict among the many factions both within and without the organization. Psychiatry has been under siege, suffering loss of prestige, status, and income. Often it has appeared that operations by the staff are more bail-out than steering a course. Survival demands a quick response and a more political orientation. Programs have been geared to realistic current concerns, while guild interests have been protected.

There has been a concentration of effort on building membership, especially among those beginning a career in psychiatry (students and residents). APA's adversarial positions and legislative lobbying have consumed much time, money, and effort.

Reorganization of the headquarters staff into highly specialized entities seems to have increased their political effectiveness and to have diminished their corporative efficiency. The complexities induced by program expansion, threats to the image and to the survival of psychiatry, budget cuts, and cost containment schemes that imperil the care of the mentally ill have put enormous stress upon the Medical Director and his staff in the 1980s. Sabshin has ably carried the great burden of leadership and has helped the organization to increase its membership, its revenues, and its power.

THE ORGANIZATIONAL ENVIRONMENT

The organizational environment is a product of many interacting forces both within and without the organization. It is more than the space and the people who occupy it. The quality of the physical and visual environment shapes behavior. The loyalty to an admired leader, high morale, and pleasant working relationships mold staff deportment. The ambience of the Parson Mansion at 18th and R Streets created a sense of quiet elegance; the 12-story glass office building at 1400 K Street seems to project impersonal efficiency.

Long-range planners within the organization underestimated the services required, as well as the space needs, for a growing association; in addition, these planners did not foresee the program and project expansion that rapidly outgrew projections. Membership growth and increase in staff is illustrated by the following:

1950:	5,856 members	14 staff
1960:	11,037 members	62 staff
1970:	18,407 members	108 staff
1980:	25,345 members	150 staff

As examples of growth of programs, not only does it require a larger staff to process membership applications and issue dues bills and directories, but communication with members has expanded in many ways. *The Bulletin*, edited for 18 months by Ann Janney, dealt with interests emerging from the Mental Hospital Institute. Under Pat Vosburgh (1951) it became a magazine (*Mental Hospitals*, and then *Hospital and Community Psychiatry*), with a growing editorial and support staff. The same was true of the *Mail Pouch* (1950). The *Mail Pouch* was started to recount the activities and travels of the Medical Director. It contained, in a packet, flyers about books, conferences, and information sheets for members. The informal pouch was replaced in the 1960s by *Psychiatric News*, with a sizable editorial staff.

Projects funded from sources other than member dues grew in number. Examples of such projects are Central Inspections Surveys, Architecture, Manpower, Insurance, and Medical Education.

From the outset, the Washington headquarters occupied buildings suited to the image of an old, established association, growing in power on the national scene. In 1948, Blain selected, for the first Medical Director's office, two rented rooms on Eye Street in a red brick Victorian mansion (which no longer exists) across the street from the Army–Navy Building. With a budget of $50,000 for salaries and expenses, it provided space for the Medical Director, his associate, Robert Robinson, and two secretaries.

Within three years the space was outgrown and the office was moved (in June 1951) to 1785 Massachusetts Avenue, N.W. The mansion had been the luxurious home of Andrew Mellon and later the headquarters of the American Council on Education. Again, within three years, pressure mounted for more space than would be available to the APA in the foreseeable future. By 1954 the staff numbered 35 (plus ten in New York and Toronto).

In 1954, members were asked to express their opinions as to the need for acquiring a central headquarters building of its own. The vote was 2 to 1 in favor. Considered as suitable locations were New York City (where many national associations were based), Philadelphia (where the Association had been founded), and Washington, D.C. (with its proximity to government and its agencies, as well as to other national organizations). Washington was chosen over Austin Davies' objection, and in spite of his determination to retain his activities in New York City.

The building chosen for the Association's first wholly owned national office was an elegant townhouse at 1700 18th Street near Dupont Circle. The APA acquired the property at a cost of $105,000 with the approval of the membership. The Association conducted a building fund drive (1954–1956) under the chairmanship of Francis Braceland, assisted by Robert Robinson, with the goal of raising $200,000. Forty-five hundred of the approximately 10,000 members voluntarily contributed an amount over the targeted goal.*

Renovation of the Parson Mansion was carefully carried out by architects and an interior decorator to recreate its original elegance at a cost of $173,000. The total cost of the building and its refurbishing was $278,000. The member donations and Association resources paid the expense without recourse to loans or mortgages (see Appendix E).

The building was occupied by staff in April 1958 and dedicated during the time of the fall committee meetings on October 31, 1958. Some 200 members, Association officers, and dignitaries attended the ceremony. It was with justifiable pride that the Association celebrated the occasion (as the press releases stated), which appropriately symbolized the significant place that psychiatry had achieved in medicine and in the fabric of American social and cultural endeavor. It was also a permanent tribute to the thousands of members who made the headquarters possible.

Arthur S. Fleming, Secretary of Health, Education, and Welfare, gave the Dedicatory Address. The souvenir booklet pictured the four-square building of Georgian design and its interior with a list of member contributors. (A description of the building, the adaptation of the space to departments, and a history of the Dupont Circle site may be found in Appendix E.)

---

* 1,006 members gave $100; they were memorialized in naming the first floor hall "The Century Room." The 50 who gave $500 had their names inscribed on a tablet in "The Modern Founders" Room, a mahogany panelled room with a fireplace that was to house an autographed collection of members' books, and a hoped-for set of portraits of the founding fathers.

In the five-year period from 1958 to 1963 during the Directorship of Matthew Ross, the collection of portraits of the leaders of American Psychiatry was begun. Around the third floor lobby were hung the pictures of APA Presidents during the Association's first 100 years. The collection was assembled by Robert Goodhammer for the centennial celebration of APA in Philadelphia (1944). Portraits of Presidents of the second hundred years were hung on the spiral staircase. Those of speakers of the Assembly and of medical directors were on the walls of the central offices on the second floor.

In the lobby was a handsome antique grandfather's clock with Westminster chimes (made in 1780 and valued at $2,000 in 1961), the gift of Dr. and Mrs. Saul Heller.

The Century Room walls were adorned by portraits of the 13 founding fathers (see Appendix F for artists and donors of these and others that followed). Above the fireplace mantel was hung a portrait of Dorothea Dix. The portrait of Adolf Meyer and his collected papers were placed in the library. Also obtained were a self-portrait of Benjamin Rush, portraits of R. Finley Gayle and Solomon Carter Fuller, the Dewey Cup, the *Journal* editor's footstool, and the President's medallion, a gift from Great Britain's Royal College of Psychiatrists.

Expansion Again

With foresight, the governing Board of the Association purchased (1960–1963) the property adjacent to the APA's headquarters, at 1807, 1809, and 1811 R Street, at costs of $42,000, $25,000, and $22,500, respectively. Later, cumbersome negotiations were pursued to secure the first option to purchase the adjacent 18th Street properties occupied by the USSR Educational Mission, contingent upon the building of a new Soviet Embassy complex in another part of the District of Columbia. Also planned was the purchase of another parcel of land behind the USSR property, to provide easy egress and additional parking. This step was never taken. An opportunity presented itself at about this time to acquire the building (owned by the National Park Service) directly across 18th Street for $225,000 in which APA was renting space. It was decided not to go ahead with this purchase.

With Barton's arrival as Medical Director in 1963, the long talked about central office became a reality with the closing of the

Toronto and New York offices. None of the personnel accepted the offer to transfer, so new personnel were hired in Washington. Growth in all aspects of APA staff activities soon filled all available space.

Planning for expansion, the House Committee extensively reviewed the options: the purchase of a 10-story building on 7th Avenue; purchase of a building on R Street; purchase of new land in Virginia, Maryland, or the District of Columbia; or the construction of a large building into which the APA could expand. Their final recommendation to the governing board was to build an annex and remain at R Street because of the desirability of the Dupont Circle area, with its good transportation and location near other national association headquarters.

In December 1963, just five years after moving into the building at 1700 18th Street, the governing Council approved the construction of a three-story building conforming to the Georgian architecture of the headquarters, to be built on the already owned R Street properties.

The same architect, engineer, builder, and interior decorator who had worked on the renovated headquarters building a decade earlier were employed. Construction was begun in 1966 and completed in 1967. Zoning restrictions forbade building offices in a residential zone, but did allow a museum and library which suited the Association's purposes to provide space for its educational activities. The building above ground was restricted to 60 percent of the land, so two floors occupying all the land were constructed below ground. During the excavation of the foundation, the long forgotten covered-over tributaries of Rock Creek (either Slash or Brown Run or, less likely, the Tiber Creek) necessitated adding six inches of concrete to the foundation slab and a battery of three pumps in the second basement to prevent any water from seeping into the structure.

The Museum Building cost, exclusive of land, was $660,000. It could not be connected to the headquarters because of zoning restrictions, although provision to connect the two buildings was built into the structure should the zoning be changed (see Appendix G).

For the dedicatory exhibit in September 1967, an attractive program guide described the Weisman collection of primitive art, an Adolf Meyer exhibit, a diorama of the founding of the Association, an exhibit of books written by the founding fathers, a history of the *American Journal of Psychiatry,* and a national art exhibit of works by mental patients.

During the years in which Robert Cohen served as curator (1967–1972), a five-year plan for a permanent exhibit on the history of psychiatry was developed, and notable exhibits were shown and enjoyed by visiting groups of students on the work of Adolf Meyer, Dorothea Dix, patient art, evaluation of ECT, and the founders of psychiatry.

At the same time the Museum Building was being constructed, the Board authorized $100,000 for renovations to the headquarters building ($94,500 was spent). This included improvement of the heating and air conditioning systems, replacement of old plumbing with copper pipes, division of the Modern Founders Library into two offices with conference room space in each for the Medical and Deputy Medical Directors (the mahogany panels and unusual lighting fixtures were matched to retain the beauty of the room); harmonizing of new draperies, refinished furniture, and new carpeting; painting of exterior and interior; and landscaping of grounds with new hedges, flowering plants, and shrubs (including a flourishing yew from a rooted cutting of one originally planted by Dorothea Dix).

Five years after the opening of the Museum Building, the projects secured with outside funding had expanded into the National Parks Building on 18th and R Streets and into rented quarters on Connecticut Avenue. The need for more space 10 years later (1977) generated so much pressure that once again the decision had to be made to either add another structure or move elsewhere.

The economic climate became worrisome in the late 1970s with recession and soaring inflation. There was a decline in the number of residents entering psychiatry. A considerable number of APA members favored curtailment of activities and retrenchment to fit available space with another building renovation. However, the majority held a more optimistic view that expansion would continue. Because of zoning restrictions at 18th and R, remaining in a residential area with piecemeal additions seemed infeasible; therefore, the directive was given to move elsewhere.

A detailed analysis was made in 1978 (by Frederick Ameling, Ph.D., a leading financial expert, and by the American Security and Trust, consultants) of the relative cost of leasing space and building an APA-owned building to cover a 30-year period. As a consequence of the study, the APA purchased land at Connecticut Avenue and Hillyer Place, N.W. (still in the Dupont Circle area) at a cost of $886,000, and contracted with Hartman-Cox Company, (architects) to draw plans for the venture, estimated to cost $6.4 million, including land. Through foresight, there was established a reserve account of $2 million for future expansion, leaving approximately $3.5 million to be raised after the sale of the APA Headquarters and Museum Buildings (which had appreciated in value to $1.5 million).

This venture came to a grinding halt when Ellen's Irish Pub, located on the site, was declared a national historical building to be preserved. The land at Connecticut and Hillyer Avenues was sold at a profit after commissions were paid ($1,046,768).

The Museum Building at 1801 R Street was sold in 1983 to the American Jewish War Veterans for $1.2 million, and the building at 1700 18th Street was sold in 1985 for $1.1 million.

Embarking on a new plan (which the Assembly and Board approved on October 20, 1979), the APA purchased land at 1400 K Street, N.W. (the site of the former Ambassador Hotel) for $5,187,470.* This was a reasonable price, for a similar site two blocks south had sold for $9.5 million. A contract was signed with a real estate developer for the construction of a modern 12-story office building of 170,000 square feet. J.B.G. Associates and A. James Clark began construction of the building with a groundbreaking ceremony on October 25, 1980. The District of Columbia Mayor, Marion Barry, delivered the welcoming address, praising the APA for participating in the development of a vital portion of the capital. Under the contract, the APA rented space (on the second, third, and fourth floors) at below market value, with provisions to add more space as needed. At the end of 45 years, the lease of J.B.G. Associates will end and the APA will own the building outright. After nearly 50 years, maintenance of an old building becomes expensive, and the space unsuited to the changes in function.

The new headquarters building has a four-story underground parking garage, and features a facade of tinted glass and architec-

---

* See Appendix H for history of this area of Washington.

tural concrete designed by architects Skidmore, Owings, and Merrill, and built by OMNI Construction Company. The approximate construction cost was $15 million. Space needs for the foreseeable future seemed solved, as the APA can expand beyond the floors filled at occupancy. Lease cost to the APA for 1982 for 48,471 square feet was $775,536 per year ($16 per square foot). In 1983 an additional 5,400 square feet on the fifth floor was leased at a cost of $125,120 per year.

Financing and building (APA land and rental) was supported by reserves, sale of the properties at Connecticut and Hillyer, at 1700 18th Street, and at 1801 R Street, and by a voluntary fund drive under the leadership of Francis Braceland. The drive fell short of its goal of $300,000, so a general assessment was levied on all members and fellows of the Association.

The organizational environment of the permanent national headquarters brought all staff components together, facilitating close working relationships in adequate space. The huge glass box of a building, similar in appearance to others close by, fronts on K Street, a busy thoroughfare with shops, hotels, restaurants, buses, and the subway. A small park can be seen from east side offices. The southern side adjoins a city area on 14th Street of porno shops and "adult" movies that cater to human lust.

The entrance to the APA building resembles any office building lobby—a hard floor with a bank of elevators and the bustle of people entering and leaving. The third floor houses a spacious library—the Dan and Logan Readers Lounge—with staff offices on the periphery and stacks of books and journals on the interior. It is on the third floor that the admission to the APA headquarters acquires distinction. Entering glass doors designating it as the American Psychiatric Association, one is greeted by a receptionist and an area decorated with attractive furnishings and Benjamin Rush's portrait. Supervisory staff and administrative offices are attractively furnished on the periphery, with staff support and work space on the interior. Fourth and fifth floor offices follow a similar pattern with ample meeting room space for business administration and program and project activities staff.

With excellent leadership in all APA staff units, superior employees who relate well to each other, and dedication to the mission of the APA, the new environment creates the impression of administrative efficiency.

THE GROWTH OF THE AMERICAN PSYCHIATRIC ASSOCIATION'S PROGRAMS

Care of Patients in the Public System

The sorry state into which care of mental patients had fallen as a consequence of staff and budget depletion due to World War II was well publicized in the media. A summary of the abysmal level of care of the mentally ill was Albert Deutsch's *Shame of the States* (11).

An aroused American Psychiatric Association made an immediate and total response to correct system defects and to improve patient care. Earlier I described the establishment of the Mental Hospital Institute (1949). A Mental Hospital Section was created in the annual meeting program of the Association; achievement awards were given to stimulate competition to make innovative improvements, and communication with the field was facilitated through the journal *Mental Hospitals* (now *Hospital and Community Psychiatry*). The Central Inspection Board was established with surveys made to improve organization and service. Contracts were drawn up and a contract survey board entered into agreement with states and institutions to advise on system changes. An Architectural Project joined the American Institute of Architects and APA to stimulate improvement in the design of hospitals. Standards for psychiatric hospitals were revised and updated. A certification process to improve the competence of hospital administrators was instituted. All of these programs and projects were products of the innovative leadership of Daniel Blain, the Medical Director during the years 1949–1958.

Planning for Service Delivery

During this burst of organizational activity, political activism stimulated Congress to pass the Mental Health Study Act (1955) which directed the Joint Commission to evaluate, analyze needs and resources, and make recommendations for a national mental health program. A vigorous effort and total commitment by the APA helped the public system to change and to improve patient care (12, 13).

Resource Development

If the level of care of patients in the public system was to be improved, there must be available psychiatrists and mental health professionals in sufficient numbers to carry out the mission. The training of professional personnel was one part of the National Mental Health Act (PL 79–487). This legislative act was the most important event in the history of the mental health movement. The act led to establishment of NIMH (1949), which arranged its major functions under Training, Clinical Services, and Research. When Congress passed the Mental Health Study Act (1955) (PL 84–182), the Joint Commission on Mental Illnesses and Health analyzed professional needs and, in *Mental Health Manpower Trends*, Vol. 3 (14), documented the complexity of the problem and the extent of the shortages in the core professions (psychiatry, clinical psychology, psychiatric social work, and nursing). Shortages were related to deficiencies in the system of secondary and higher education, and to the public perception of mental health professionals with its impact upon the stimulation of bright young students to choose a career in the mental health field. The brightest must complete college studies before going to medical school or to other professional schools. The teaching of psychiatry and the quality of supervised practice in the mental health system helped to determine the selection of psychiatry, clinical psychology, psychiatric social work, or psychiatric nursing over the competitive interests of other medical specialties or other professional fields. Albee (14) stated, "sufficient professional personnel to eliminate glaring deficiencies in our care of mental patients will never become available if the present population trend continues without a commensurate increase in the recruitment and training of mental health manpower" (14, p. 259).

The formation of a National Manpower Council (1957), an APA Committee on Manpower (1960), and a National Commission on Mental Health Manpower were indicative of broad interest in professional development. In 1963, the APA established a Division of Manpower Research under Robert F. Lockman, which published three informative reports that established the essential data base for psychiatry.

A national survey of all identifiable psychiatrists was undertaken. Three publications summarized the findings: *The Nation's Psychiatrists* (15); *Psychiatric Services, System Analysis, and Man-*

power Utilization (16); and *The Nation's Psychiatrists: 1970 Survey* (17). An NIMH symposium held in 1967 at Airlie House led to the publication of *Manpower For Mental Health* (18); a 1966 Macy Conference on *Women in Medicine* was followed by a volume of the same title (19). The APA and the National Commission on Mental Health Manpower, with the help of Roche Laboratories, published *Careers in Psychiatry* in 1968 (20).

The APA joined the Coalition for Health (AAMC, AMA, and others) to lobby for adequate budgets for the public mental health system. Also formed was a coalition of national organizations on manpower issues, and a Liaison Group on Mental Health to inform each participant group on positions to be taken on pending legislation (and to work toward a consensus, if possible). This flurry of activity in the 1960s was highly successful in gaining support both in fiscal and social policy formation, with direct benefit to the mental health field.

Community Mental Health Centers

The American Psychiatric Association has played a central role in the Community Mental Health Center Movement, from its ancestry, conception, birth, growth and development, and turbulent adolescence, to its present state of rebellion against its origin (21–27). In order to better explain the background of community mental health centers, I will trace some of the history surrounding family and community care, already mentioned in Chapter 6.

As I have already mentioned, community care of the mentally ill in 18th- and early 19th-century America was replaced by institutional care. Wretched neglect and an inhumanity in the community gave way to compassionate care in asylums, with discipline and structured activity in rural settings away from stressful family interrelationships. Moral treatment restored many persons in the early period of small institutions.

Not all mental hospital superintendents accepted the institutional care system for all patients. In 1853, John M. Galt II outraged Kirkbride, Earle, and Ray, his fellow members in the Association of Medical Superintendents of American Institutions for the Insane. He called New England asylums "mere prison houses" and said "the insane are susceptible of a much more extended liberty than they are now allowed" (28). He proposed the placement of some residents on a farm or in a family home (as in use at Gheel for 500 years), where the chronically insane might work "to tend toward restoration of sanity" (28).

It took 30 years (1885) until a large-scale application of Galt's premise was tested in Massachusetts, with the beginning of a family care program (31). Other states were slow to follow, for it was not until the 1930s–1950s that family placement became an accepted model as an alternative to the mental hospital.

Adolf Meyer contributed the view of the patient as a whole person with social as well as biologic and psychologic constructs; with his wife as social worker, visits were made to the patient's home. In 1915, Meyer advocated an integrated program of prevention, treatment, aftercare, participation by family physicians, and the organization of care within defined geographic areas (32).

The National Committee for Mental Hygiene made a significant contribution to the Community Mental Health Movement with its insistence on involvement of nonmedical personnel in patient care, and in the use of interdisciplinary personnel in clinics (32). This concept was put into practice in the Child Guidance clinics of the early 1900s.

Thomas Salmon's advocacy of screening recruits upon induction and early treatment of psychiatric disorders during World War I was later incorporated into community mental health center practice (1960–1970).

Other significant advances in community care were the psychopathic hospital (1902) and the general hospital psychiatric unit (1930s). Essential elements in the concept of community care of patients were: the development of the halfway house (1879); aftercare (1880s); the day hospital (1935); social clubs (1944); Amsterdam's district plan (1930, with home visits and supervision in the community) and The Acre (a prototype of the Community Mental Health Center in the 1950s); the Worthing Plan of England's Graylingwell Hospital; and the rise of outpatient psychiatry (29, 30).

Also needed for an understanding of the ancestry of community mental health centers is an understanding of the change in social philosophy. Social Darwinism and the belief in an irrevocable heredity were rejected in favor of the belief that the social, economic, and political environment had a significant effect upon the individual. "Crucial elements in individual maladjustment were the social and legal matrix in which illness or instability occurred" (33). Environmental manipulation, a better social setting, a job, housing, and absence of discrimination were steps that could be taken to alleviate stress on the individual, and to ease emotional and psychological problems.

Eric Lindemann developed "crisis theory." Group therapy became widely practiced, and Maxwell Jones popularized the therapeutic community. Social studies of communities documented the link between environment and health, and research in hospitals demonstrated the importance of social factors on the health of the disadvantaged—the poor and the alienated. The federal government responded with funded programs to correct inequities.

The idea of the Community Mental Health Center Movement was conceived at a time when socio-political liberalism was associated with the belief that "social conditions cause mental illness, so [one must] change social conditions" (32–34).

The parents of the Community Mental Health Center Movement were the APA's Kenneth Appel, AMA Council on Mental Health's Leo Bartemier, and their associates, who formed the Joint Commission on Mental Illness and Health in 1955 with the 36 participating organizations. The recommendations of that group in *Action for Mental Health* (35) led Robert Felix (head of NIMH), with some help from the Braceland Committee, to draw up the blueprint for the CMHC Movement. The APA leaders at the time were Felix (President, 1961); Barton (President, 1962); Branch (President, 1963); Ewalt (President, 1964); with those already mentioned— Leo Bartemier (President, 1952), Kenneth Appel (President, 1954), and Francis Braceland (President, 1957). Dan Blain, George Tarjan, and Karl and William Menninger were active behind the scenes to insure implementation of the proposed program. NAMH joined in national and state programs to reach policy and opinion molders. The APA brought state mental health officials, political leaders, organization heads (AMA–AHA), and key congressmen together to insure action.

When President Kennedy, in the first mental health message to Congress in 1963, announced "a bold new approach" with a shift in patient care from hospitals to community centers, swift passage of legislation PL 88–164 (1963) followed to give birth to the Community Mental Health Center Movement. Later amendments (from 1965 on) and federal regulations would provide support and staffing money for defined essential services.

The widely heralded birth was followed by APA–NAMH studies (with NIMH help) to foster healthy growth and development. The Joint Information Service (APA–NAMH) under Raymond Glasscote issued a series of informative reports calling attention to models of successful practice (21–23).

The *American Journal of Psychiatry*, and, in particular, APA's *Hospital and Community Psychiatry*, carried many articles on community mental health centers in the 10-year span from 1965–1975. Annual meeting programs and Hospital and Community Psychiatry Institutes featured studies, reported progress, and gave achievement awards to innovative community programs.

The APA Task Force on Community Mental Health Services (1980), the Group for the Advancement of Psychiatry (1983), and others (Barton and Sanborn in 1977) made critical comments on performance (32, 36, 37). The increasing dominance of the mental health professions in the community mental health centers, with a reduction in the role of psychiatrists, disturbed the APA. Often the physician was relegated to signing insurance forms in order to secure funding, and to prescribing drugs (sometimes without seeing the patient). Responsibility for diagnosis and treatment was often taken by nonmedical personnel, and the medical model rejected for a social one.

Nine major assumptions on which the community mental health center program was based were examined by GAP (32). These assumptions were that community care is 1) less expensive; 2) better; 3) comprehensive and beneficial; 4) continuous in care; 5) essential and accessible; 6) largely due to an environment that produces mental illness; 7) enhanced by designating a catchment area for provision of services; 8) favorable to preventive efforts to reduce the incidence and prevalence of mental illness; and 9) aided by local responsibility and local control. Most of the assumptions, GAP concluded, were unproven, with little evidence of validity.

There were additional goals of community mental health centers cited by Barton and Barton (38): early detection and early application of treatment seeking to restore individuals to the highest possible level of independent activity; strengthening of health producing factors and diminishing of health inhibiting factors; and being responsive to both community and individual health needs.

The community mental health centers were launched with enthusiasm and high hopes. Twelve years later, in 1975, critics called the movement a failure, with most psychiatrists expressing doubts and pessimism about its future (38).

The events that produced obstacles to the success of the community mental health centers may be summarized as follows:

- The 1965 Amendments to the Community Mental Health Centers Act changed the original stipulation that directors be psychiatrists, and channeled federal funds directly to communities (to satisfy the AMA and the Republican party), by-passing state mental health authorities.
- NIMH lost its constituency and found no new one in communities.
- Responsible community control was not to be expected, as facts attested. There were local power struggles: catchment areas didn't match local political districts; the size of the CMHC budget dislocated the local budget; and the state continued to influence policy under their broad mandates. In addition, directors lacked administrative skills (36).
- An APA Task Force on CMHCs (Task Force Report #4, 1972) was strongly supportive of the purpose of the CMHC and endorsed the CMHC as a major response to changes in medical practice. It called for integration of services in the catchment area with active treatment and rehabilitation, and for close working relationships between the medical community and the human service delivery system. It further urged return to physician–psychiatrist directors of CHMCs.

The APA, under Perry Talkington (President, 1972–1973), and Smith, Kline and French President's Fund Grant, developed the project "closing the gaps," in which findings published in *Delivery of Mental Health Service* (37) state that it is essential to improve: accessibility and quality; aftercare; emergency services; scope of services to children, adolescents, and elderly; and public education.

The U.S. General Accounting Office evaluated CMHC services in 1977, with the following findings:

- The reputed census drop in state mental hospitals due to CMHC activities was refuted as only a phenomenon due to transfer to nursing homes and board-and-care homes.
- Rather than care for the deinstitutionalized population, CMHCs provided services to those with normal problems in living. There

was no evidence that CMHCs were less costly than mental hospitals.

- NIMH had only limited ability to influence local programs.
- Extensive fragmentation of services existed (36).

Social and political activism (for better housing, jobs, welfare entitlements, education, recreation, voting rights, antidiscrimination, and even street crossing-signals) dissipated scarce health dollars without reducing either incidence or prevalence of mental illness. With psychological and social factors seen as causative, the biological factors were downplayed. Mental health professionals selected the troubled and worried, and avoided the chronically and seriously mentally ill.

Threats of cuts and reduction in federal support made funding of CMHCs unstable. In the economic squeeze, survival sometimes skewed patient selection to those who could pay for psychotherapy, with the result being neglect of the poor.

One response to the growth of a nonmedical mental health system was a rapid expansion of general hospital psychiatric units (to over 1,000 as compared with 700 federally funded CMHCs). The general hospital could provide emergency service, inpatient, outpatient, and day hospital care, as well as consultation services to patients either in hospital or in outpatient clinics. As more psychiatrists abandoned the mental health center, they sought general hospital appointments.

In the decade from 1975–1985, psychiatry moved closer to medicine; community medicine departments were established; emergency medicine became a specialty area of practice; and ambulatory care was the favored setting for therapy.

The Community Mental Health Center provided an early model for health care delivery. The opportunity existed for utilizing the health agencies in the community coordinated to serve patient needs. The wisdom of planning to meet a community's health needs was illustrated, and responsibility for the catchment area seen as feasible, albeit with boundaries more flexible and based upon more than geography and numbers alone.

Financing Patient Care Through Insurance Programs

The APA contributed significantly to the inclusion of psychiatric benefits in insurance plans (39). Insurance coverage for mental illness was a priority area for APA effort for 27 years (1957–1984).

In the years 1957–1958, the APA sponsored a session at its annual meeting in May (1957) entitled "Health Insurance and Psychiatric Coverage" (40); and the Council on Mental Health of the AMA held a national conference entitled "Coverage of Mental Illness in Blue Shield Plans" (November 1957). Discussion in the following year provided the ferment that led to a joint study by Group Health Insurance (GHI) of New York, the APA, and the National Association of Mental Health, to answer the question, "Is short-term psychiatric treatment insurable?"

With the help of an NIMH grant, a sample of 76,000 GHI subscribers was covered for up to 15 outpatient treatment sessions and up to 30 days of inpatient care without additional charge. This study was made in New York City at a time when the state Blue Cross plan excluded care for mental illness, and at a time when over 130 million people in the U.S. had insurance coverage for medical and surgical illnesses.

The findings of the study, begun in July of 1959 and reported by Helen Avnet in *Psychiatric Insurance* (41), demonstrated that three out of four patients seen were recovered or improved under the provided benefits in an average of 10 outpatient visits or an average hospital stay of 23 days. Because approximately one-half of the patients treated in the office used the maximum benefit (mostly under psychoanalytic therapy) and one-half of these continued treatment after termination of the benefits, the cautious conclusion was "In the present stage of acceptance of psychiatry there appears to be little danger that the costs of insuring the extent of covering offered by the Project would be prohibitive if spread over an average cross section of the 1960 population" (41, p. 258).

The Chairman of the GHI study, Harvey J. Tomkins (Advisory Committee), and John M. Cotton (APA District Branch Committee) would continue to be central figures in APA actions on behalf of insurance coverage for mental illness.

In 1963, Daniel Blain (APA's President-Elect), with Harvey Tompkins, John Cotton, Perry Talkington, and others, joined in a series of exchanges between the union (Melvin Glasser, Director of Social Security Department, UAW) and management of the automobile industry that led to securing (in 1966) the first dollar coverage for psychiatric disorders for 4.2 million workers.

In 1965, Blain and Barton secured an NIMH grant to fund Phase I of a three-phase research project. Phase I (1965–1967), based at APA (under Robert Pfeiler, assisted by Linda Loy), studied patterns of referral, utilization (under- or overutilization), and the characteristics of users. With the help of an APA Task Force on Prepaid Insurance and the UAW staff (Melvin Glasser, Karl Kirshman, and Thomas McPartland), and APA Assembly liaison representatives, visits were made to 30 cities with concentrations of UAW workers, and contacts were made in 47 other cities to familiarize those concerned with the terms of the UAW benefit package and to conduct data collection on preutilization.

Phase II of the project (1967–1971) was solely the responsibility of the Michigan UAW staff—they collected data on utilization as well as on characteristics of users of the benefit package.

During Phase I and II, and before Phase III began, APA was involved in three highly significant activities that profoundly influenced the field (production of guidelines, inclusion of benefits in Medicare and Medicaid, and Joint Information Service data).

An APA workshop (Cotton, Talkington, and others) brought together psychiatrists and agencies such as the National Association of Private Psychiatric Hospitals and the National Association of State Mental Program Directors in 1965, and developed APA's *Guidelines for Psychiatric Services Covered Under Health Insurance* (42). To discuss and elaborate the APA position, insurance companies, self-insured corporations, and interested others were convened, which led to wide adoption and to revision of the original guidelines. This document and the process to insure implementation did profoundly influence the third parties.

The APA actively worked to introduce coverage for mental illness into federal legislation in Medicare and Medicaid (1965–1966). At the outset, APA representatives (Walter Barton, Robert Gibson, Stuart Gould, Howard Rome, Harold Visotsky, John Donnelly, and Leonard Ganser) were told the pending legislation was too important to risk failure by adding psychiatric benefits. It is certain that without the extraordinary effort made by the APA, psychiatric benefits would not have been included as they were when the legislation was finally passed.

Phase III of APA's Insurance Project began in 1970 with a grant from NIMH. Louis S. Reed, Ph.D., a distinguished health economist and authority on mental health insurance, accepted the post of principal investigator. Assisted by Patricia Scheidemandel* and Evelyn Meyers of the APA staff, and a consultant panel of the country's leading experts in health insurance, *Health Insurance and Psychiatric Care* (43) was published in 1972. The book was the most comprehensive collection of data on the utilization and cost of psychiatric services under public and private insurance programs ever compiled.

The research study revealed that admission rates for mental conditions were from three to five per 1,000 population. The mental health benefit costs ranged from three to six percent of the total costs for all conditions covered by health insurance. In-hospital services, under the high option plan for federal employees, provided a conservative estimate of 5.6 admissions per 1,000 population. Costs (in 1969) were $4.13 per person and equal to 6.3 percent of benefit costs for all conditions. Outpatient costs (1969) were $2.16 per individual (43). The data demonstrated the feasibility of coverage for conditions and provided the basis for APA's slogan "Equal Coverage for Mental Disorders." Copies of the study with a summarizing pamphlet were sent to all Congressmen as an educational tool to facilitate implementation into social policy.

The APA's interest in third party financing of patient services did not end with the completion of the study. The APA, at the federal level, and its District Branches, at the state level, pressed for legislation to include mental health coverage in all health insurance plans. Reed updated the basic data in 1974 (44), and the APA published various additional studies in 1975 (45) and updated the information again a decade later in 1983 (46) and 1984 (47). By the 1980s virtually all health insurance plans offered some coverage for psychiatric service. Approximately 64 percent of insurance programs for hospital service had equal coverage for mental as for other conditions. Nearly all plans had coverage for outpatient services, but only in six percent was it the same for psychiatric services as for other medical service.

---

* Scheidemandel, Charles Kano, and Raymond Glasscote of the APA–NAMH Joint Information Service were co-authors of *Health Insurance for Mental Illness,* with a foreword by the Hon. Earl Warren, Jr.—President of NAMH—published by the APA in 1968.

Treatment

Treatment of the patient and patient care issues became a priority concern of the APA when John Talbott became president in 1984. While the Association, from its founding, was always interested in clinical problems, these had been submerged since the 1970s in the dominant concern with legal, political, social, and guild issues.

Electroconvulsive therapy (ECT) was the subject of the Group for the Advancement of Psychiatry's first report (1947). ECT was the first truly effective therapy producing dramatic results. GAP's Report #1 (48) was directed at the indiscriminant use and abuse of ECT. The report was revised in 1950 (49) to provide indications for usage. The APA issued a Task Force Report on the subject (1978) to reiterate its value as a therapeutic agent when cities and states, badgered by antipsychiatry adherents, pressed for abolition of the use of ECT (50).

The APA issued statements on the efficacy of psychotherapy (51), on biofeedback (52), on treatment planning (53), and on the topic that had been on the 1844 agenda of its first meeting—restraint and seclusion (54).

To keep members abreast of current treatments and other issues in psychiatry, the APA introduced in 1982 a track in its annual meeting program and an annual volume, *Psychiatry Update: The American Psychiatric Association Annual Review* (55).

One of the APA's most ambitious undertakings in the area of therapy was the presidential project (Smith Kline and French Presidents Fund grant) of Jules Masserman (President 1978–1979): the establishment of an APA Commission on Psychiatric Therapies. *The Psychiatric Therapies* (56) was five years in preparation and was the landmark end-product of the Commission's work. Some 45 experts contributed to this state of the art of therapy in 1984.

Confidentiality

When the legitimate right of insurance companies to some information about a patient covered by its benefits threatened the traditional confidentiality of the psychiatrist–patient relationship, the APA issued a policy statement, as noted earlier in this chapter, the *Problems in Confidentiality* (57). Five years later, the APA Task Force's *Report on Confidentiality and Third Parties* (58) expanded and clarified the issues, outlining principles and actions essential to preserving confidentiality.

The dynamic growth of computer technology and the enormous amount of personal information fed into data-gathering machines that could be linked and possibly leak information, thereby violating privacy, threatened to destroy confidentiality. In 1973, a widely publicized break into a psychiatrist's office to steal confidential data from a patient's (Daniel Ellsberg's) record, and the testimony by a White House staff member at Senate hearings that "anybody in a white coat could walk on a hospital ward and look at records," shocked the medical community into joining psychiatrists for corrective action.

The APA took the leadership in inviting representatives of the medical specialty organizations, insurance companies, computer experts, medical record librarians, the AHA, NAMH, mental health lawyers, and consumer groups—50 in all—to a conference entitled Confidentiality of Health Records, November 6–9, 1974, in Key Biscayne, Florida. The report, *Confidentiality* (59), alerted all concerned parties to the threats to privacy and the need for system change. The short volume remains, a decade later, the best and most comprehensive statement on the subject.

A National Commission for the Preservation of Confidentiality of Health Records was formed at the suggestion of Walter Barton (60). The Commission was an information exchange on abuses, promoted guidelines and protective legislation, and encouraged educational activities. The Commission (under Natalie Springgarn as Executive Director) had problems in financing and survived only a few years.

Quality Control

The decade of the 1970s was one of accountability, and marked the beginning of the effort to control health costs that were soaring beyond the inflationary spiral of other cost increases. The Social Security Amendments of 1972 (PL 92–603) "contained an attempt to control costs that required physicians to review the necessity for and to determine the appropriateness of services provided under all federal health care programs" (61, p.175).

The medical profession had long ago developed methods to check on the quality of its services. Weekly clinical pathology conferences in hospitals reviewed accuracy of diagnosis, as did tissue committees. Before the flurry of activity that followed the Social Security Amendments of 1972, Donald Hammersley, of the APA staff, produced a manual in 1968: *Psychiatric Utilization Review* (62).

The AMA attempted to persuade Congress to delete the section on Professional Service Review Organization (PSRO) (PL 92–603). Although it failed in the attempt, it did succeed in making major changes. The American Hospital Association developed a quality assurance program in 1972 (63). In 1973, APA issued policy statements on peer review (64) and on PSRO (65). District Branches were urged to form peer review committees and to join the local medical society's review components on a consultant basis. The APA ad hoc Committee on PSROs developed model criteria sets (66). The *American Journal of Psychiatry* featured a special section on peer review (67), and the APA issued the *Manual on Psychiatric Peer Review* (68). Robert Gibson (APA President 1976–1977) chaired an APA conference and edited the report *Professional Responsibilities and Peer Review in Psychiatry* (69).

The APA entered into contractual agreements to serve as peer review for CHAMPUS, Aetna, and Blue Cross programs. In 1985, it extended its contractual endeavors for related activities. Assurance of quality care in a time of cost containment and budget reductions was a priority issue in the 1980s. This concern was particularly manifested as more psychiatric hospitals and services were drawn into investor-owned for-profit corporations.

Care of Patients with Chronic Mental Disorders

It took approximately 20 years for the backlash resulting from deinstitutionalization to begin, when public clamor aroused the profession to do something about this problem. The APA appointed a Task Force on the Chronic Mental Patient under the leadership of John Talbott. The Group for the Advancement of Psychiatry and the President's Commission on Mental Health also called attention to the problem, and Congress included the chronic patient in Title 1 of the Mental Health Systems Act (70–73).

Talbott advocated programs for the chronic mental patient that included psychopharmacological therapy with monitoring of medication, psychotherapy, socialization, proper housing, rehabilitation, and case management in the following settings: public and private mental hospitals, VA hospitals, nursing homes, community mental health centers, community agencies, and other ambulatory services. Groups to be included were children, adults, the elderly, and those living in rural as well as urban areas. The plight of the homeless mentally ill—the street people—was also the subject of an APA report (74). Awareness of the problem was achieved by the APA, but this was only the beginning of action to better the condition of the chronic patient (by the mid-1980s).

A related problem, essential to patient care, has been the significant loss of psychiatrists working in the public service delivery system. Psychiatrists are difficult to recruit and retain in the state's Departments of Mental Health. They are but a small minority among the Commissioners. No longer are psychiatrists directors of community mental health centers, and only a few continue to work in mental health centers in a subordinate role. Psychiatrist state hospital superintendents have been replaced by mental health professionals or nonmedical managers. The voice of psychiatry in shaping public policy is being lost (13). To study the problem and make recommendations, the APA appointed a Task Force on Psychiatric Leadership in Public Mental Health Programs under the chairmanship of Kenneth Gaver. The ad hoc committee (1982–1983) developed a series of surveys to produce the background data, which demonstrated the flight of psychiatry from the public system and the noted lack of APA or District Branch support. In 1983 the ad hoc committee was disbanded and a committee of the same name formed under the chairmanship of Steven Katz. The group functioned under the Council of Medical Education and Career Development. (The final report has not been published as of this writing.)

Growth of the Profession

The remarkable growth in the numbers of psychiatrists attests to the success of the program for manpower development. Psychiatry has been transformed from a profession isolated from the rest of medicine (in the late 19th century) into a medical specialty (in the first half of the 20th century), and into a major area of instruction in medical schools (after 1950). The series of APA conferences on medical education, at decade intervals, has improved teaching of psychiatry in the medical schools and developed quality education for residents. The APA was one of the first medical organizations to stress the need for continuing medical education, to articulate policy, and provide a mechanism for continued self-assessment to increase clinical competence.

A great deal of effort has been expended to develop a standardized classification of mental disorders. The APA's *Diagnostic and Statistical Manual of Mental Disorders, First Edition (DSM-1)* was the first attempt by any organization in the world to issue an official manual of diagnostic terms in psychiatry. Its successive revisions have demonstrated the move from a symptom oriented typology toward a more etiological focus as scientific discovery permitted. The editors of the *Diagnostic and Statistical Manual of Mental Disorders* (particularly *DSM-III*) have made important contributions, worldwide, to the growth of the profession. The latest revision of this *Manual, DSM-III-R*, will be published in the spring of 1987.

The APA's communication with the field of psychiatry has improved in extent and in quality. From a start without funds, the library of the APA has grown to a modest resource facility. The library started on shelves in the Medical Director's office with books donated and autographed by APA member-authors. By 1967, the library had grown into a small but valuable reference library under John O'Meara and later Jean Jones. The large space in the building at 1400 K Street enabled the library and its head, Zing Jung, to expand its collection, particularly of archival books and materials on the history of psychiatry. The advancement of technology in the field of library science has tied a small resource into a larger one, making retrieval of nearly all significant literature readily available.

Manpower Development

At the end of World War II there were 3,634 psychiatrists in the United States; by 1952, the number had increased to 7,500, and, a decade later, to 13,000. When the APA's leaders Dan Blain, Howard Potter, and Harry Solomon created the Manpower Commission (1960), its studies would document the growth in nationwide surveys. I have already cited the publications in the section entitled "Advances in Psychiatry," so only a few statistics will be given here. The 1965 survey identified 18,740 psychiatrists, of whom 75 percent were born in the United States; approximately 13 percent were women. The 1970 survey identified 25,755 psychiatrists, of whom approximately five percent were non-Caucasian. Psychiatry was third (behind pediatrics and internal medicine) among medical specialties in the proportion of women in the field. The percentage of women in psychiatry and in all of medicine is still increasing in the 1980s.

By 1985 the number of psychiatrists who were members of the APA was over 31,000. Of this number, over 200 were medical student members, and nearly 14 percent of the total membership—4,220 out of 5,100 (82.6 percent)—were members-in-training (residents in psychiatry).

Medical Education

The landmark contributions made by the APA's (1952) medical education conferences have been detailed in Chapter 6, as have been the pioneering ventures in continuing medical education. In the 1980s, the improvement of teaching in the medical schools and in the period of residency training has become the responsibility of two organizations that began informally with meetings (in the 1970s) during the APA's annual meeting: the American Association of Chairmen of Departments of Psychiatry, and the American Association of Directors of Psychiatric Residency Training.

In the late 1960s the APA initiated the first Psychiatric Knowledge and Skills Self-Assessment Program (PKSAPI). After initial experimentation at shorter intervals, the successive offerings (PKSAP III–V), at approximately five-year intervals, attracted an ever increasing number of psychiatrists. The program evolved into a major test program with a large syllabus, variations in test procedures, and feedback on performance. Approximately 75 percent of the several modules dealt with current developments, and 25 percent dealt with basic knowledge.

In the early 1970s, the APA became a partner with the Association of University Programs in Health Administration (AUPHA) in developing a curriculum, continuing education program, and materials for teaching administrative psychiatry. The APA also expanded its annual meeting program to include one-half day as well as full day courses in many areas, including administrative psychiatry for continuing education. More than one hundred courses on many subject areas have been given each year so far in the 1980s.

Communication within the Field of Psychiatry

American Psychiatric Association annual meetings have attracted about 10,000 individuals each year to participate in a rich scientific smorgasboard of current topics. The change in programming in the 35 years from 1950 to 1985 has been truly remarkable. Throughout the years of transition, the psychiatrist has demonstrated motivation to learn. Social and recreational attractions of host cities did not pull many away from the crowded meeting rooms. Political and organizational activities have not expanded significantly, but the scientific aspects have. From Sunday through Friday of the week-long sessions, from early morning until late at night, psychiatrists partake of the offerings: annual reviews, tracks on a subject area, special lectures, panels, debates, new research, symposia, films, videos, breakfast meetings, and after-dinner special sessions.

The quality of its journals (the *American Journal of Psychiatry* and *Hospital and Community Psychiatry*) have continued to improve, with the editors enjoying the privilege of selecting a few "best" papers from hundreds submitted. *Psychiatric News* has been followed by many other regularly published newsletters targeted to selected groups of members: legislative matters both federal and state, public affairs, residents, spouses, ethical issues, minority affairs, and many more, to enhance information exchange of a diverse membership with special interests.

I have already noted that an area of significant achievement was the classification of mental disorders. The *Diagnostic and Statistical Manual of Mental Disorders, First Edition (DSM-I)* emerged out of the perceived need for an official classification by military psychiatrists during World War II. After the APA modified the military's classification, it was published in 1952 and reprinted 20 times. The *Diagnostic and Statistical Manual of Mental Disorders, Second Edition (DSM-II)* appeared in 1967, and was even more widely circulated with sales so large that it could support other, less popular, APA publications. The *Diagnostic and Statistical Manual of Mental Disorders, Third Edition (DSM-III)* (1980) was an even more ambitious venture involving many individuals over several years, and many subcommittees, with extensive field testing before finalization.

DSM-I utilized, in its classification, the term "reactions," reflecting the influence of Adolf Meyer's views of mental disorders as reactions of the personality to psychological, social, and biological factors. When *DSM-II* was developed an attempt was made to simplify universal coding by relating it to the International Classification of Diseases (ICD–8). The term "reaction" was replaced with terms in general use, without implying any particular theoretical allegiances. While APA collaborated on the ICD–9, a decision was made to develop an official manual for the United States that would not only be a clinical standard, but would also be useful in research and administration. This was to become the *DSM-III*. New knowledge was incorporated when research data attested to its validity. Disorders were described in great detail and generally without regard to etiology. A multiaxial evaluation system was introduced in *DSM-III*, assigning personality and development disorders to Axis II, physical disorders to Axis III, severity to Axis IV, and highest level of adaptive capacity to Axis V.

Insufficient time has elapsed to judge the impact of *DSM-III*. It appears that because of promotional and educational endeavors it has been a worldwide best seller and a standard guide to clinical diagnosis.

THE LOCUS OF POWER IN THE ORGANIZATION: POLICY DEVELOPMENT

The locus of power within the organization was to shift, and the structure to dramatically change, during the second half of the 20th century.

It is fortunate that the legacy of John C. Whitehorn (President, 1950–1951) clarified APA structure of governance and APA process of policy formation in a *Manual of Organization and Policies* (1951). Whitehorn was Professor of Psychiatry and occupied the Chair formerly occupied by Adolf Meyer at Johns Hopkins University. As a laboratory biochemist and superb clinician and academician, his flair for administration was unexpected.

The power in the organization (1951) resided within the governing Council, whose spokesman was the President. There were 16 councilors—4 officers and 12 councilors (officers were elected annually and councilors served a three-year term). The Council, and its designated officers, were virtually unchanged from the time of the second constitution and reorganization of the APA in 1892.

A new power base developed with the Medical Director and his support staff. With the appointment of Dan Blain, a strong leader, it took but a few years to accumulate prestige and authority to set APA's course. In his 1946 Presidential Address at the 102nd annual meeting, Karl Bowman (President, 1944–1946) called for the appointment of a full-time psychiatrist as Medical Secretary rather than a Medical Director, warning "having both a Medical Director and a President would create a great deal of confusion as to just who is the head of the Association" (*New Directions*, pp. 15–31, 1946). Bowman's suggestion went unheeded.

The high visibility of the Medical Director, who traveled throughout the country, visited local societies and hospitals, communicated directly with members via *The Bulletin* and *Mail Pouch* and later in all APA publications, represented the Association at meetings other than APA's, formed working relationships with medical specialty associations, developed projects, answered queries from the news media and the public, and possessed the detailed information upon which the governing bodies depended for their decision-making, inevitably filled the role as Association leader. Furthermore, the Medical Director was continuous in office over a span of years, while the other officers changed at regular intervals.

A third base of power—the Assembly—took over 20 years to mature. The desire to make the Association a more democratic organization grew along with an expanding membership in the Association. The "town meeting" style of the annual meeting (at which officers and councilors were elected from a single slate of candidates presented by the Nominating Committee, and at which Council actions were reviewed by assembled members) was no longer acceptable. For example, in 1946, only 300 votes were cast at the annual business meeting when the membership approached 5,000.

The Reorganization Committee, appointed by President Karl Bowman in 1944 (under the Chairmanship of Karl Menninger), after four years of study, reported its recommendations at the annual meeting in Washington, D.C., in 1948. The carefully studied plan had been formulated after reviewing the governance of other similar organizations, including the American College of Physicians and the American Medical Association. The so-called Menninger Plan followed the AMA model. To make the Association a representative one, it was proposed to form a House of Delegates made up of representatives of the entire membership elected by their local constituent District Branches. The House of Delegates (Legislative) would choose the Association's officers and determine policy, while a Board of Trustees (Executive) would become the administrative arm.

The reception to the report was mixed: some approved, others were suspicious, a few anxious, and the majority hostile; and so they voted their disapproval. The passion and unfortunate rhetoric that characterized the election of officers at the Washington meeting (mentioned in Chapter 5) was the subject of unfavorable publicity.

The Reorganization Committee had expected thorough discussion of their plan. During the years of study, as I have mentioned earlier, only eight percent of members responded to the Committee's questionnaire survey.

Why, then, was there an emotional rejection of a plan that would, 25 years later, be the one the Assembly would fight to attain? It is not enough to say it was ahead of its time. Karl Menninger as Chairman of the Reorganization Committee was also a member of the Group for the Advancement of Psychiatry. Some of the hostility toward that "elitist" leadership group (whose membership represented a veritable "who's who" in psychiatry) was displaced from GAP to the Menninger Plan. The Group for the Advancement of Psychiatry was seen as pushing APA in the direction of broader involvement in social issues by those who saw psychiatry in the position of liaison between medicine and society. To accomplish this, objective change in both attitudes and the organizational structure was essential to facilitate response to social issues and a consultant liaison role. As I have already noted, many of those opposed would join "Robbie's Rangers" to preserve standards—the priority of providing clinical services to patients.

The proposed reorganization plan was seen not only as a move in the direction of greater involvement of psychiatry in social issues, but as the adoption of an AMA model. From 1946–1950, the AMA was not held in high esteem by psychiatrists, and few were APA members. The AMA House of Delegates was perceived as ultra-

conservative, whereas psychiatry was perceived as liberal in orientation. Underscored was the attitude of indifference of the APA (as
distinct from the APA leadership group embroiled in the display of
emotion) to organizational squabbles, for members had enough
problems in their clinical practices to consume all of their energies.

The Reorganization Committee, under the chairmanship of D.
Ewen Cameron, went back to the drawing board and came up with
a revised plan (its final report) at the 1949 annual meeting in
Montreal. Cameron, with the skills of negotiation and bargaining,
built on the existing constitutional provision to establish District
Branches. He proposed the creation of an Assembly of District
Branches, whose representatives, elected locally, would meet to
consider matters sent to it by the Council. While limited in power,
it would, Cameron suggested, be a place for training the future
leaders of the APA. The members assembled at the annual business meeting voted for adoption of the plan.

The accumulation of power by the Assembly was a slow process
that took place over two decades. It was a happy coincidence that
the principal architect of the Assembly, D. Ewen Cameron, was
then President of the APA (1952–1953), and was the one who
called to order the first meeting of the Assembly in 1953. Cameron
told the assembled delegation from 16 District Branches, "There is
a time for a bold and unyielding stand; there is a place for the slow
waiting and patient persistence at the birth of new custom . . .
Many things that ultimately become valuable and constructive
parts of our daily living were repeatedly rejected by a social
structure not ready to incorporate them. . . . [the idea of an
organization structure for local representatives elected by the
members had been rejected.] Courage, wisdom, and never-ending
persistence are essential" (75).

The Assembly elected as its first Speaker Joseph Abramson and
as its first Recorder, John Saunders. Much early effort of the group
went into the development of a structure, procedure, and the
stimulation of local areas and states to build new branches. Soon
afterward, dissatisfaction arose with the expressed view that "it
was no more than a debating society." In 1955 the Council agreed
that the Assembly could present issues to the Council on its own.
When President Harry Solomon (1957–1958) suggested that the
Assembly might take on some of the duties of the Council, the
prompt response was to ask for the transfer of the membership

processing function to District Branches. This was accomplished three years later.

The rebirth of the idea that the Assembly should be the legislative arm (as in the Karl Menninger Plan) began in 1960. When the Council rejected the change, it was attuned to the indifference of the membership to further change at the time.

The further unfolding of the Assembly's struggle to attain power is tied into the changes brought on by the policy retreats of the Board of Trustees. These retreats brought into being a fourth power base—the Reference Committee.

Efforts to make the organizational components more effective were begun by William Menninger, who, in 1949, was dissatisfied with the inactivity and lack of productivity of the committees. Whiteborn continued the effort with the establishment of an Oversight Coordinating Committee for better planning and clearer objectives for each component.

As these efforts were being made, the expanding power of the Medical Director's office made it possible to give increasing support to APA's committee structure. In 1963 the Council transferred many of its routine decision-making responsibilities on administrative matters (crank-turning operations)—within broad policies—to the Medical Director. This shift, which continued in the next 20 years, increased the power of the Medical Director's office.

The Council (later the Board of Trustees), since its formation in 1892, had always been the policy making body. As the issues on which policy decisions had to be made multiplied with the growth of the Association, and as the complexity of the issues became greater (requiring more background data), the Council first formed a Long Range Planning Committee (1956–1963) to assist in the study of current issues and to bring to it recommendations. A brief summary of some of its many recommendations will give the flavor of its diverse menu of topics considered:

1956

- Develop working relationships with hospitals and departments of psychiatry in the Caribbean and Central America
- Publish a Spanish edition of the *Newsletter* (only one was prepared and received with favor)
- Hold a bilingual divisional meeting in either Florida or Texas, to which Spanish-speaking colleagues would be invited (one was held in Miami with very poor attendance; it was judged a failure)

1961

- Form a liaison committee with Pan American countries to work out relationships (with a possible goal of establishing a Pan American Psychiatric Association)

President Walter Barton, in his Toronto address (*New Direction*, pp. 241–255), suggested APA become a U.S. national organization, and that the psychiatric associations in the defined territory in APA's constitution become a federation, closing the District Branches of APA in Canada. (The Canadian Psychiatric Association, and the psychiatric associations in other countries, were to be autonomous.) Neither Pan American nor Canadian APA members liked the idea. Only a trickle of leaders in psychiatry from other countries joined the APA, with little growth of the APA beyond the U.S. borders. (The APA continued to issue policies that applied only within the U.S., and not within its constitutionally defined areas.)

1963

A special charge was given to answer the question "What should APA be doing five years from now?" The committee chaired by Francis Gerty replied:

- Establish no new affiliate societies—work toward their becoming District Branches
- Give the Assembly authority to set up its own committees
- Have regional representation on Council
- Relate Assembly Policy Committee to Council
- Encourage newsletters in District Branches
- Redirect *Mental Hospitals* magazine for broader audiences: general hospitals, clinics, and CMHCs
- Weed out inactive committees
- Suggest that Chairman of the Coordinating Committee form a steering committee with committee chairman
- Suggest that the APA develop its own continuing medical education (CME) program
- Push for more active APA support for legislation it favors in Congress

Many of the 1963 recommendations of the Long Range Policy Committee were subsequently put into action.

The Council responded to President Blain's (1964–1965) call for a special session (a policy retreat) to answer the question "Is the APA organized to play its appropriate role in dealing with existing problems and pressures which confront the profession of psychiatry as a whole; and if not, what changes are indicated?" The retreat was held at Airlie House (Warrenton, Virginia) on September 11–13, 1963. In addition to the Council and past APA Presidents, invited were the past Speaker and Speaker-Elect, Chairman of the Budget Committee, and a guest—Leo Simmons, a sociologist. The deliberations were divided into goals and priorities, and the structural changes essential to attain them. Thirty-eight Airlie House Propositions emerged, which were widely disseminated for discussion in Assembly and in District Branches before action was taken. It was 2½ years later (January 1966) that the propositions were edited and circulated to all members (76). The proposed structural changes came into being five years after the Airlie House Retreat, when the Council became the Board of Trustees (1969). Structural change was a slow process requiring alteration of the constitution (achieved in 1968).

Propositions dealing with Association goals were more exhortation than action oriented (for example: the objectives of the Association are directed to the people of the United States; we should establish working relationships with associations in other countries; we ought to establish appropriate types of corresponding members; we should avoid nuclear war; we should study ways to prevent war). Some recommendations were modified in the study process, as the following propositions indicate: prohibit District Branches in other countries (some had been already established in Canada); allow no more than one District Branch in a state (some had several); subdivisions within a state should be chapters of the District Branch (where more than one chapter exists, establish a liaison group with authority to speak for the entire state with one voice). A proposition recommended that the Medical Director's Office be the sensor for emerging issues. This was implemented with the creation of an additional body, the Committee on Emerging Issues. Proposition 5 stated that the primary function of the Board of Trustees should be the formulation of basic policies. The wish was expressed that it be relieved of administrative detail. Another recommendation was that the Medical Director develop a manual, *Official Policy Statements*. This was done. Strong local associations were seen as essential in the years ahead (Proposition 25), with a role in support, at the community level, of members and psychiatric facilities.

The most significant outcome of the Airlie House Retreat was the structural reorganizational plan that revamped the committee system, creating the Reference Committee with the authority to accept, reformulate, or reject policy recommendations emerging from groups of experts.*

By the second day of the Retreat, rumor had spread that the Medical Director, Walter Barton, had in his pocket a plan for structural change that might be the sought-after solution. The agenda was cut short to hear the proposal. The purpose of the proposed reorganization plan was to strengthen the role of the Assembly by expanding what was the Council into a Board of Trustees (25 members), which would include the Speaker of the Assembly and the area Trustees nominated and elected by the members in the area. Because a sizable proportion of the total membership was not, at the time, covered by District Branches, their members were to be represented by nationally elected Trustees-at-Large. To provide leadership continuity, the three immediate past presidents would each serve a three-year term on the Board. Five officers (President, President-Elect, Vice-President, Secretary, and Treasurer) comprised the remainder of the Board.

The revamped Committee structure was organized under six Councils, each with a chairman. The six chairmen plus the President-Elect, the Speaker-Elect, and the Medical Director were organized as a Reference Committee. The Reference Committee dealt with overlapping concerns of its Councils and referred matters to and from the Board of Trustees.

Each Council of five members (with a five-year term, one appointed each year by the President with no second term) was assigned an area of responsibility and had under its control Task Forces (the component to be the preferred and usual method to

---

* John K. Galbraith, in his best-selling *The New Industrial State* (Boston, Houghton Mifflin, 1967), insightfully said "briskly conducted meetings invariably decide matters already decided . . . working parties, Task Forces [are the means developed by executives to avoid the disastrous consequences of making decisions themselves] make decisions . . . the product not of individuals but of groups." (Thus the power to make decisions rests in groups.)

deal with an issue) with a clearly defined objective and a time designated in which to meet it. Where necessary, standing committees could still be appointed in the fashion established in the constitution. The original six councils were: 1) Medical Education and Career Development; 2) Mental Health Services, later Psychiatric Service; 3) Research and Development; 4) National and International Affairs (it would later be split into two councils); 5) Professions and Associations (this would later be abolished and its concerns dealt with in a variety of ways); and 6) Internal Organization. In the 1980s, the Councils numbered 11, with: 7) Aging; 8) Children and Adolescents and their Families; 9) Psychiatry and Law; 10) Standards and Economics of Health Care; and 11) as noted above in International Affairs.

The reorganization plan was adopted with a new constitution in 1968. As the Reference Committee had time to study recommended policy, and with the Speaker-Elect (a member who brought issues to the attention of the Assembly for review), the approval process, when brought to the Board by the President-Elect, was expedited. In time (as I have noted) the Reference Committee became the fourth base of power.

A second planning conference was held at the APA offices, December 13–14, 1968. Four objectives were set: to seek consensus on the questions relating to delivery and financing of services; to study ways to involve the Association more actively in the legislative process; to develop a mechanism for establishing an APA position on specific legislation; and to set priorities in appointment of Task Forces.

Participants included not only the ones represented at Airlie House, but also the six Coordinating Councilors, the Assembly Policy Committee, Task Force Chairman on Models of Delivery of Psychiatric Service, Chair of Public Information, the President, President-Elect of the Canadian Psychiatric Association, and six consultants (77).

The format followed by the Conference allowed four keynote speakers to highlight the points made in a paper distributed to attendees for study beforehand. Then summaries were made of the discussions of work groups that met after each presentation.

While the awareness level on the issues was raised in all participants and the deliberations made available to interested readers of the *Journal,* perhaps the most action-oriented outcome was in the area of APA's legislative activities. The recommended legislative liaison officer was appointed—Caesar Giolito. As head of the APA's Government Affairs Department, he would prepare legislative positions which, after review, would be presented at Congressional hearings by selected APA leaders. A network of legislative representatives, with one in each state, was brought to Washington for an annual training seminar, and on-the-job training with visits to their legislators.

Also established were relations with AMA's Washington office, where analyses of pending legislation were shared. A Liaison Group of Mental Health Agencies was formed, composed of those associations that testified on federal legislation. Consensus, if possible, was agreed upon or differences in positions made explicit.

Approximately 50 leaders of the APA participated in the third Trustees Policy Meeting, March 17–20, 1971, held again in Washington, D.C. The format was similar to that used at the 1968 policy retreat. The four topics presented and discussed in small groups were: Should APA establish a separate Political Action Group?; Should APA establish a Peer Group Program for Quality Control?; Does APA have a responsibility to police its members when ethical, moral, incompetent, or negligent matters are suspected?; What should be psychiatry's role in social issues? Also on the agenda was a review of the consequences of the Airlie House Reorganization and possible changes in APA's annual meeting.

The sessions allowed leaders to discuss in depth several pressing current issues and to share their deliberations with the membership via the *Journal* (78). The formation of a political action group was rejected at the time (it would be formed as the Corporation for the Advancement of Psychiatry (CAP), with a Political Action Committee (PAC) in 1981).

The topic on Peer Review and Quality Control produced a recommendation for a Task Force (it was formed, policy statements on both Peer Review and on Professional Service Review Organizations were later issued, model criteria sets developed, and an active APA role in review for CHAMPUS and third party insurers defined).

The agenda items on policy concerned with moral, ethical, and conduct of members led to the recommendation that APA issue Ethical Guidelines and investigate complaints; a hearing was to be the responsibility of the local District Branch, with an appeal mechanism to a national Ethics Committee. The third Trustees

Policy Meeting also reaffirmed APA adherence to the AMA Code of Ethics. *The Principles of Medical Ethics, With Annotations Especially Applicable to Psychiatry,* was issued by the APA in 1973. It detailed the procedures to be followed. The pamphlet was widely disseminated beyond the membership, to educate the field in using the mechanisms when appropriate. Interest in ethical matters accelerated, as did the number of ethical complaints.

The topic on the role of psychiatry in social issues was endorsed as presented by L.J. West in a resolution. It contained 11 points, such as: meeting the public's needs for service; permissiveness and authority in child rearing; the revolt of blacks against segregation; rebellion of students; crime and law-and-order; the change in sexual mores; pollution of the environment; experimentation on humans; and prevention of war. The upshot of the discussion was that the *APA had a responsibility to provide the evidence* when it commented on the mental health aspects of a social issue. The wisdom of accompanying position statements on social issues, providing evidence that referred to scientific theories or experiences establishing the relevance of a particular social issue to mental illness and health, was not always followed in the years after 1971.

The informal agenda at the Third Trustees' Policy Meeting did produce another significant development. A Commission on Legislative Affairs was established to educate members and guide the staff Department on Government Affairs in its formulation of APA positions presented at Congressional hearings.

In 1973, a Policy Retreat was held February 1–3 in Atlanta, Georgia. The agenda was divided into two parts, Internal Affairs and External Affairs (79).

The review of the Association's Internal Affairs noted the increasing influence of the Reference Committee on policy formulation, and also the role of the Medical Director and his staff on policy development. The Assembly did provide a place for discussion of problems, but needed to speed up its ability to respond and to improve its communication with the Board of Trustees. The latter body was viewed as not as efficient as desired.

Perhaps the most significant outcome of the Atlanta Policy Retreat emerged from the deliberations on External Affairs. Noting that it had been 12 years since the publication of the Joint Commission's *Action For Mental Health*, the need for a second joint study was put forward by Perry Talkington (President,

1972–1973). Major changes had occurred in service delivery and in financing. The need for study and for a plan for the future was evident to those assembled (Dr. Talkington reiterated in his Presidential Address, in May of 1973, the need for a new national study). In March of 1974, Bertram Brown, Director of NIMH, and Philip B. Hallen, President of the Maurice Falk Medical Fund, convened a broad cross-section of leaders in New York City to explore the need. In October of that year, a similar group was convened under the auspices of the Robert Wood Foundation. In November 1974, Elliott Richardson spoke of the need for a new commission at the annual meeting of the National Association for Mental Health. A consensus of need for a new study was assumed. With Dale Farabee as head of a planning group (January 1, 1975), there emerged, on April 16, 1975, the Public Corporation for Mental Health. The goals of the group were research programs on the current national system of delivery; definition of problem areas; work with DHEW and appropriate state agencies to improve service; making available to Congress and HEW's Secretary its plan for the best possible mental health service.

It was the ferment in the political process, with the planning and stimulation of the Public Corporation, that led President Carter to appoint the President's Commission on Mental Health, mentioned earlier in this chapter. Translation of recommendations of the study Commission into the Mental Health Systems Act was completed when passed by both houses of Congress and signed into law by the President. However, no funds were appropriated to implement the Act and the effort came to naught.

In March (20–23) of 1975, what was to be called the "Key Conference" was held in Key Biscayne (80). The APA's President was John Spiegel (1974–1975). The President-Elect was Alfred Freedman, who served as Chairman of the Conference. The stated objectives for the policy retreat were:

- To review the internal organization of the APA
- To develop a structure to determine priorities (in a new way— not the one in use at the time, which was a retreat in the summer at a resort area where elected officers, the Speaker, and the Speaker-Elect could informally decide upon priorities for the year)
- To develop more vigorous legislative advocacy

- To explore innovative methods to insure maximum participation of members in APA affairs

The hidden agenda was the goal of shifting power in the organization to the Assembly. The overrepresentation of attendees from the Assembly skewed the outcome. The organization of the conference also shaped the result. Discussion over three days was to be in small groups organized into three coordinating groups: Objectives, Assembly-Board relationships, and Implementation, with the latter having eight groups on the following topics: decision-making, special interests, fiscal, obstacles, staff, Assembly–Reference Committee relations, District Branch, and Area Councils. The first coordinating group was reluctant or unable to grapple with objectives, goals, and how best to attain them, and plunged into the design of a structure to shift power to the Assembly as the "grass roots" representative of members. The Association's mission and objectives were accepted as given, and no modification seemed necessary. A 1974 survey of Council's Committees and Task Forces had turned up few problems, so no changes were suggested. In the style of Assembly procedure, a series of action papers emerged along with 109 propositions. Warren Williams, Speaker of the Assembly (1973–1974), struggled valiantly with the support of his constituency present to gain power and prestige for the Assembly, with the Assembly occupying a central role in the governance of the Association.

A consolidated version of the deliberations was prepared out of the mass of paper, raw data, and tape transcription (80). To deal with it, an ad hoc committee was appointed in December 1975. This body was replaced shortly thereafter by a Joint Conference Committee with equal representation from the Board and the Assembly. For two years they argued and debated the various models of governance. Three designs received the most attention:

Unicameral Assembly: the governing body with an Executive Committee meeting frequently and APA officers to be elected by the Assembly

Bicameral Assembly: lower house, the legislative branch with the Board; upper house, nationally elected, as the executive branch

Reciprocal–Collaborative Assembly and Board: with policy originating in either body to be approved by the other. Differences were to be settled by a referendum. Some components were to report to Assembly, and some to Trustees.

The final report of the Joint Conference Committee was made to the Board of Trustees in December 1977. It proposed a unified system with the Assembly as the primary decision-making body. The Assembly was to be structured with authority over two subdivisions: Area Councils—each headed by an APA Vice President (District Branches and members were under this rubric); and the Executive Board—composed of President, President-Elect, the Immediate Past President, Secretary, Treasurer, and Vice Presidents (the Reference Committee, Councils, and their components were included under this structure).

The APA leadership was out of touch with membership during the three-year struggle, as the Massachusetts Psychiatric Society correctly noted in its call for defeat of the proposal. The amendment to the constitution failed to receive the required two-thirds vote. Members were concerned with problems in practice, indifferent to the power struggle, convinced that "you don't fix it if it ain't broke."

The Association made no radical change in its structure. The Assembly did gain power and prestige. Matters of policy were simultaneously sent to the Assembly and to the Board. Power, by reason of expertise, in the Reference Committee was diluted as Chairmen of Councils were replaced by an equal number of Assembly and Trustee representatives. The Assembly became more democratic with more proportional representation (retaining one vote for 500 members), minority groups were given representatives, and mandatory reporting to constituencies was required.

In the troubled years of the 1960s issues surrounding civil rights, powerlessness, and discrimination intruded into the APA. There were disruptions of sessions at annual meetings, protest marchers, and sit-in protesters who commandeered microphones to make statements. At the Miami meeting in 1969 President Raymond Waggoner (1969–1970) gave black minority members a voice in policy making by designating Observer-Consultants to APA components. Homosexuals sought APA support for help in securing rights. This led to heated debates of the Board regarding the scientific versus political aspects, a referendum, change in *DSM-II*, and a Committee on Gay and Lesbian Issues in the Council on National Affairs.

Women's concerns about representation in governance, and their belief that annual meetings should be held in states ratifying the Equal Rights Amendment, were major concerns in the 1970s. The APA responded with the election of women to the Board, a Committee on Women, a representative in the Assembly, endorsement of the Equal Rights Amendment, and, finally, in the 1980s, the election of a woman Secretary of the APA (Elissa Benedek) and the first woman President (Carol Nadelson, 1985–1986).

The image of psychiatry has become a concern of the Association during the late 1970s and 1980s. For years after World War II, psychiatrists rode the crest of the wave of public optimism, and their dreams of prevention of mental illness, system changes to improve care, reduction of social stress, and even prevention of wars were supported by society. In the present climate of cost containment, there has been a decline in public perception of all physicians. The physician has become the scapegoat for the escalating cost of health care, which has soared to heights well above the inflation rate. When public disapproval of the high cost of therapeutic care began to extend to treatment modalities and the service delivery system, the Association set about image-building.

In the late 1970s the Association began to expand its efforts to improve the public image of psychiatry. A Joint Commission on Public Affairs was established to monitor public image problems and to develop and implement strategies to combat them. Beginning in 1981, the Division of Public Affairs expanded its media relations activities and began formal establishment of a public affairs network. By the end of 1985, public affairs representatives had been identified in all District Branches, and public information committees formed. Local media contacts by District Branches increased, and a national news and feature service was started. The Division of Public Affairs responded promptly to adverse media stories. By 1986, there had been a measurable increase in stories about mental illness and psychiatry in newspapers, magazines, and on television. But as this is written, no evaluation has been undertaken to determine whether this increased attention has changed public attitudes for the better.

Other actions were taken by the Association to improve image. Fees were voluntarily frozen and ethical complaints were promptly investigated through a revision of the ethics complaint process. Ties to medicine and other medical specialty organizations were strengthened. The Medical Director (Dr. Sabshin) and staff (especially Drs. Hammersley, Robinowitz, Sharfstein, and Spurlock) have participated in activities with AMA, AHA, American College of Physicians, Council of Medical Specialty Organizations, Academy of Psychiatry and Religion, Forensic Psychiatry, and National Mental Health Association. In addition, liaison representatives have been designated to many organizations whose activities have touched upon psychiatry's professional concerns, such as the American Academy of Child Psychiatry, the Academy of Family Practice, the American Association of Medical Colleges, the American Bar Association, the American College of Emergency Physicians, the American Women's Medical Association, and many, many others.

Psychiatry and its organizations have struggled to keep abreast of transforming forces during the last 15 years of the 20th century. The pressures for change have been greatest in the setting or environment of care and treatment, in the ties of psychiatry to medicine and its advancing technology, in shifts of emphasis in medical education, and in the authority of the psychiatrist.

The setting of treatment has shifted from the state mental hospital to the "community." The welfare system has become the largest system for care of the mentally ill, with little or no treatment offered. The correction system (usually with no treatment) cares for the mentally ill "when not dangerous to self or others," but when damaging to property or troublesome to society. Psychiatry has abandoned the nonmedical community mental health center system in favor of the general hospital. The latter offers emergency care, outpatient, day treatment, and inpatient care in a medical setting. Ambulatory status has become the principal setting for psychiatric care, with a short stay on a psychiatric unit.

Ties of psychiatry to technology have been extended with new diagnostic tools (such as CAT and PET) and laboratory tests for blood levels of drugs. Research promises a breakthrough in the understanding of the causation of affective disorder and schizophrenia.

Medical education has been under pressure to adjust to ambulatory care as the primary mode of service delivery, with greater emphasis upon administrative, ethical, legal, and rehabilitative knowledge and skills.

The glut of physicians makes it likely that an even greater number of mental disorders will be treated by the general practitioner, adding to the growing number of mental health professionals competing with psychiatrists, and diverting more patients away from psychiatric specialists. Guild interests of the profession demand greater attention. Marketing services and public relations now became useful tools in meeting competition.

The economic crunch and preoccupation with reducing costs of health care have made psychiatrists anxious, as the methods proposed for control do not appropriately fit psychiatric patients' problems. The struggle to maintain quality of care in the face of these pressures has become very real.

Psychiatrists are apprehensive since the investor-owned, for-profit corporations have made major inroads into the public and private hospital sector. Returning in a new form were the old moral concerns: "Who would care for the poor mentally ill?" and "Would the psychiatrist be the advocate of the patient or of the corporation that paid his or her salary?"

The authority of the psychiatrist has been diminished. No longer omnipotent and accepted as "the doctor knows best," now the psychiatrist has to convince the patient that a suggested therapy is the best available among alternatives. The sharing of decision-making with the mentally disabled has many unresolved problems. The challenges to the authority of the psychiatrist by mental health professionals has convinced many legislatures, some courts, and a segment of the public that there "is no difference in the knowledge or skills" between psychiatrists and any mental health professional. These challenges have impelled psychiatry to increase its public education endeavors and have moved it toward a closer association with the rest of the medical profession.

It remains the task of the historian in the next century to unravel the impact of the forces pressing upon psychiatry at this time.

APPENDIX

Appendix A

BENJAMIN RUSH (1746–1813)*

John and Susanna Rush came to America in 1683 and settled in
Byberry, Pennsylvania, on a 500-acre farm 12 miles from Philadelphia. Five generations of Rushes lived on this land. Benjamin
was born there on January 4, 1746. He graduated from Princeton
at the age of 15, served a five-year apprenticeship, and completed
his medical education abroad at Edinburgh and in Paris. In 1769,
he began medical practice (at the age of 23) in Philadelphia. By
choice, much of his work was with the poor. A revolutionary in
politics, he joined the Continental Army as Surgeon in 1777. He
was a signer of the Declaration of Independence. In 1783 he
joined the staff of the Pennsylvania Hospital, where in the next 30
years of service he influenced thousands of students.

---

* In order to better understand the basis for Rush's recognition as the Father
of American Psychiatry, I cite a few facts but advise interested readers to extend
their knowledge by reading the brief summary in Farrar CB: Benjamin Rush and
American Psychiatry, Am J Psychiatry 100:3–15, 1944; and Binger C: Revolutionary Doctor: Benjamin Rush, 1746–1813. New York, W.W. Norton, 1966.
The latter volume contains references to other biographies and to Rush's
writings.

Rush's radical spirit inspired innovation and social reforms: He was a founder of the American Antislavery Society and he advocated rights for all. He led an antialcoholism crusade in 1783, worked for prison reform, and urged advanced education for women. He promoted public schools and a national university to train public servants, and was a founder of Dickinson College.

Rush had broad medical interests in obstetrics, pediatrics, geriatrics, tuberculosis, and ethics. It was his book *Medical Inquiries and Observations Upon Diseases Of The Mind* (Philadelphia, Kimber and Richardson, 1812) that went through many editions and was the dominant textbook for nearly 70 years. Madness, in Rush's view, was an arterial disease affecting the blood supply to the brain. Antimony, bloodletting, and mercury were the remedies he used, along with diet, rest, exercise, hydrotherapy, occupational therapy, diversion, and travel. Rush didn't advance the science, but he made the study of the mind his major interest.

Rush was in active practice on April 14, 1813, seeing patients as usual. That night he developed a cough, chills, and fever with chest pains that rapidly progressed to difficulty in breathing and extreme weakness. His attending physician thought he had typhus. Rush believed that his old pneumonary tuberculosis had become acute. His biographer, Carl Binger, guessed that he had pneumonia. Rush died five days after the onset, on April 19th, at the age of 67.

The American Psychiatric Association, in 1965, placed a bronze tablet on his grave with the inscription:

Benjamin Rush
1746–1813

Father of American Psychiatry
Signer of the Declaration of Independence
Heroic Physician, Teacher, Humanitarian
Physician General of the Continental Army
Physician to the Pennsylvania Hospital
Professor of Physic, University of Pennsylvania

The American Psychiatric Association uses the likeness of Benjamin Rush as its symbol, on its seal, banner, stationery, and newspaper.

Appendix B

THE FOUNDING FATHERS: BRIEF BIOGRAPHICAL SKETCHES*

Samuel Bayard Woodward (1787–1850)

When I was a resident at Worcester State Hospital, a majestic bust of Dr. Woodward stood in the library. It portrayed a handsome, heroic figure who looked like George Washington. Woodward was 6 feet, 2 inches tall and weighed 260 pounds. His hair was white; he moved with graceful vigor, was dignified, deeply religious, and projected cheerfulness and unquenchable optimism.

Woodward was born June 10, 1787, in Torrington, Connecticut, and died in Northampton, Massachusetts, January 3, 1850 at the age of 63. He studied medicine under his physician father's tutelage and began to practice at the age of 21 in Weathersfield, Connecticut.

His rise to prominence was swift, for he soon became secretary of the state medical society and its examiner at Yale. In 1830 he was elected state senator. He was involved in the founding of Hartford Retreat, in the choice of the site, and in raising of funds; later, he was one of its visiting physicians.

His interest in mental disorders developed out of his experiences with patients seen in his medical practice, and in those of fellow physicians who sought his advice. In September 1832 he

---

* Short biographies of the original 13 founders can be found in references to Chapter 2.

For Amariah Brigham and John S. Butler, see Braceland FJ: The Institute of Living: The Hartford Retreat, 1822–1972. Hartford, Connecticut, The Institute of Living, 1972.

Additional references to individual founders will be cited in the biographical material. A valuable insight is provided by Jones RE: Correspondence of the APA founders. Am J Psychiatry 119:1121–1134, June 1963.

Extensive commentary on the 13 founders of the APA is given in Chapter 3 of McGovern CM: Masters of Madness: Social Origins of the American Psychiatric Profession (Hanover, New Hampshire, University Press of New England, 1985). Her notes on pages 199–205 are a rich source of references to the founders.

was appointed Superintendent of the Worcester (Massachusetts) State Insane Asylum, a post he held for 14 years until he resigned for reasons of health on June 30, 1846.

The Worcester Asylum was a model of state responsibility and of humane, enlightened care. Its annual reports were widely read, as 3,000 copies were circulated by order of the legislature. Woodward's optimistic treatment outcomes stimulated other states to develop similar institutions and therapeutic programs. Woodward also advocated medical care and an institution for the care of inebriates.

Woodward was the first President of the Association and served in that post for four years until May 11, 1848. After completing his duties he moved to Northampton, where he died in 1850. He was well suited for the initial leadership role, for he brought to it a national reputation, more than 10 years of successful experience as an administrator, and the enthusiasm, energy, and promotional skills needed to launch the new organizaton.

For further details see:

Chandler G: Life of Dr. Woodward. American Journal of Insanity 8:119–135, Oct 1851

Grob GN: The State and the Mentally Ill: A History of the Worcester State Hospital in Massachusetts, 1830–1920. Chapel Hill, University of North Carolina Press, 1966

Woodward SB: Collected Papers. Worcester, Massachusetts, American Antiquarian Society

Samuel White (1777–1845)

White was the most eminent specialist in mental disorders in New York State and was President (1844) of the New York State Medical Society. This organization already was involved in catalyzing the development of a national medical association.

White was born in Conventry, Connecticut, on February 23, 1777. He died on February 10, 1845, only four months after the Association of Medical Superintendents' first meeting.

White was a tall, slender man with iron gray hair and a dignified and grave countenance, who was able to relate well to others. He studied medicine under a distinguished surgeon in the Revolutionary Army. He began his practice in Hudson, New York, in 1792 at the age of 20, and soon had an extensive practice. Dr. White achieved fame when he removed a swallowed spoon from the intestines of a mental patient (before the discovery of anesthesia). His surgical skills led to calls often long distances away from home. In 1808, he was appointed Professor of Obstetrics and Practical Surgery in the Berkshire Medical School in Pittsfield, Massachusetts. In 1830, he established a private lunatic asylum in Hudson, New York that was recognized as outstanding.

White was President (1843–1844) of the New York State Medical Society when he delivered an address on insanity and its treatment. Curwen, commenting on the address in 1885, said it was "one of the best synopses of our knowledge of insanity, especially of its treatment, which has ever been published" (see Farrar CB: Foreword to the Centennial Issue, Am J Psychiatry, 100, 1944).

White's comments in his 1844 address advocated minimum restraint, an open door policy, and humane treatment, an approach which would return again in the reforms of the 20th century.

The Hudson Lunatic Asylum, after Dr. White's death in 1845, became first a home for wayward girls, then a home for orphans, and, finally, the Hudson Public Library.

Thomas S. Kirkbride (1809–1883)

No other individual among the founders contributed more than Dr. Kirkbride to the developing Association, for he served as an officer for 26 years.

Thomas Kirkbride was one of the younger men in 1844. He was of medium height and slight build, with straight brown hair, a high forehead, and an under-the-chin beard. He was pleasant, quiet with winning charm, and a strong sense of duty. Added to these traits were tenacity of purpose, impulsiveness, and obsessiveness.

Kirkbride was born in Brick's County, Pennsylvania, on July 31, 1809, and began his education in a Friend's school. He served a medical apprenticeship at the age of 18 under a Trenton physician, graduated from the University of Pennsylvania in 1832, and then served one year as physician at Friend's Asylum after which he entered the practice of surgery.

Inspired by Woodward's accomplishments at the Worcester Asylum and by Bell's work at McLean, he accepted the post of physician-in-chief of the Department of the Insane of the Pennsylvania Hospital when it was offered in 1840. An able administrator, he spent his entire career as Chief Executive of the Pennsylvania Hospital's Department of the Insane acquiring national prominence for his development of standards—then called propositions—for his advocacy of good nursing care and for his expertise in hospital organization and construction. His basic plan for mental hospitals is still known as the Kirkbride Plan. It describes a central core for administrative services with lateral wings extending from the core for the classification of patients in wards.

Kirkbride's best-known publication is his book *On the Construction, Organization and General Arrangements of Hospitals for the Insane* (Philadelphia, Lindsay and Blakeston, 1854). Dr. Kirkbride was one of a group (along with Earle, Ray, and Nichols) who served as friends and advisors to Dorothea Dix in her crusade for improved care of the mentally ill. Kirkbride died in 1883, giving 39 years of service to the Association and a lifetime of service to his hospital. Of the original 13 founders, only Pliny Earle and Butler lived longer than he did.

For further details see:

Bond ED: Dr. Kirkbride and His Mental Hospital. Philadelphia, J.B. Lippincott, 1947
Kirkbride TS: Papers. Philadelphia, Institute of the Pennsylvania Hospital

William MaClay Awl (1799–1876)

William Awl was one of the original nucleus of individuals whose opinion was crucial in the decision to hold the meeting in 1844 from which the Association emerged. He was chosen to be Vice-President of the Association to fill the vacancy created by White's untimely death. Awl held this post until he became President of the Association in 1848, and served until his resignation from the Association in 1851.

Awl was born in Harrisburg, Pennsylvania, on May 24, 1799. His mother was proud of her lineal descent from John Harris, founder of the city of Harrisburg, and of her father, William MaClay, the first U.S. senator from Pennsylvania.

Awl was raised on a farm. When he was 15 he attended Northumberland Academy. He studied medicine as an apprentice to a physician, and then attended a course of lectures (1819–1820) at the University of Pennsylvania. Later in life, he received an honorary M.S. from Jefferson College.

It seems unusual to us, but not remarkable in the 1830s, that Awl walked from Lancaster, Pennsylvania, to Columbus, Ohio. There he established a successful general practice. Local notice of a surgical operation that he performed helped his practice grow.

In 1853 he helped organize a medical convention to take measures to improve the care of the insane and the education of the blind. Later he was appointed a trustee to assist in the building of the two institutions in Ohio for the blind and the insane. To learn more, he visited asylums along the east coast. In 1838 he resigned as trustee and was appointed Superintendent of the Ohio Lunatic Asylum in Columbus.

Awl was a man of medium height, with a large head, bald on top, rimmed with bushy hair over the ears and back. He has been described as having a strong character, and as being an innovator with an abundance of common sense. Although appearing grave and determinedly earnest, he loved to beguile his associates with a joke. He was dead serious in his outspoken opposition to bleeding as a treatment of acute mania (1845).

Awl was a victim of the political system that characterized Ohio for so many years. In 1850 he was forced out of his post as superintendent by the system of political appointment. When he accepted a similar post in the institution for the blind, being out of the field, he resigned as President of the Association in 1851. Awl lived another 25 years before his death on November 19, 1876.

Luther V. Bell (1806–1862)

Luther Bell was a handsome, brilliant leader, formally trained in medicine, who had a broad knowledge of mental disorders. He was a skilled diagnostician who brought to the Association experience in the political system. He was born in Francestown, New Hampshire, on December 30, 1806 into a distinguished family. His great grandfather had been a state senator. His father served in both houses of the New Hampshire legislature, and was governor and later U.S. senator. His brother was chief justice of the state supreme court.

Bell was a precocious adolescent, entering Bowdoin College at the age of 13, and earning a medical degree from Dartmouth Medical School (1826) at the age of 20. After six years of general practice in Derry, New Hampshire, he found time to fulfill family tradition with service in the state legislature. He played an active part in establishing the asylum at Concord, New Hampshire. In 1834 he won the annual Boylston Prize for a dissertation on dietetics and smallpox. He later was to receive honorary degrees in civil law and a doctor of laws.

In 1837 he was elected Superintendent of the McLean Asylum and held the post for 19 years, until 1856. He was a friend and advisor of Dorothea Dix. He was known as an expert in the medical aspects of mental disorders, in legal matters, in spiritualism (to the dismay of some of his colleagues), and in the coercive administration of food to the insane who refused to eat. Known also as an expert in heating and ventilation of buildings, that was the subject of his presidential address to the Massachusetts Medical Society in 1857. With Ray, he assisted in the founding of the Butler Hospital in Providence, Rhode Island.

Bell was an active participant in Association affairs for 12 years. He served as Vice-President from 1850–1851, and as President from 1851–1855. His description of acute mania was so able that the disorder was called "Bell's Disease" for some years.

He resigned his post at McLean because of ill health, but had enough energy to volunteer as Surgeon to the 11th Massachusetts Regiment in 1861. He was promoted to Division Medical Director of General Hooker's troops. He died in camp on February 11, 1862. He was the only one of the founders to serve in the Civil War.

John S. Butler (1803–1890)

John Butler devoted 46 years to the work of the Association of Asylum Superintendents, serving as Vice-President for eight years (1862–1870) and as its President for three (1870–1873). He was an honorary member of the Royal Medico-Psychological Association of Great Britain.

Butler was born in Northampton, Massachusetts, in 1803. After receiving a master's degree at Yale, he was apprenticed to two Northampton physicians. He attended some lectures at Harvard and was granted an M.D. degree from Jefferson Medical College in Philadelphia in 1828. This was followed by 10 years of practice in Worcester. There he met Dr. Woodward, who permitted him to follow one of his patients through to successful recovery in the Worcester State Asylum.

When the city of Boston's Lunatic Asylum was opened in 1839, on the strong recommendation of Dr. Woodward, Butler became its first superintendent. He found politics so unpleasant in Boston that he resigned in 1842, intending to go into practice. At that time, Brigham left an opening at the Hartford Retreat when he moved to Utica, New York. Butler elected to fill the vacancy in Hartford. He stayed on for 40 years, contributing to the growth, stability, and preeminence of the Retreat.

Butler was a stout man, of medium height, with a high forehead and gray hair. He wore an under-the-chin beard and steel rimmed glasses. A strong, energetic administrator, he was also a warm person who spoke with clarity and radiated optimism. He was a staunch advocate of individualized treatment and saw each of his patients daily. He was the first person in the United States to propose that mental disorders be included in the realm of public health and in the field of preventive medicine.

Upon retiring from the Retreat, Butler entered private practice and served as the president of the first State Board of Health (in Connecticut, in 1873), a post he held until his death in Hartford, at the age of 87, on May 21, 1890.

Amariah Brigham (1798–1849)

Amariah Brigham lived for only five years after the founding of the Association, but assured his place in history by establishing the *American Journal of Insanity,* which he started as a personal venture at the Utica Asylum.

Brigham was six feet tall but weighed only 130 pounds. He had small features, blue, expressive eyes, thin brown hair, and a soft melodic voice. He possessed a superior, well cultivated intellect, was self-possessed, sociable, kind, and generous. He was born in Marlborough, Massachusetts, on December 26, 1798. He was raised on a farm, one of six children. His father died when he was 11 years old. At that time he was sent to live with his uncle—a physician—and began his education in New York. Two years later his uncle died, leaving him adrift again. At 14 he got a job in a bookstore and used this opportunity to read everything he could. Later he taught school, saved his money, and went to New York to study at the College of Physicians and Surgeons. After an apprenticeship, he settled in Greenfield, Massachusetts and practiced there for seven years. He traveled abroad, visiting medical centers in Edinburgh, Paris, and Europe (1828–1829).

In 1831 he began to write *The Influence of Mental Cultivation and Mental Excitement on Health* and *The Influence of Religion on Health*. He wrote about epidemic cholera, and about brain and spinal cord function. He was known to be an excellent lecturer when he was appointed professor of anatomy and surgery at his alma mater.

Brigham was respected as a fine clinician, an excellent teacher, and an independent thinker. He read widely (with a 2,000-volume personal library) and was the author of the popular book, *The Influence of Mental Cultivation and Mental Excitement on Health* (1832). He wrote to Eli Todd about prospects for practice in Hartford. He moved to Hartford on Todd's advice.

When the post became vacant, he was appointed the third superintendent of the Hartford Retreat—not without some reservations—for he had been denounced from local pulpits as an infidel for his views on religion.

In the brief two years during which he headed the Hartford Retreat, he demonstrated his able administrative skill, he centralized authority, and he introduced the latest scientific methods. He stressed early detection and early treatment, occupation, and industry to divert the mind into healthy productivity.

When the very large new asylum was ready for use in Utica, New York, Brigham accepted the challenge to be its chief executive. It was there, two years later in July of 1844, that he inaugurated the first psychiatric publication in the English language—the *American Journal of Insanity.* When the Association of Asylum Superintendents was formed, he noted the event in the *Journal's* pages. Through the years the *Journal* noted the actions and progress of the Association and carried articles by distinguished specialists at home and abroad. The *Journal* became a cohesive force, holding the young Association together, and became the principal scientific voice of psychiatry in America in the years to come.

Nehemiah Cutter (1787–1859)

Nehemiah Cutter, along with Samuel White, operated a private mental asylum. He was interested and active in the Association and was a regular attendant of its meetings. He was a stout man of medium height with a square face, light, curly hair, and dark eyes. Described as even-tempered, affable, energetic, and well liked, he was known for his good character and successful administration of the Cutter Retreat.

Cutter was born in Jaffrey, New Hampshire on March 30, 1787, graduated from Middlebury College in 1814, and received formal training and a medical degree at Yale in 1817. After a time in general practice in Pepperell, Massachusetts, he saw an increasing number of mental patients. At first (1822) he cared for these patients in his own house. In 1834 he built the asylum.

Originally it was a one-story building to which later another story was added, making accommodations for 40 patients. Dr. Cutter was assisted in his work by Dr. Charles E. Parker and, occasionally, by Dr. James S.N. Howe, general practitioners. On May 1, 1853 the Retreat burned to the ground. There was no loss of life, but one patient would have perished had she not been carried down a ladder.

Following the fire, Drs. Cutter and Howe divided patients between them. Cutter's new residence was enlarged to care for patients, a venture that proved unsuccessful financially. After Cutter's death on March 15, 1859, the building was purchased by Dr. Jonathan Shattuck for a boys' school. The building was twice moved on rollers until, finally, it occupied the site of the original Cutter Retreat, where it stood until 1921 (when it was torn down, as it no longer met building codes).

Upon his death, the memorial (Am J Insanity 16:42–46, 1859–1860) described him as having "remarkable zeal in the objects of our Association," as an active discussant of papers presented at the meetings, and as one who worked for the advancement of the Association.

Pliny Earle (1809—1892)

Pliny Earle was to outlive the other 12 founders, to contribute more to the literature than any of the others except Ray, to teach, to distinguish himself as an able administrator, and to be a force in the development of the Association over a span of 41 years. He served as the Association's Vice-President (1883—1884) and as President (1884—1885). He was also an organizer of the American Medical Association and of the New York Academy of Medicine. For 48 years he was an honorary member of the Royal Medico-Psychological Association in Great Britain.

Earle was a dynamic, good-looking man, with a high forehead topped with graying hair. He wore a short beard. He was born into a Quaker family in Leicester, Massachusetts, on December 31, 1809. He attended Friends' School in Providence, after which he taught school for several years. He earned an M.D. degree from the University of Pennsylvania in 1837. He spent the next two years in Europe visiting mental institutions and the leaders in medicine—Lister, Tuke, and Esquirol. Upon his return he began his practice of medicine in Philadelphia.

In 1844, Earle was appointed superintendent of the Bloomingdale Asylum in New York, where he remained for five years. After a second European tour, particularly in Germany and Austria, he familiarized his colleagues, through his writings, with the work being done in these countries, work that had hitherto been neglected in the United States. Upon his return from Europe he expected that he would be named a superintendent; and was despondent when he was not.

For the next 15 years Earle devoted most of his time to consultation, study, writing, and serving as visiting physician to the Government Hospital for the Insane (St. Elizabeths Hospital in Washington, D.C.), and as visiting physician to the New York State Lunatic Asylum. He also served as professor of psychological medicine at the Berkshire Medical Institution at Pittsfield, Massachusetts (1863).

In 1864, Earle was appointed Superintendent of the State Lunatic Hospital at Northampton, Massachusetts, a post he held until his retirement at the age of 76 in 1885. His skill in administration won him praise from the Massachusetts Board of Charities.

Scarcely a year went by without Earle's writing a published article. Some of his titles are surprisingly modern—*The Psycho-*

pathic Hospital of the Future (1867) and *Psychological Medicine: Its Importance as Part of the Medical Curriculum* (1866). His most important book was *The Curability of Insanity* (1877), in which he exposed the statistical errors of his colleagues whose "hopes had outlived their judgment" (see Curwen J: The Original Thirteen Members of the AMSA. Warren, Pennsylvania, E. Corwan Co., 1885).

Earle was an advocate of small hospitals, separate asylums for chronic patients, regular exercise for patients, family care, state rather than county responsibility for care, occupation for patients, and efficient administration of institutions. He vigorously opposed bleeding, blistering, and the "douche" for punishment.

For further details see:

Earle P: Collected Papers. American Antiquarian Society, Worcester, Massachusetts
Earle P: Statistics of insanity. American Journal of Insanity 6:141–145, 1849
Earle P: Curability of Insanity. Philadelphia, J.B. Lippincott, 1887
Sanborn FB (Ed): Memoirs of Pliny Earle. Boston, Damrill and Upham, 1898

John Galt (1819–1862)

John Galt was the youngest of the original 13, and the most scholarly. He was fluent in several European languages and read Greek and Arabic. His reading of the foreign languages led to a summary of the pertinent literature on contemporary mental care in the book *The Treatment of Insanity* (New York, Harper and Brothers, 1846). He was a frequent contributor to the *American Journal of Insanity* and to magazines for the public as well.

Galt was born in Williamsburg, Virginia, on March 19, 1819 into a dynasty associated with institutional administration of the insane. His great uncle was the first "keeper"—administrator—of the oldest mental hospital in the colony at Williamsburg, Virginia (1773). Both his grandfather and father had been attending physicians there. John M. Galt was the institution's first medical superintendent.

Galt attended William and Mary College, receiving an AB degree in 1838. He received his M.D. degree from the University of Pennsylvania in 1841, after which, at the age of 22, he was appointed to head the Williamsburg Asylum.

Galt was an advocate of moral treatment, occupation, recreation, bibliotherapy, and music therapy as a means of preventing withdrawal and encouraging involvement in daily activities.

Galt kept abreast of developments abroad. His interest in a farm at St. Anne's, France, an experiment of the French hospital Bicetre, and in the family care system in Gheel, Belgium, led him to make a series of suggestions (*Am J Insanity* 11:352–357, 1855; and *Annual Reports of Hospital*, 1855–1857) that could have modified the existing hospital system. The following is a summary of his suggestions:

- Chronic patients should be placed as boarders in families in communities adjacent to the hospital.
- Selected patients should be paroled to live and work in the community.
- Every institution should have a farm attached, with cottages for convalescent and chronic patients.
- There should be a single controlling power in the institution— the medical superintendent.
- There should be more extended liberty for patients.

Galt came under severe attack for these expressed views at the 1855 annual meeting of the Association, when he was critical of contemporary institutions as "mere prison houses notwithstanding their many internal attributes of comfort and elegance" (Am J Insanity 11:352–357, 1855).

A few days after federal troops occupied Williamsburg during the Civil War (on May 6, 1862), Galt died at the age of 43 from what was described as a violent attack of indigestion. He was buried in the Bruton Parish churchyard in the town in which he lived all his life.

Isaac Ray (1807–1881)

Perhaps the most outstanding of the group of founders was Isaac Ray. An original thinker, he was a prolific writer whose medical-legal contributions are still quoted more than 100 years later. Ray was active in the Association for 23 years, serving as Vice-President (1851–1855) and as President (1855–1859).

Isaac Ray was born in Beverly, Massachusetts, on January 16, 1807. He attended Phillips Andover Academy and Bowdoin College. He was then apprenticed to Dr. Shattuck of Boston before completing his studies at Harvard Medical School (1827). After a year abroad in England and France he practiced in Portland and Eastport, Maine.

In 1841, he accepted the post of Medical Superintendent at the State Hospital for the Insane in Augusta, Maine. He stayed there only until 1845, when Butler Hospital trustees invited him to become that hospital's first superintendent, an institution which he and Luther Bell had helped to plan. Before taking the job he again traveled extensively in Europe. Ray remained at Butler in Providence, Rhode Island, for 20 years (1867). He resigned for reasons of health but continued to write and do some consulting in Philadelphia, where he had chosen to live in retirement. He died on March 31, 1881.

Ray was an able and progressive administrator, a nationally renowned medico-legal expert, a teacher who lectured at Brown University and at the University of Pennsylvania, and who founded the Social Service Association. He was the first to use and define the term "mental hygiene" in a book (1863). His most widely acclaimed and quoted book (1838), *Medical Jurisprudence of Insanity*, went through six editions.

For further details see:

Quen JM: Isaac Ray and mental hygiene. Ann NY Acad Sci 291:83–93, 1944

Stearns AW: Isaac Ray, psychiatrist and pioneer in forensic psychiatry. Am J Psychiatry 101:573–584, 1945

Charles H. Stedman (1805–1866)

Charles H. Stedman was a surgeon who, primarily, was in the right place at the right time to be remembered in the history of psychiatry. He is remembered as a founding father of APA and as the recipient of glowing praise from Charles Dickens.

Stedman was born in Lancaster, Massachusetts, on June 17, 1805. He attended Yale but did not graduate. He graduated from Harvard Medical School in 1828 and shortly thereafter became the resident surgeon at Chelsea (Massachusetts) Naval Hospital. During his 10 years in that post he edited a translation of Spurzheim's book on the anatomy of the brain. It was popular enough to warrant a second edition.

In 1840 he began the practice of surgery in Boston. Two years later, when John Butler resigned his post, he became the Superintendent of the Boston Lunatic Asylum and also physician to the adjacent correction and welfare institutions.

By 1851 Stedman had enough of institutional administration, and he returned to private practice in Boston. He found time to be the first state coroner, a state senator, and a member of the Governor's Council. When the Boston City Hospital was opened in 1864 he was a visiting surgeon, and was its senior surgeon when he died on June 7, 1866. Dr. Henry P. Stedman, Charles' son, for many years operated a private mental hospital in Boston.

Francis T. Stribling (1810–1874)

We have at last come to the founder who, with Woodward, gave birth to the idea that led to the historic organizational meeting in 1844. Stribling attended meetings of the Association for 30 years. He was never an officer.

Stribling was born January 20, 1810 in Staunton, Virginia, and lived all of his professional life in that town. A clerk in the office of his father—the county clerk—Stribling, after several years, determined that he wanted to be a physician. He was apprenticed while in his teens to a local doctor, then attended the University of Virginia, and later spent a year at the University of Pennsylvania earning his medical degree in 1830 at the age of 20.

He practiced in Staunton until 1836 when, at the age of 26, he was appointed the Medical Superintendent of the Western Lunatic Asylum in Staunton. He was an able administrator who pressed for adequate appropriations to carry out the goals of the institution. He favored moral treatment, small institutions, and the training of attendants.

Stribling did not regularly attend Association meetings. Although he had been a cofounder, after the 1844 meeting he did not attend again until 1852. McGovern wrote that he returned when "the pressures of asylum administration in Virginia increased to the point where he once again sought support from his professional colleagues" (McGovern, p. 73).

Stribling favored "greater precision" and "more uniformity in reporting statistics" (McGovern, p. 72). He may have expressed his disappointment in the report of the Committee on Statistics by his nonattendance. Stribling regarded John Galt as a rival rather than a colleague.

Stribling died at Staunton on July 23, 1874, at the age of 64.

References

McGovern CM: Masters of Madness: Social Origins of the American Psychiatric Profession. Hanover, New Hampshire, University Press of New England, 1985

Appendix C

DOROTHEA DIX (1802—1887)

Dorothea Dix was born in Hampden, Maine, in 1802. Her father was a ne'er-do-well, existing at the poverty level, and fanatically religious. When she was 12 years old Dorothea was sent to Boston to live with her grandmother, who impressed on the child a sense of duty and spartan discipline as essential life forces. At the age of 14, Dorothea Dix opened a school for little children in Worcester, Massachusetts. It failed. She went back to Boston for further education and tried again. This time her boarding school was highly successful. She became known as an excellent teacher with a keen mind, enriched in summer association with the friendship of William Ellery Channing.

Always in frail health, in 1836 she was unable to continue teaching. She went to England for convalescence and there invested her time visiting York Retreat and met Tuke. She returned refreshed to resume her teaching. She became sought as a consultant in education.

Dix's career as a reformer followed an invitation to teach a class of inmates one Sunday in the East Cambridge jail. She was revolted by the filth, neglect, and brutality, and by the placement of insane residents in unheated cells. It was bitter cold, so she asked for heat in the cell block. The warden ridiculed the notion, for "everyone knows the insane are insensitive to temperature." The rebuff became a challenge to action and revealed her tenacity for a cause. She got the heat turned on in the jail with a court order. That was only the beginning, for she next surveyed all the jails, prisons, and receptacles for holding the mentally ill in the state. With a well organized report and documented facts, she initiated a pattern of action that was to be repeated many times. Having made what we call a needs assessment, she consulted many leading experts to gain their critical comment, advise on strategy, and to enlist their support.

In Massachusetts, she turned to Luther Bell, Pliny Earle, Horace Mann, and Samuel Gridley Howe for advice. Having prepared a "Memorial to the Legislature," she next made personal contact with key legislators and citizens to mobilize support. Her action in Massachusetts took place in 1843, and in New York in

January 1844, before the Association of Medical Superintendents was founded in October 1844.

So successful was her strategic planning that she initiated the action with local support and aided the development of a public institutional system under the policy of state responsibility for the insane. Butler Hospital in Providence, St. Elizabeths in Washington, D.C., and 30 public mental hospitals were opened as a consequence of her crusade. She campaigned for improved care in Nova Scotia and Newfoundland, revised Scotland's system, and developed an institutional plan for Italy.

She was one of the first management consultants: at Bloomingdale Asylum, she settled a dispute and advised correction for overcrowding, improved supervision, heating, and toilet facilities. She was known throughout the world as an apostle for humane care of the insane.

Dix was the catalyst for an action that often was delayed; but she did succeed in broadening the role of government in the care of the mentally ill. She was always a strong, tenacious person with singular devotion to her cause—the improvement of the care for the mentally ill. She was accurate in her observations but not above exaggerating them to gain a point. She was a controversial figure—a sensationalist, some called her—and some said she was a distorter of truth, a meddler, and often "a foreigner."

During the Civil War she served as a supervisor of women nurses. Another outstanding woman reformer, Florence Nightingale, had demonstrated that cleanliness, hygienic practices, supply control, and good management could reduce infection and wound mortality in 1854 during the Crimean War. Utilizing these principles, a Civil War hospital was built on Dix's suggested plan (see Bordley J, Harvey AM: Two Centuries of American Medicine. Philadelphia, W.B. Saunders, 1976).

Dix continued her active work for nearly three decades, from the 1840s through the 1870s. In 1881, at nearly 80 years of age, she retired to live out her life in an apartment arranged for her at a hospital she founded—the New Jersey State Hospital in Trenton. She died in 1887 at the age of 85, and was buried in Mt. Auburn Cemetery in Cambridge, Massachusetts. Many memorials to her memory were erected, among them Dixmont State Hospital in Clenfield, Pennsylvania, and Dix Hall Hospital in Raleigh, North Carolina. Samuel Bell Waugh (1814–1885), a prominent portrait artist and landscape painter from Philadelphia, made a portrait of

Miss Dix in 1865, the original of which hangs in Dixmont Hospital. An exact and most satisfactory duplicate of that painting was painted in 1966 by Eleanor Thompson, a Pittsburgh artist. This portrait hangs in the APA headquarters building. A yew tree planted by Miss Dix at Trenton State Hospital was the source for a cutting of the flourishing yew that graces the grounds at 1700 18th Street, Washington, D.C. (Perhaps someone will grow a cutting for the lobby of the APA at 1400 K Street to preserve her memory in a living plant originally started by her own hand.)

Appendix D

THE MEDICAL DIRECTORS OF APA

Daniel Blain (1898–1981), the first Medical Director, served in that capacity for 10 years, from 1948 to 1958. He was born of missionary parents in Kashing, China. Tutored at home by his mother until the age of 11, he was then sent to boarding school in Shanghai. At the age of 13 he came to America, a stranger in his own country. He adapted well and was proud to be the fifth generation to attend Washington and Lee College. After pre-medical training at the University of Chicago, he attended Vander-bilt Medical School, graduating with an M.D. degree in 1929. His internship was in Boston's Brigham and City Hospitals. His train-ing in psychiatry was in Stockbridge, Massachusetts, and Silver Hill, Connecticut. In 1936 he married Logan Starr, the member of an old Philadelphia family. They had one child. Logan was truly the first lady—campaigning for support of travel of wives of presidents and serving as a gracious hostess to entertain digni-taries and APA leaders at her lovely country estate in the center of Philadelphia, "Belfield."

After a brief period of private practice in New York City, Dr. Blain joined the U.S. Public Health Service. He was the first American Board Diplomate in the U.S. Public Health Service. With the rank of Captain, he was appointed Medical Director of the War Shipping Administration. In that role he organized treat-ment and rehabilitation for casualties in the Merchant Marine. In 1945 he was named Chief of the Department of Psychiatry at the Veterans Administration, where he was instrumental in creating the residency training program in psychiatry, mental hygiene clinics, and psychiatric units in all VA general hospitals; he planned (with Paul Hahn) the design and construction of new VA psychiatric hospitals.

In 1948 he was appointed APA Medical Director. Blain's health handicapped him and after 10 years in office he asked to be relieved of his duties. Surgery helped him to regain his energies and led him briefly to be Director of Mental Hygiene in California. From there he went to the Institute of the Pennsylvania Hospital and while in that job became the APA's 93rd President (1964–1965). The Airlie House Conference was his major contribution of that period, for he issued the call to make the organizational changes essential to a speedier response. In 1966 Blain became Director of the Philadelphia State Hospital. After his third retirement, he remained actively engaged in writing a psychiatric history of the 25 years after World War II, a project funded by grants but never completed. In 1975 the New York Academy awarded him its Solomon Medal and in 1980 he won the Distinguished Service Award of the APA. He died suddenly in 1981.

Matthew Ross (1917–   ), the second Medical Director, served for four years, from 1958 to 1962. He received his M.D. degree from Tufts University Medical School in Boston in 1942. His internship was at Kings County Hospital in Brooklyn, New York. His psychiatric training was obtained at the Brentwood VA Hospital in Los Angeles. He went into private practice in 1948 and enrolled in the L.A. Psychoanalytic Institute, completing his training in psychoanalysis in 1951.

In 1953 Ross was a founder and the first President of the Southern California District Branch of the APA. He was a professor of psychiatry at UCLA from 1953 to 1958.

From 1956 to 1957, Ross was Speaker of APA's Assembly. After his four years as Medical Director and a brief sojourn as a Fulbright Research Scholar in the Netherlands, Ross returned to the private practice of psychiatry in Newport Beach, California, and to teaching as clinical professor of psychiatry (1974–   ) at the University of California at Irvine.

Walter Barton (1906–   ), third Medical Director, served for 11 years, from 1963 to 1974. Barton was born in Oak Park, Illinois, a suburb of Chicago, and lived there and in Elmhurst, Illinois, until he went to the University of Illinois at Urbana and its Medical School in Chicago (B.S., M.D. [1931]). His internship was served at the West Suburban Hospital (Oak Park, Illinois) and his residency at Worcester State Hospital, Massachusetts.

After a tour in Neurology at the National Hospital at Queen Square in London as clerk of F.M.R. Walshe, he returned to Worcester and climbed through the ranks to Acting Superintendent when he entered the military service. He served in the Surgeon General's Office organizing its occupational therapy department and the army's rehabilitation program, and also served overseas as a Lt. Colonel in the 126 general and 116 station hospitals (in the latter as a commanding officer).

While still in the Army, he began service at Boston State Hospital as its Superintendent. (The Governor of Massachusetts, a friend of the army's Surgeon General, made the arrangement possible to solve a management crisis at the state hospital.)

Barton served the APA in many capacities during his superintendency of the Boston State Hospital: Rehabilitation Committee (chairman) (1948–1952); Section Council for Mental Hospitals (1949–1952); delegate from Massachussetts in the Assembly at its time of organization; Coordinating Council for Technical Aspects of Psychiatry (1950–1953); on its Governing Council and Executive Committee (1952–1955); Chairman of the Internal Management Committee; Representative to the Joint Commission on Mental Illness and Health; President-Elect and President of the APA, 1960–1962.

Dr. Barton served as a Director of the American Board of Psychiatry (1962–1970) and was its President. He was on the Residency Review Committee for Psychiatry and Neurology and for 20 years was the APA's representative to AMA's Council on Mental Health.

Barton also served many other organizations as president, such as the Group for the Advancement of Psychiatry, the Massachusetts Psychiatric Association, and the American College of Mental Health Administration. He has been a clinical professor of psychiatry at Boston University (1954–   ), and professor of psychiatry (active emeritus) at Dartmouth Medical School from 1974 to the present.

The APA granted Barton its Distinguished Service Award (1975) and its first award in administrative psychiatry (1983).

Barton's wife, Elsa, served as Logan Blain had done, as hostess to foreign dignitaries, welcomer of APA's new members, new staff, and new leader's wives to insure their comfort and to help them know they were appreciated. She was affectionately called APA's "Den Mother."

Melvin Sabshin (1925–   ), the fourth Medical Director, assumed his post in 1974 (and continues, as this is published, in 1986). Dr. Sabshin received his medical education at Tulane University School of Medicine (M.D., 1948), served his internship at Charity Hospital in New Orleans, and served his residency at Tulane (1949–1953). He completed psychoanalytic training (1955–1961) at the Chicago Institute.

In 1953 Dr. Sabshin joined the staff of Michael Reese Hospital (Chicago). By 1955 he was its Associate Director until 1961, when he was appointed Professor and Head of the Department of Psychiatry at the University of Illinois College of Medicine (Abraham Lincoln School of Medicine). He was Acting Dean of the Medical School (1973–1974) when he assumed the post of Medical Director of the APA.

Dr. Sabshin had long served the APA in various capacities: Chairman, Council on Research and Development; Chairman, Program Committee; Editorial Board—*American Journal of Psychiatry;* President, Illinois Psychiatric Society; and as an elected member of the Board of Trustees.

Edith Goldfarb Sabshin, his wife, is a Fellow of the APA, a training psychoanalyst and supervisor, with an active clinical teaching and consultation practice. She has been Assistant Dean of the Chicago Psychoanalytic Institute and Secretary of the American Psychoanalytic Institute.

As a team they bring broad interests in psychiatry into the organization and share their extensive contributions in books and articles in the scientific literature.

Appendix E

THE HEADQUARTERS AT 1700 18TH STREET

Renovations designed to restore the building at 1700 18th Street were under the direction of Horace W. Peaslee, assisted by Frank Cole, architects. Elizabeth Stetson-Adams was the interior decorator, Wilberding Co., the engineers, and William P. Lipscomb, the builder. The cost of renovation was $173,000. The total cost of $278,000 was paid by the Association from the fund drive donations and its own resources without recourse to loans or mortgages.

A dignified entrance led to an imposing hall with a graceful curving staircase. Visitors were welcomed by a receptionist in the hall; business offices were to the right, and to the left the Century Room, a spacious hall for receptions and meetings. The second floor featured the beautiful panelled Modern Founder's Room as a Library, with the center available as an officer's room. The adjacent offices housed Public Affairs and secretarial staff. The third floor provided space for the Medical Director, membership, and journal staff. On the fourth floor were offices for *Mental Hospital* magazine and service staff, and the Physician's Education Project staff.

History of the Site of the First Permanent Home

The Washington territory patents were secured from the King of England and from Lord Baltimore. The land rose in terraces from the basin of the Potomac River and its tributaries to a height of 90 feet at Dupont Circle. In 1664, Slash Run and Brown Run traversed the area on their way to join Rock Creek.

In 1796, what is now Florida Avenue was then Boundary Street, marking the edge of the city. Connecticut Avenue was a dirt road ending at Dupont Circle. P Street was a principal road from the Circle to Georgetown. Massachusetts Avenue was barely a trail. The land north of M Street and west of 16th Street was a worthless cypress swamp (as excavations for the Mayflower Hotel confirmed, when tree trunks were discovered 30 feet below the surface). Small game was plentiful and the area was a popular hunting ground.

In a landscape painted in 1844, the artist William MacLeod viewed the United States Capitol's low dome from the area. The foreground of the picture is a rural scene with a boy on a horse, two cows, and a stretch of farmland.

Anthony Trollope, the British novelist, on a visit to America in 1862 described Slash Run and Brown Run as running blood-red from an adjacent slaughterhouse which permeated the area with an insufferable stench. Trollope called the area an undrained wilderness, where one wades in a bog, knee-deep in mud. In 1870 the streams were covered over.

There was only one house on Massachusetts Avenue, west of 17th Street, in 1871. It belonged to a fortune teller, Madame D. In the same year a farm at the north end of the city was purchased by two individuals. Senator William M. Seward owned half (bounded by New Hampshire, Connecticut, and Florida Avenues) and Curtis Hillyer the other (bounded by Connecticut, Florida, and Massachusetts Avenues). A brickyard (1875) was located at what is now 20th and P Streets.

Dupont Circle—once called Pacific—by the 1900s became a fashionable section of the rapidly expanding capitol city. At Number 15 Dupont Circle was built a 40-room marble mansion designed by Sanford White for "Sissy" Patterson. Evelyn Walsh McLean lived at 2020 Massachusetts Avenue, and Christian Henrick's (a Washington brewer) mansion was at 1518 New Hampshire Avenue. Fashionable strollers walked around the Circle and artists relaxed there, enjoying the sun.

It was at 1704 18th Street in 1910 that Arthur Jeffrey Parsons built his town house.* After his death, Paul Warburg, a member of the Federal Reserve Board, lived in the house. During the period when Parsons resided in the building, it was a gathering place for artists, authors, and officials of government. After Parsons returned to Dublin, New Hampshire, in 1913 he lived only a short time and the property was vacant until Warburg rented it. As Vice President of the newly created Federal Reserve Board, he brought

---

* Parsons was a scholar, connoisseur of the arts, a gentleman of means who served as honorary consultant to the Library of Congress. He founded the print collection and was Chief of the Division of Prints. At his death in 1915, his rare book collection commanded top price at auction. The house was owned by Parsons' estate until 1942. (A.J. Parsons, building permit 3655 December 2, 1909, Lot 159, square 133. Cost in 1942, $75,000. Architect, Hornblower and Marshall; builder, Frank Wagner.)

into the library members of the banking industry, as Warburg was a board member of many financial institutions (he was also a trustee of Tuskegee College and on the board of Juilliard School of Music. Mrs. Warburg, the former Nancy Loeb, was a talented violinist and held musicals and concerts in their home. † Later it was rented to the Brazilian Embassy, and for a time it served as the Hungarian legation. In the 1940s it became a boarding house. The library and ballroom were partitioned into bedrooms and baths to house 73 boarders, mostly women government workers. The French administrative mission occupied the building after the APA purchased it, until the renovation and restoration began in the spring of 1957.

Occupants of 1700 18th Street

Arthur J. Parsons	1910–1913	
Paul M. Warburg	1915–1918	Member, Federal Reserve Board; Father of Bettina Warburg, a New York psychoanalyst
Emory Winship	1919–1921	Commander, U.S. Navy; appointed by President Wilson to the Bureau of Navigation
Vacant	1921–1923	
Albert D. Lasker	1923	Chairman, Shipping Board
David A. Reed	1924	U.S. Senator
Robert M. Thompson	1924–1928	President, Navy League
Gurgel do Amaral	1928–1931	Ambassador from Brazil
Mrs. Bryce J. Allans	1933	
John Pelenys and the Hungarian Legation	1934–1939	Minister to U.S. from Hungary

---

† The source for this history is the pamphlet *SLA Moves to Washington,* in which a section entitled "A History of the Building Fund Search and New Headquarters for SLA" was prepared by Jane Brewer Armann on the occasion of the purchase of the building by the Special Libraries Association, May 31, 1985.

Mr. and Mrs. William H. Kechner	1940–1941	Named building Stuart Hall Converted to a boarding house for young federal workers. Library and ballroom remodeled into living quarters
Leo G. Sheridan	1942–1943	Administrative Services
French Mission	1948–1957	
APA Headquarters	1958–1982	
APA Peer Review Project	1983–1984	

The Special Libraries Association outgrew its headquarters at 235 Park Avenue South in New York City. It began a search for larger space in 1981. The Special Libraries Association purchased the building at 1700 18th Street for $1.1 million on May 31, 1985. What began as Parsons' home housing a rare books collection, once again, as the cycle turned, became the home for books.

Appendix F

PORTRAITS AND GIFTS TO THE AMERICAN PSYCHIATRIC ASSOCIATION

Portraits

Benjamin Rush: This portrait was the gift of Dan and Logan Blain in 1961. It was commissioned in 1960 at a cost of $1,000. It is a copy of the Peale portrait that hangs in Independence Hall in Philadelphia. However, the artist is said to have copied Rush's hands from the portrait by Sully.

Benjamin Rush: This self-portrait was the gift of Dr. Bernard L. Diamond in 1962. It was purchased from the Argosy Bookstore and Galleries in New York City. The portrait was exhibited in the Philadelphia Museum in the early 19th century as a self-portrait; however, attempts to authenticate this painting as a self-portrait have been unsuccessful.

Founding Fathers: The Council (April 25, 1959) authorized the House Committee—Zigmond Lebensohn, Chairman—to secure portraits and specified their size (24″ wide and 24″ high) and framed with gilded frames not wider than 4″ with no need that portraits be uniform in style or medium and that originals, if available, were desired.

Thomas Kirkbride: This portrait was the gift of the Kirkbride family in 1959 (Mrs. Lydia B. Kirkbride of New Canaan, Connecticut, her son, and the Kirkbride sisters, including Miss Elizabeth of Albany, New York). The artist was Phillips. A copy of the original hangs in the Institute of The Pennsylvania Hospital.

William MaClay Awl: This portrait was the gift of Dr. and Mrs. Philip Rond of Columbus, Ohio in 1960. The purple hue of the face did not please Dr. Rond, so a second portrait was painted by the unknown artist and accepted in 1961.

Samuel Bayard Woodward: This portrait was the gift of the Eastern Psychiatric Research Association (Dr. David J. Impastato) in

1961. The artist, Oppenheimer, painted this copy of an original in the possession of Woodward's great-granddaughter, Dr. Katherine Woodward of New York City. Dr. Woodward planned to donate the original, but a problem arose in getting family members to relinquish their claim. (The Worcester State Hospital also has a portrait of Dr. Woodward and an early photograph (blast type), as well as a classic style bust.)

Amariah Brigham: This portrait was the gift of the Institute of Living (Dr. Francis Braceland) in 1961. The artist is unknown. This painting was copied from an original portrait that hangs in the Institute of Living, Hartford, Connecticut.

John S. Butler: This portrait was the gift of the Hartford Psychiatric Society (Dr. Edward B. Swain) in 1961. The artist is unknown, but appears to be the same artist as the one who painted the portrait of Brigham. The painting was copied from the original portrait lent by the Institute of Living in Hartford, Connecticut.

Isaac Ray: This portrait was the gift of the Butler Hospital, Providence, Rhode Island (Dr. Charles Jones) in 1962. The artist is unknown. It is a copy of an original that hangs in Butler Hospital.

Nehemiah Cutter: This portrait was the gift of the National Association of Private Psychiatric Hospitals (Dr. John Saunders) in 1968. The artist was Ralph S. Lawton, who worked for the Armed Forces Institute of Pathology preparing portraits from photographs. This technique was used to paint the portrait of Dr. Cutter.

Charles H. Stedman: This portrait was the gift of the Northern New England District Branch (Dr. Benjamin Simon) in 1968. The artist was Byrd Farioletti, who painted it from a framed picture of Dr. Stedman that hangs in the Boston State Hospital. The Countway Library in Boston has another original portrait (reproduced in the APA's *100 Years of American Psychiatry*).

John Minson Galt, II and *Francis Taliaferro Stribling:* These portraits were gifts of the Neuropsychiatric Society of Virginia (Dr. Howard W. Asbury) in 1963. The artist was Mrs. Francis White, who painted these portraits from photographs in the APA archives.

Luther Bell: This portrait was the gift of the McLean Hospital (Dr. Francis de Marniffe) in 1967. The artist was K.A. Smith-Brunet, who painted it from an original by Weght (made a century earlier) that hangs in the McLean Hospital.

Samuel White: This portrait was the gift of the Mid-Hudson District Branch (Dr. Herman Snow) in 1969. The artist was Ralph Lawton, who painted it from a photograph of a painting by Sarah Relyea that hangs in the State Capital at Albany, New York (the photograph is in the APA archives).

Pliny Earle: This portrait was the gift of Gralnick Foundation (Dr. Alexander Gralnick) in 1969. The artist was Joseph Kelley. The original was painted from a photograph of a tintype picture now in the National Library of Medicine. The picture used in APA's *100 Years of American Psychiatry* is a photograph taken in 1880, some 36 years later than the one used by the artist. Portraits of Dr. Earle hang in the Northampton (Massachusetts) State Hospital and at the Westchester Division of the New York Hospital.

Other Gifts

Adolf Meyer, portrait, *Collected Papers* and his *Psychobiology,* gift of Mrs. Adolf Meyer, 1958

"Grandfather" English clock, gift of Dr. and Mrs. Saul I. Heller, 1958

Late 18th-century (about 1780) mahogany Westminster chimes crest over arched and glazed door, carved floral motif moon phases; door, $6' \times 27''$, value $1,500

Dorothea Dix portrait, gift of Dixmont State Hospital (1963): copy by E. Thompson of an original painted in 1865; presented to the hospital by an anonymous donor

Solomon Carter Fuller (1872–1953), portrait of the first black psychiatrist: Boston neurologist, psychologist, and psychiatrist, on faculty of Boston University; gift of Dr. and Mrs. Charles Prudhome (1971); Artist: Naida Willette Page, staff artist of the *Journal of the National Medical Association*

R. Finley Gayle, Jr. (President, APA, 1955–1956): gift of Southern Psychiatric Association, 1960

Dewey Cup (a silver pitcher) and editor's footstool in memory of Richard Dewey, Editor, *American Journal of Psychiatry* (1894–1897), presented to Dr. Dewey in 1898 on the occasion of his retirement: presented to Dr. Farrar by Francis Gerty, APA President, on his retirement at the annual banquet (1965). He in turn presented it to Francis Braceland, incoming Editor, who gave it to the APA Museum. (Dr. Gerty came into possession of the cup in 1961 from Dr. Dewey's daughter.)

Presidential Medallion: gift of the Royal Medico-Psychological Association (later the Royal College of Psychiatrists); (with a field of blue and 13 stars representing APA's Founding Fathers, surrounding a center engraving of Benjamin Rush) was the gold medallion presented to APA President Henry W. Brosin in May 1968 at the opening session of the annual meeting (a joint meeting with the British association) by President H.V. Dicks of the Royal Medico-Psychological Association.

Appendix G

MUSEUM BUILDING

The Museum Building fronted R Street and blended with the adjacent headquarters. The small grounds were tastefully landscaped (Ladybird Johnson, wife of President Lyndon B. Johnson, awarded a prize—given at a White House ceremony—to the APA for the beautification project).

The entrance hall was just large enough for a receptionist to control entrance and for a wall exhibit case. The curator's office to the left also had a galley to provide food service for meetings. A handsome conference room with seating for 24 around a huge table was adjacent. The museum occupied the rest of the floor. For the dedicatory exhibit in September of 1967 an attractive program guide described the Weisman collection of primitive art, an Adolf Meyer exhibit, a diorama of the founding of the Association, an exhibit of books written by the Founding Fathers, a history of the *American Journal of Psychiatry*, and a national art exhibit of works by mental patients.

The second floor of the museum building housed the *Psychiatric News* staff, the Joint Information Service, and the Government Relations and Public Affairs departments.

The third floor provided space for two major publications, the *American Journal of Psychiatry* and *Hospital and Community Psychiatry*.

The large first level below ground housed the Association Library, with reference section, study booths, stacks, and a periodicals area. The office of the librarian was adjacent to a large work area, and to an archives and rare book storage vault with climate control.

The second level basement provided space for duplication, mail room, publications inventory, and a general storage area for both museum and archival materials.

After the removal of the staff to the new headquarters building at 1400 K Street, the museum building was purchased in December 1983 by the American Jewish War Veterans for $1.2 million.

Appendix H

THE HEADQUARTERS AT 1400 K STREET

Before the District of Columbia was established, what is now
14th and K Streets was part of a large tract of land called "Pont
Royal" owned by the Pearce family. It was sold to the Davidson
family in 1791.

As the 19th century began, the area north of what is now F
Street was open land. The fields were dotted by a few scattered
frame dwellings. A spring, arising in what is now Franklin Square,
provided the drinking water for those few families living in the
area. From the spring a small creek was formed that meandered
through the adjacent fields.*

By 1864 there were but few changes, as Harriet Riddle Darow
described in *Civil War Recollections of a Little Yankee*. She recalled
that her father's home on 13th Street was "almost in the country, so
nearly did it touch the outlying hills." Animals ran at large—
cows, pigs, goats, and geese, and pastured in anyone's front yard.
She said Franklin Square was an open field—an unkempt,
grassless common, surrounded by a white wooden fence with gaps,
here and there, in the boarding. There were only a few houses
facing the square, the most imposing of which belonged to the
Secretary of War, Stanton. Darow recalled seeing many soldiers fill
their canteens at the spring in Franklin Square.

Gradually the city expanded, after the end of the Civil War, with
residences being built north from F Street and Lafayette Square.
Impressive homes were built along K Street. By the end of the 19th
century it was a prestigious residential area. At 13th and K was the
large brick Mexican Legation where General U.S. Grant visited
the minister, Romero, several times. Also on K Street (at 1321) was
a mansion built by John Sherman, a Secretary of State, and
occupied by the Japanese Ambassador (Viscount Aoki). The names
of the owners of houses in the area can be found in Hal H. Smith's
Historic Washington Houses.

Within another 50 years the commercial growth of the city
crowded out the residences and expanded to include all of K

---

* The source of this material is Hines C: Recollections of Washington City.

Street. (One of the architectural gems—the General Warder House—was moved from 15th and K to upper 16th Street to make way for an office building.)

The Ambassador Hotel was built at 14th and K in about 1930. Forty years later, hard times caused it to close in 1975. The hotel building was torn down and upon that site the new APA building was constructed.*

---

* The above material was supplied by the Columbia Historical Society of Washington, D.C., with photocopies of structures by Marjorie S. Belcher of the Collections Unit.

Appendix I

OFFICERS AND MEETING PLACES OF THE AMERICAN PSYCHIATRIC ASSOCIATION

Presidents of the Association

1844–1848	1	Samuel B. Woodward
1848–1851	2	William MaClay Awl
1851–1855	3	Luther V. Bell
1855–1859	4	Isaac Ray
1859–1862	5	Andrew MacFarland
1862–1870	6	Thomas S. Kirkbride
1870–1873	7	John S. Butler
1873–1879	8	Charles H. Nichols
1879–1882	9	Clement A. Walker
1882–1883	10	John H. Callender
1883–1884	11	John P. Gray
1884–1885	12	Pliny Earle
1885–1886	13	Orpheus Everts
1886–1887	14	H. A. Buttolph
1887–1888	15	Eugene Grissom
1888–1889	16	John P. Chapin
1889–1890	17	W. W. Godding
1890–1891	18	H. P. Stearns
1891–1892	19	Daniel Clark
1892–1893	20	J. B. Andrews
1893–1894	21	John Curwen
1894–1895	22	Edward Cowles
1895–1896	23	Richard Dewey
1896–1897	24	Theophilus O. Powell
1897–1898	25	Richard M. Bucke
1898–1899	26	Henry M. Hurd
1899–1900	27	Joseph G. Rogers
1900–1901	28	Peter M. Wise
1901–1902	29	Robert J. Preston
1902–1903	30	G. Alder Blumer
	31	A. B. Richardson (died before taking office)
1903–1904	32	A. E. Macdonald

1904–1905	33	T. J. W. Burgess
1905–1906	34	C. B. Burr
1906–1907	35	Charles G. Hill
1907–1908	36	Charles P. Bancroft
1908–1909	37	Arthur F. Kilbourne
1909–1910	38	William F. Drewry
1910–1911	39	Charles W. Pilgrim
1911–1912	40	Hubert Work
1912–1913	41	James T. Searcy
1913–1914	42	Carlos F. MacDonald
1914–1915	43	Samuel E. Smith
1915–1916	44	Edward N. Brush
1916–1917	45	Charles G. Wagner
1917–1918	46	James V. Anglin
1918–1919	47	Elmer E. Southard
1919–1920	48	Henry C. Eyman
1920–1921	49	Owen Copp
1921–1922	50	Albert M. Barrett
1922–1923	51	Henry W. Mitchell
1923–1924	52	Thomas W. Salmon
1924–1925	53	William A. White
1925–1926	54	C. Floyd Haviland
1926–1927	55	George M. Kline
1927–1928	56	Adolf Meyer
1928–1929	57	Samuel T. Orton
1929–1930	58	Earl D. Bond
1930–1931	59	Walter M. English
1931–1932	60	William L. Russell
1932–1933	61	James V. May
1933–1934	62	George H. Kirby
1934–1935	63	C. Fred Williams
1935–1936	64	Clarence O. Cheney
1936–1937	65	C. Macfie Campbell
1937–1938	66	Ross McC. Chapman
1938–1939	67	Richard H. Hutchings
1939–1940	68	William C. Sandy
1940–1941	69	George H. Stevenson
	70	H. Douglas Singer (died before taking office)
1941–1942	71	James King Hall
1942–1943	72	Arthur H. Ruggles

1943–1944	73	Edward A. Strecker
1944–1946	74	Karl M. Bowman
1946–1947	75	Samuel W. Hamilton
1947–1948	76	Winfred Overholser
1948–1949	77	William C. Menninger
1949–1950	78	George S. Stevenson
1950–1951	79	John C. Whitehorn
1951–1952	80	Leo H. Bartemeier
1952–1953	81	D. Ewen Cameron
1953–1954	82	Kenneth E. Appel
1954–1955	83	Arthur P. Noyes
1955–1956	84	R. Finley Gayle, Jr.
1956–1957	85	Francis J. Braceland
1957–1958	86	Harry C. Solomon
1958–1959	87	Francis J. Gerty
1959–1960	88	William Malamud
1960–1961	89	Robert H. Felix
1961–1962	90	Walter E. Barton
1962–1963	91	C. H. Hardin Branch
1963–1964	92	Jack R. Ewalt
1964–1965	93	Daniel Blain
1965–1966	94	Howard P. Rome
1966–1967	95	Harvey J. Tompkins
1967–1968	96	Henry W. Brosin
1968–1969	97	Lawrence C. Kolb
1969–1970	98	Raymond W. Waggoner
1970–1971	99	Robert S. Garber
1971–1972	100	Ewald W. Busse
1972–1973	101	Perry C. Talkington
1973–1974	102	Alfred M. Freedman
1974–1975	103	John P. Spiegel
1975–1976	104	Judd Marmor
1976–1977	105	Robert W. Gibson
1977–1978	106	Jack Weinberg
1978–1979	107	Jules H. Masserman
1979–1980	108	Alan A. Stone
1980–1981	109	Donald G. Langsley
1981–1982	110	Daniel X. Freedman
1982–1983	111	H. Keith H. Brodie
1983–1984	112	George Tarjan
1984–1985	113	John A. Talbott

| 1985–1986 | 114 | Carol C. Nadelson |
| 1986–1987 | 115 | Robert O. Pasnau |

Vice Presidents of the Association

1958–1959	William Terhune
1958–1959	David C. Wilson
1959–1960	S. Spafford Ackerly
1959–1960	Franklin Ebaugh
1960–1961	D. Griffith McKerracher
1960–1961	Raymond W. Waggoner
1961–1962	Henry W. Brosin
1961–1962	Titus H. Harris
1962–1963	Alfred Paul Bay
1962–1963	John R. Saunders
1963–1964	Hugh T. Carmichael
1963–1964	M. Ralph Kaufman
1964–1965	Addison M. Duval
1964–1965	Aldwyn B. Stokes
1965–1966	Marion E. Kenworthy
1965–1966	Frank Luton
1966–1967	Alfred W. Auerback
1966–1967	Ewald Busse
1967–1968	George Tarjan
1967–1968	Cecil L. Wittson
1968–1969	Paul V. Lemkau
1968–1969	Philip B. Reed
1969–1970	Hamilton F. Ford
1969–1970	Edward O. Harper
1970–1971	Herbert S. Gaskill
1970–1971	Charles Prudhomme
1971–1972	Viola W. Bernard
1971–1972	Herbert C. Modlin
1972–1973	Judd Marmor
1972–1973	Milton Greenblatt
1973–1974	Harold M. Visotsky
1973–1974	Mildred Mitchell-Bateman
1974–1975	June Jackson Christmas
1974–1975	Jules H. Masserman
1975–1976	Jack A. Wolford

1975–1977	Daniel X. Freedman
1976–1978	Alan A. Stone
1977–1979	Donald G. Langsley
1978–1980	Lewis L. Robbins
1979–1981	Peter A. Martin
1980–1982	Robert J. Campbell
1981–1983	Carol C. Nadelson
1982–1984	Robert O. Pasnau
1983–1985	Elissa Benedek
1984–1986	Irwin N. Perr
1985–1987	Paul J. Fink

Secretaries of the Association

1844–1852	Thomas S. Kirkbride
1852–1854	H. A. Buttolph
1854–1858	Charles H. Nichols
1858–1893	John Curwen
1893–1897	Henry M. Hurd
1897–1904	Charles B. Burr
1904–1906	Emmett C. Dent
1906–1909	Charles W. Pilgrim
1909–1915	Charles G. Wagner
1915–1918	Henry C. Eyman
1918–1921	Henry W. Mitchell
1921–1924	C. Floyd Haviland
1924–1928	Earl D. Bond
1928–1933	Clarence O. Cheney
1933–1938	William C. Sandy
1938–1941	Arthur H. Ruggles
1941–1946	Winfred Overholser
1946–1950	Leo H. Bartemeier
1950–1954	R. Finley Gayle, Jr.
1954–1958	William Malamud
1958–1961	C. H. Hardin Branch
1961–1965	Harvey J. Tompkins
1965–1969	Robert S. Garber
1969–1972	George Tarjan
1972–1975	Robert W. Gibson
1975–1977	Jules H. Masserman
1977–1981	H. Keith H. Brodie

1981–1983	Harold Visotsky
1983–1985	Shervert Frazier
1985–	Elissa Benedek

Treasurers of the Association

1947–1954	Howard W. Potter
1954–1958	Jack R. Ewalt
1958–1959	Robert H. Felix
1959–1963	Addison M. Duval
1963	Walter H. Obenauf
1963–1968	Dale C. Cameron
1968–1973	Hayden H. Donahue
1973–1976	Jack Weinberg
1976–1980	Charles B. Wilkinson
1981–	George H. Pollack

Editors of the American Journal of Psychiatry

1844–1849	Amariah Brigham
1849–1854	T. Romeyn Beck
1854–1886	John P. Gray
1886–1894	G. Alder Blumer
1894–1897	Richard Dewey
1897–1904	Henry M. Hurd
1904–1931	Edward N. Brush
1931–1965	Clarence B. Farrar
1965–1978	Francis J. Braceland
1978–	John C. Nemiah

Speakers of the Assembly

1953–1954	Joseph L. Abramson
1954–1955	Crawford N. Boganz
1955–1956	Addison M. Duval
1956–1957	Mathew Ross
1957–1958	David C. Wilson
1958–1959	Walter H. Obenauf
1959–1960	Alfred Auerback
1960–1961	John R. Saunders
1961–1962	Edward G. Billings

1962–1963	G. Wilse Robinson, Jr.
1963–1964	Robert S. Garber
1964–1965	Philip B. Reed
1965–1966	Duncan Whitehead
1966–1967	Hamilton Ford
1967–1968	John R. Adams
1968–1969	Malcolm J. Farrell
1969–1970	Perry C. Talkington
1970–1971	John S. Visher
1971–1972	Harry H. Brunt, Jr.
1972–1973	James C. Johnson
1973–1974	Warren S. Williams
1974–1975	Robert B. Neu
1975–1976	Miltiades L. Zaphiropoulos
1976–1977	Irwin N. Perr
1977–1978	Daniel A. Grabski
1978–1979	Robert J. Campbell III
1979–1980	Robert O. Pasnau
1980–1981	Melvin M. Lipsett
1981–1982	Lawrence Hartmann
1982–1983	William R. Sorum
1983–1984	Harvey Bluestone
1984–1985	Fred Gottlieb
1985–1986	James M. Trench
1986–1987	Roger Peele

Recorders of the Assembly

1953–1959	John R. Saunders
1959–1962	Lester E. Shapiro
1962–1965	Hamilton F. Ford
1965–1967	Malcolm J. Farrell
1967–1968	Perry C. Talkington
1968–1969	John S. Visher
1969–1970	Harry H. Brunt, Jr.
1970–1971	James C. Johnson, Jr.
1971–1973	Robert B. Neu
1973–1975	W. Payton Kolb
1975–1976	George L. Mallory
1976–1977	Robert J. Campbell III
1977–1978	John H. Houck

1978–1979	Melvin M. Lipsett	
1979–1980	Jack B. Kremens	
1981–1982	Howard Gurevitz	
1982–1983	Harvey Bluestone	
1983–1984	James M. Trench	
1984–1985	Aron Wolf	
1985–1986	Irvin M. Cohen	

Meeting Places of the American Psychiatric Association (formerly known as the Association of Medical Superintendents of American Institutions for the Insane and the American Medico-Psychological Association)

1844	1st	Philadelphia, Pa.
1845		No meeting held
1845	2nd	Washington, D.C.
1847		No meeting held
1848	3rd	New York, N.Y.
1849	4th	Utica, N.Y.
1850	5th	Boston, Mass.
1851	6th	Philadelphia, Pa.
1852	7th	New York, N.Y.
1853	8th	Baltimore, Md.
1854	9th	Washington, D.C.
1855	10th	Boston, Mass.
1856	11th	Cincinnati, Ohio
1857	12th	New York, N.Y.
1858	13th	Quebec, Canada
1859	14th	Lexington, Ky.
1860	15th	Philadelphia, Pa.
1861		No meeting held due to the disturbed condition of the country.
1862	16th	Providence, R.I.
1863	17th	New York, N.Y.
1864	18th	Washington, D.C.
1865	19th	Pittsburgh, Pa.
1866	20th	Washington, D.C.
1867	21st	Philadelphia, Pa.
1868	22nd	Boston, Mass.
1869	23rd	Staunton, Va.
1870	24th	Hartford, Conn.

1871	25th	Toronto, Canada
1872	26th	Madison, Wis.
1873	27th	Baltimore, Md.
1874	28th	Nashville, Tenn.
1875	29th	Auburn, N.Y.
1876	30th	Philadelphia, Pa.
1877	31st	St. Louis, Mo.
1878	32nd	Washington, D.C.
1879	33rd	Providence, R.I.
1880	34th	Philadelphia, Pa.
1881	35th	Toronto, Canada
1882	36th	Cincinnati, Ohio
1883	37th	Newport, R.I.
1884	38th	Philadelphia, Pa.
1885	39th	Saratoga, N.Y.
1886	40th	Lexington, Ky.
1887	41st	Detroit, Mich.
1888	42nd	Fortress Monroe, Va.
1889	43rd	Newport, R.I.
1890	44th	Niagara Falls, N.Y.
1891	45th	Washington, D.C.
1892	46th	Washington, D.C.
		New Constitution adopted. Name changed to American Medico-Psychological Association
1893	47th	Chicago, Ill.
1894	48th	Philadelphia, Pa.
		Fiftieth year since Founding. Semi-Centennial.
1895	49th	Denver, Colo.
1896	50th	Boston, Mass.
1897	51st	Baltimore, Md.
1898	52nd	St. Louis, Mo.
1899	53rd	New York, N.Y.
1900	54th	Richmond, Va.
1901	55th	Milwaukee, Wis.
1902	56th	Montreal, Canada
1903	57th	Washington, D.C.
1904	58th	St. Louis, Mo.
1905	59th	San Antonio, Tex.
1906	60th	Boston, Mass.
1907	61st	Washington, D.C.
1908	62nd	Cincinnati, Ohio

1909	63rd	Atlantic City, N.J.
1910	64th	Washington, D.C.
1911	65th	Denver, Colo.
1912	66th	Atlantic City, N.J.
1913	67th	Niagara Falls, Canada
1914	68th	Baltimore, Md.
1915	69th	Fortress Monroe, Va.
1916	70th	New Orleans, La.
1917	71st	New York, N.Y.
1918	72nd	Chicago, Ill.
1919	73rd	Philadelphia, Pa.
1920	74th	Cleveland, Ohio
1921	75th	Boston, Mass.
		New constitution adopted. Name changed to American Psychiatric Association.
1922	76th	Quebec, Canada
1923	77th	Detroit, Mich.
1924	78th	Atlantic City, N.J.
1925	79th	Richmond, Va.
1926	80th	New York, N.Y.
1927	81st	Cincinnati, Ohio
1928	82nd	Minneapolis, Minn.
1929	83rd	Atlanta, Ga.
1930	84th	Washington, D.C.
1931	85th	Toronto, Canada
1932	86th	Philadelphia, Pa.
1933	87th	Boston, Mass.
1934	88th	New York, N.Y.
1935	89th	Washington, D.C.
1936	90th	St. Louis, Mo.
1937	91st	Pittsburgh, Pa.
1938	92nd	San Francisco, Calif.
1939	93rd	Chicago, Ill.
1940	94th	Cincinnati, Ohio
1941	95th	Richmond, Va.
1942	96th	Boston, Mass.
1943	97th	Detroit, Mich.
1944	98th	Philadelphia, Pa.
		Centennial Meeting
1945		No meeting held
1946	99th	Chicago, Ill.

1947	100th	New York, N.Y.
1948	101st	Washington, D.C.
1949	102nd	Montreal, Canada
1950	103rd	Detroit, Mich.
1951	104th	Cincinnati, Ohio
1952	105th	Atlantic City, N.J.
1953	106th	Los Angeles, Calif.
1954	107th	St. Louis, Mo.
1955	108th	Atlantic City, N.J.
1956	109th	Chicago, Ill.
1957	110th	Chicago, Ill.
1958	111th	San Francisco, Calif.
1959	112th	Philadelphia, Pa.
1960	113th	Atlantic City, N.J.
1961	114th	Chicago, Ill.
1962	115th	Toronto, Canada
1963	116th	St. Louis, Mo.
1964	117th	Los Angeles, Calif.
1965	118th	New York, N.Y.
1966	119th	Atlantic City, N.J.
1967	120th	Detroit, Mich.
1968	121st	Boston, Mass.
1969	122nd	Miami (Bal Harbour), Fla.
1970	123rd	San Francisco, Calif.
1971	124th	Washington, D.C.
1972	125th	Dallas, Tex.
1973	126th	Honolulu, Hawaii
1974	127th	Detroit, Mich.
1975	128th	Anaheim, Calif.
1976	129th	Miami, Fla.
1977	130th	Toronto, Canada
1978	131st	Atlanta, Ga.
1979	132nd	Chicago, Ill.
1980	133rd	San Francisco, Calif.
1981	134th	New Orleans, La.
1982	135th	Toronto, Canada
1983	136th	New York, N.Y.
1984	137th	Los Angeles, Calif.
1985	138th	Dallas, Tex.
1986	139th	Washington, D.C.
1987	140th	Chicago, Ill.

Notes and References

Chapter 1

1. Ramon Parres of Mexico City, distinguished psychiatrist and psychoanalyst, supplied this information. See also his History of Psychiatry in Mexico, World Studies in Psychiatry, vol. 2, no. 3. Northfield, IL, Medical Communications, 1979
2. LaFay H: The Maya, children of time. National Geographic 148:729-767, December 1975
3. Stuart GE: Riddle of the glyphs. National Geographic 148:768-791, December 1975
4. Coe WR: Resurrecting the grandeur of Tikal. National Geographic 148:792-798, December 1975
5. Hall AJ: A traveler's tale of ancient Tikal. National Geographic, 148:799-811, December 1975
6. Calder R: Medicine and Man. New York, Signet, 1958
7. Belsasso G: History of psychiatry in Mexico. Hosp Community Psychiatry 20:342-344, 1969
8. McDowell B: The Aztecs. National Geographic 158:704-751, December 1980
9. Molino-Montez AF: The building of Tenochtillan. National Geographic 158:753-775, December 1980
10. Josephy AM: The Indian Heritage of America. New York, Alfred Knopf, 1968
11. The story of the Iroquois is taken mostly from Farb P: Iroquois primitive democracy, in Man's Rise to Civilization: As Shown by the Indians of North America from Primeval Times to the Coming of the Industrial State. New York, E.P. Dutton Company, 1940
12. Longfellow HW: The Song of Hiawatha. New York, Walter J. Black, Inc., 1932
13. Driver HE: Indian wealth: is it only a myth? The American Way 4:22-28, October 1971
14. The Bible: Deuteronomy 28:28; Leviticus 20:27; I Samuel 21:13-15; Daniel 4:33

15. Alexander FG, Selesnick ST: The History of Psychiatry. New York, Harper and Row, 1966
16. Zilboorg G, Henry GW: A History of Medical Psychology. New York, W.W. Norton, 1941
17. Deutsch A: The Mentally Ill in America. Garden City, New York, Doubleday Doran, 1937
18. Bryan WA: Administrative Psychiatry. New York, W.W. Norton, 1936
19. Richards DW: Hippocrates of Ostia. JAMA 204:1049-1056, 1968
20. Tuchman BW: A Distant Mirror: The Calamitous 14th Century. New York, Ballantine, 1978
21. Escolano G: Decado Primera de la Historia de la Insigne y Coronada Ciudad y Reyno de Valencia. Valencia, Pedro Patrico, May 1610
22. Chamberlain AS: Early mental hospitals in Spain. Am J Psychiatry 123:143-149, 1966
23. Bassoe P: Spain as the cradle of psychiatry. Am J Psychiatry 101:731-738, 1945
24. Boardley J, Harvey AM: Two Centuries of American Medicine. Philadelphia, W.B. Saunders, 1976
25. King LS: American Medicine Comes of Age, 1840–1920. Chicago, American Medical Association, 1984
26. A search by the National Library of Medicine identified Jacob Varrvanger as practicing medicine in New York, 1647–1652, and the founder of the Dutch Hospital which was torn down 24 May 1680
27. Viets HR: The first medical publications. N Engl J Med 268:600-601, 1963
28. Wesley J: Primitive Physics: Or An Easy and Natural Method of Curing Most Diseases. 1747. Reprint edition, London, The Epworth Press, 1960
29. Buchan W: Domestic Medicine, or the Family Physician, second edition. Philadelphia, 1771
30. Gunn JC: Domestic Medicine. Knoxville, 1830
31. Starr P: The Social Transformation of American Medicine. New York, Basic Books, 1982
32. Grob GN: Mental Institutions in America: Social Policy to 1875. New York, The Free Press, 1973
33. Gardner RD: The bicentennial of the Eastern State Hospital, in American Psychiatry: Past, Present and Future. Edited by

Kriegman G, Gardner RD, Abse DW. Charlottesville, University Press of Virginia, 1973
34. Henderson DK, Gillespie RD: A Textbook of Psychiatry, fourth edition. London, Oxford University Press, 1937
35. Rush, Benjamin: see Appendix A

Chapter 2

1. Freud S: New introductory lectures on psychoanalysis, in Complete Psychological Works, Standard Edition, vol. 17. Translated and edited by Strachey J. London, Hogarth Press, 1964
2. Minnigerode M: The Fabulous Forties, 1840–1850: A Presentation of Private Life. New York, G. Putnam, 1924
3. Starr P: The Social Transformation of American Medicine. New York, Basic Books, 1982
4. Shyrock RH: Medicine and Society in America, 1660–1860. New York, New York University Press, 1960
5. Estes JW: Hall Jackson and the Purple Foxglove: Medical Practice and Research in Revolutionary America, 1760–1820. Boston, University Press of New England, 1980. Excerpts, Medical Care at the Siege of Boston, Centerscope (Boston University) 2:24-32, 1980
6. Cash P: The phoenix and the eagle: the founding of the Boston and Massachusetts medical societies in 1780 and 1781. N Engl J Med 305:1033-1039, 1981
7. Hurd HM: The Institutional Care of the Insane in the United States and Canada. Baltimore, The Johns Hopkins Press, 1916
8. Rothman D: The Discovery of the Asylum: Social Order and Disorder in the New Republic. Boston, Little Brown and Co., 1971
9. Franklin B: Some Accounts of the Origin of the Pennsylvania Hospital from Its First Rise. Philadelphia, 1754
10. Deutsch A: The Mentally Ill in America. New York, Doubleday Doran, 1937
11. Shosteck R: Notes on an Early Virginia Physician. American Jewish Archives 23:1-15, 1971
12. Kriegman G, Gardner RD, Abse DW (Eds): American Psychiatry, Past, Present and Future. Charlottesville, University Press of Virginia, 1975

13. Hamilton JM: Acting Superintendent of Spring Grove State Hospital, personal communication, January 16, 1973

14. Carlson ET: Uses of the Past Hospitals and Modern Psychiatry. Mental Hospitals 9:25, 1958

15. Brigham A: Am J Insanity 1:1, July 1844

16. Brill H, Zitrin A: Personal communication with investigation, 1966

17. Fisher TW: The new Boston Insane Hospital. American Journal of Insanity 50:1-10, July 1883

18. Hall JK, Zilboorg G, Bunker HA: One Hundred Years of American Psychiatry—1844–1944. New York, Columbia University Press, 1944

19. Griffin J: Personal communication, 1985

20. Bordley J, Harvey AM: Two Centuries of American Medicine. Philadelphia, W.B. Saunders, 1976

21. King LS: Medical education: the AMA surveys the problem. JAMA 248:3017-3021, 1982

22. Ebaugh FG: History of psychiatric education in the United States from 1844–1944. Am J Psychiatry 100:151-160, 1944

23. Brigham A: Remarks on the Influence of Mental Cultivation Upon Health. Hartford, Connecticut, F.J. Huntington, 1832

24. King LS: American Medicine Comes of Age. Chicago, American Medical Association, 1984

25. Musto D: History and psychiatry's present state of transition. Arch Gen Psychiatry 12:385-392, 1970

26. King LS: The founding of the American Medical Association. JAMA 248:1749-1752, 1982

27. King LS: Medical sects and their influence. JAMA 248:1221-1224, 1982

28. Kett JH: The Formation of the American Medical Association. Westport, Conn., Greenwood Press, 1968

29. Kaufman M: Homeopathy in America. Baltimore, The Johns Hopkins Press, 1971

30. Bockhoven JS: Concepts of schizophrenia in the writing of Benjamin Rush. Compr Psychiatry 1:112-120, 1960

31. Rush B: Medical Inquiries and Observations Upon the Diseases of the Mind. Philadelphia, Kimber and Richardson, 1812

32. Dain N: Concepts of Insanity. New Brunswick, New Jersey, Rutgers University Press, 1964

33. From the Historical Exhibition (1963) on the occasion of the 120th anniversary of the founding of the Royal Medico-Psychological Association, held in the Welcome History Library, London

34. Grob GN: Samuel B. Woodward and the Practice of Psychiatry in Early Nineteenth Century America. Bulletin of History 36:420-443, Sept–Oct 1962

35. Galt JM: The Treatment of Insanity. New York, Harper and Brothers, 1846

36. Bond ED: A mental hospital in the fabulous forties. Am J Psychiatry 4:527-536, 1925

37. Grob GN: The State and the Mentally Ill: A History of the Worcester State Hospital in Massachusetts, 1830–1920. Chapel Hill, University of North Carolina Press, 1966

38. Earle P: Memoirs as quoted in Deutsch A: The Mentally Ill in America. New York, Doubleday Doran, 1937

39. Curwen J: The Original Thirteen Members of the Association of Medical Superintendents of American Institutions for the Insane. Warren, Pennsylvania, E. Corwan & Co., 1885

40. Association Meeting, Washington, DC: American Journal of Insanity 3:87-92, July 1846

Chapter 3

1. Mitchell SW: Address on the occasion of the 50th anniversary of the founding. Proceedings of the American Medico-Psychological Association, Philadelphia, May 1894

2. Channing W: Some remarks on the address delivered to the American Medico-Psychological Association by S. Wier Mitchell, M.D. American Journal of Insanity 51:170, 1894

3. Beard CA: A Basic History of the United States. New York, Doubleday Doran, 1944

4. Naylor CD: The role of medicine: an appraisal. Forum on Medicine 3:725-730, 1980

5. Deutsch A: The Mentally Ill in America. New York, Doubleday Doran, 1937

6. Howells JG (Ed): World History of Psychiatry. New York, Brunner/Mazel, 1975

7. Zilboorg G, Henry GW: A History of Medical Psychology. New York, W.W. Norton, 1941

8. Dain N, Carlson ET: Moral Insanity in the United States, 1835–1866. Am J Psychiatry 118:795-801, 1962

9. Jarvis E: Insanity and Idiocy in Massachusetts. Report of the Commission on Lunacy, 1855, with a Critical Introduction by Gerald N. Grob. Cambridge, Harvard University Press, 1971

10. American Journal of Insanity 12:94-97, 1855

11. Vandenberg JH: The Changing Nature of Man. New York, W.W. Norton, 1961

12. Ebaugh FG: The history of psychiatric education in the United States from 1844–1944. Am J Psychiatry 100:151-160, 1944

13. Deutsch A: Military psychiatry: the Civil War, 1861–1865, in One Hundred Years of American Psychiatry. Edited by Hall JK, Zilboorg G, Bunker HA. New York, Columbia University Press, 1944

14. Shapiro JS: In Line of Duty: A History of Psychiatry and the Combat Soldier from the Civil War to Viet Nam. Washington, DC, American Psychiatric Museum Association, July, 1974

15. Barton WE: Life and Works of S. Wier Mitchell. Unpublished thesis written for degree at University of Illinois, 1930. S. Wier Mitchell, who, as the leading neurologist in 1894, was to use his role as invited lecturer to the Association of Medical Superintendents to castigate its members, was an amazing man. He was a great teacher, an able mechanic, an outstanding clinician, a sensitive poet, writer of children's stories, and a popular novelist. Offered the post of first president of the American Neurologic Association, he turned it down. He wrote about his Civil War experience in the novels *The War Years* and *Westways*, but also in the professional books *Gunshot Wounds and Injuries of the Nerves* and *Reflex Paralysis* and *Fat and Blood* and *How to Make Them* (1877). His "rest cure" prescribed isolation from the stress of everyday living to build up strength. Mitchell also advanced the knowledge of atropine (for muscle spasm), morphine (for pain relief), cannabis, and snake venom. Erythromelagia, which he described, was known as "Mitchell's Disease." When Mitchell died in 1913 he had authored 246 scientific articles and books, 30 short stories and poems, and 18 volumes of other literary works.

16. Ebaugh FG: History of psychiatric education in the United

States from 1844 to 1944. Am J Psychiatry 100:151-160, 1944

17. Grob GN: Mental Institutions in America: Social Policy to 1875. New York, The Free Press, 1975

18. Binger C: Revolutionary Doctor, Benjamin Rush (1746–1813). New York, W.W. Norton, 1966

19. Bockhoven JS: Moral Treatment in American Psychiatry. New York, Springer, 1963

20. Brigham A: Moral treatment. American Journal of Insanity 4:1-15, 1847

21. Braceland FJ: The Institute of Living: The Hartford Retreat 1822–1972. Hartford, Connecticut, The Institute of Living, 1972

22. Cheney CO: Dorothea Lynde Dix. Am J Psychiatry Centennial Anniversary Issue 100:61-68, 1944. For a brief biography, see Appendix C

23. Grob GN: Mental Illness and American Society, 1875–1940. Princeton, Princeton University Press, 1983

24. Himelhoch MS, Shaffer AT: Elizabeth Packard: 19th century crusader for the rights of mental patients. Journal of American Studies 13:343-375, 1979

25. Grob GN: The State and the Mentally Ill. Chapel Hill, University of North Carolina Press, 1966

26. Tucker GA: Lunacy in Many Lands: Being an Introduction to the Reports on the Lunatic Asylums of Various Countries Visited, 1882–5. Sydney, Australia, C. Potter, 1887

27. Journal of Nervous and Mental Diseases 6:343, 1879

28. Jones RE: Correspondence of the APA founders. Am J Psychiatry 119:1121-1134, 1963

29. Kline GM, Thom DA, Wallace GL (Eds): Bulletin of the Massachusetts Department of Mental Diseases, Fernald Memorial Issue, vol. 14, April, 1930

30. Alexander FG, Selesnick ST: The History of Psychiatry. New York, Harper and Row, 1966

31. Cytryn L, Lourie RS: Mental retardation, in Comprehensive Textbook of Psychiatry II. Edited by Freedman A, Kaplan HI, Saddock BJ. Baltimore, Williams & Wilkins, 1975

32. Baker BW: History of the care of the feebleminded. Bulletin of the Massachusetts Department of Mental Diseases, Fernald Memorial Issue 14:19-29, 1930

33. Sloan W, Stevens HA: A Century of Concern: A History of American Association on Mental Deficiency. Washington, DC, American Association on Mental Deficiency, 1976

34. Haskell RH: Mental deficiency over 100 years. Am J Psychiatry 100:107-118, 1944

35. American Association on Mental Deficiency was founded under the name Association of Medical Officers of American Institutions for Idiots and Feebleminded, and followed the pattern of the early APA in many ways: its name was similar, its membership was restricted, its program at annual meetings featured reports from the states, it instituted presidential addresses in 1886 (the APA did this in 1883) and it was severely criticized in 1894 by Osborne, as the APA was criticized by Mitchell. In 1926 the association met at the same time and place of the APA annual meeting, and in that year the question of amalgamation with APA was debated. Because of the very different membership mix of educators, criminologists, sociologists, and psychologists, as well as psychiatrists, amalgamation was deemed inadvisable. Ten years later, instead of meeting every year with the APA, the associations began to meet together every third year. Another effort to establish closer relationships developed in 1956, when Gail Walker was made chairman of the APA Committee on Mental Deficiency. Walker had been president of the AAMD the year before. The APA Committee recommended liaison representatives to both associations, APA recognition of AAMD institutions for training psychiatrists, and inspection of schools for the retarded by APA surveyors.

36. Bunker HA: American psychiatry as a specialty, in One Hundred Years of American Psychiatry. Edited by Hall JK, Zilboorg G, Bunker HA. New York, Columbia University Press, 1944

37. Curwen J: History of the Association of Medical Superintendents of American Institutions for the Insane. Warren, Pennsylvania, E. Cowan Co., 1885

38. Farrar C (Ed): Centennial Issue. Am J Psychiatry 100:1-198, 1944

39. Callender JH: History and Work of the Association for Medical Superintendents of American Institutions for the Insane. American Journal of Insanity 40:1-32, 1883

40. Starr P: The Social Transformation of American Medicine.

New York, Basic Books, 1982

41. Proceedings of the American Association of Medical Superintendents of Institutions for the Insane, 1866. American Journal of Insanity 23:61-62, 1866. See also Callender JH: History and work of the Association. American Journal of Insanity 40:1-32, 1983. The Proposition was developed over a period of years, beginning in 1854.

42. Overholser W: An Historical Sketch of St. Elizabeths Hospital in Centennial Papers; St. Elizabeths Hospital, 1855–1955. Washington, DC, St. Elizabeths Hospital Centennial Commission, 1956

43. Hamilton SW: American mental hospitals, in One Hundred Years of American Psychiatry. Edited by Hall JK, Zilboorg G, Bunker HA. New York, Columbia University Press, 1944

44. Hurd H: Institutional Care of the Insane in the United States and Canada. Baltimore, Johns Hopkins Press, 1916

45. Zilboorg G: Legal aspects of psychiatry, in One Hundred Years of American Psychiatry. Edited by Hall JK, Zilboorg G, Bunker HA. New York, Columbia University Press, 1944

46. Overholser W: The founding and the founders of the association, in One Hundred Years of American Psychiatry. Edited by Hall JK, Zilboorg G, Bunker HA. New York, Columbia University Press, 1944

47. Ray I: A Treatise on the Medical Jurisprudence of Insanity. Boston, Little, Brown, 1838. Reprint edition, Cambridge, Massachusetts, Belknap Press, 1962

48. Quen JM: Isaac Ray and Charles Doe: responsibility and justice, in Law and the Mental Health Professions. Edited by Barton WE, Sanborn CJ. New York, International Universities Press, 1978

49. Dunton WR: The second half-century of the Journal. American Journal of Psychiatry 100:41-60, 1944

50. Ray I: American Journal of Insanity 7:217, 1850

51. Ray I: American Journal of Insanity 32:345, 1861

52. Ray I: American Journal of Insanity 35:354, 1864

53. Pollock HM, Wiley ED: A contribution to the history of psychiatric expert testimony. Am J Psychiatry 100:119-133, 1944

54. Chapin JB: Presidential address. American Journal of Insanity 46:1-21, 1889

55. Meyer A: Letter to Stanley Hall, President of Clark University,

Worcester, Massachusetts, December 7, 1895. Reproduced for APA members on the occasion on the 100th anniversary of the birth of Adolf Meyer. Nutley, New Jersey, Roche Laboratories

56. Tucker BR: Silas Wier Mitchell. Am J Psychiatry 100:80-86, 1944
57. Bunker HA: Psychiatric literature, in One Hundred Years of American Psychiatry. Edited by Hall JK, Zilboorg G, Bunker HA. New York, Columbia University Press, 1944
58. Whitehorn JC: Psychiatric research, in One Hundred Years of American Psychiatry. Edited by Hall JK, Zilboorg G, Bunker HA. New York, Columbia University Press, 1944
59. Deutsch A: History of mental hygiene, in One Hundred Years of American Psychiatry. Edited by Hall JK, Zilboorg G, Bunker HA. New York, Columbia University Press, 1944

Chapter 4

1. Furnas JC: The Americans: a Social History of the United States: 1587–1914. New York, Putnam, 1969
2. Grun B: The Timetables of History. New York, Simon and Schuster, 1975
3. Bordley JB, Harvey AM: Two Centuries of American Medicine 1776–1976. Philadelphia, W.B. Saunders, 1976
4. Grob GN: Mental Illness and American Society, 1875–1940. Princeton, Princeton University Press, 1983
5. Starr P: The Social Transformation of American Medicine. New York, Basic Books, 1982
6. For additional information on Beers, see Dain N: Clifford W. Beers: Advocate For The Insane. Pittsburgh, University of Pittsburgh Press, 1980
7. Griffin JD: The amazing careers of Hincks and Beers. Can J Psychiatry 27:668-671, 1982
8. Deutsch A: The Mentally Ill in America. Garden City, New York, Doubleday Doran, 1937
9. Deutsch A: The history of mental hygiene, in One Hundred Years of American Psychiatry. Edited by Hall JK, Zilboorg G, Bunker HA. New York, Columbia University Press, 1944
10. Ridenour N: Mental Health in the United States. Cambridge, Massachusetts, 1961

11. Hunter RC: Personal communication, December 2, 1983
12. Kenworthy ME: Contributions to social work, in Psychoanalysis Today. Edited by Lorand S. New York, International Universities Press, 1944
13. Alexander F: Development of ego psychology, in Psychoanalysis Today. Edited by Lorand S. New York, International Universities Press, 1944
14. Jelliffe, SE: Psychoanalysis and internal medicine, in Psychoanalysis Today. Edited by Lorand S. New York, International Universities Press, 1944
15. Eisenbud J: Mental hygiene, in Psychoanalysis Today. Edited by Lorand S. New York, International Universities Press, 1944
16. Quen JM, Carlson ET (Eds): American Psychoanalysis: Origins and Development. New York, Brunner/Mazel, 1978
17. Jones E: The Life and Works of Sigmund Freud. 3 vols. New York, Basic Books, 1955
18. D'Amore, ART: William Alanson White—pioneer psychoanalyst, in William Alanson White: The Washington Years, 1903–1937. Edited by D'Amore ART. Washington, DC, US HEW–NIMH, 1976
19. Alexander FG, Selesnick ST: The History of Psychiatry. New York, Harper and Row, 1966
20. Gardner GE: History of child psychiatry, in Comprehensive Textbook of Psychiatry II. Edited by Freeman AM, Kaplan HL, Saddock BJ. Baltimore, Williams & Wilkins, 1975
21. Gardner GE: In Memoriam: William Healy, M.D. Am J Orthopsychiatry 34:960-964, 1964
22. Bulletin of Massachusetts Department of Mental Diseases, Fernald Memorial Issue. vol. 14, nos. 1 and 2, April 1930
23. Ryan WC: Mental hygiene in the schools. Am J Psychiatry 100:144-146, 1946
24. Bullis HE: Human Relations in the Classroom. 2 vols. Wilmington, Delaware, Delaware State Society For Mental Hygiene, 1947
25. Shakow D: Reflections on a do-it-yourself training program in clinical psychology. Journal History of Behavioral Sciences 12:14-30, 1976
26. Brown R: Social Psychology. New York, The Free Press, 1965
27. For histories of psychology, see: Reisman JM: A History of Clinical Psychology (covers period 1890 to 1959). New York,

Irvington, 1976; APA Task Force Report No. 15: The History of American Psychiatry: A Teaching and Research Guide. Washington, DC, American Psychiatric Association, 1979

28. Deutsch A: The convergence of social work and psychiatry: an historical note. Mental Hygiene 24:92-97, 1940

29. Steward IM: The Education of Nurses: Historical Foundations and Modern Trends. New York, MacMillan, 1944

30. Muller TG: The Nature and Direction of Psychiatric Nursing. Philadelphia, J.B. Lippincott, 1950

31. Sivadon PD: Occupational Therapy in France: 100 Years Ago and Today. St. Elizabeths Hospital Centennial Papers, 1855–1955. Washington, DC, St. Elizabeths Hospital, 1956

32. Dunton WR, Licht S: Occupational Therapy: Principles and Practice. Springfield, Illinois, Charles C Thomas, 1950

33. Deutsch A: The Story of GAP. New York, Group for the Advancement of Psychiatry, 1959. This account relates the origins, goals, and activities. GAP has continued into the present, not as a political organization, but as an authority on issues important to psychiatry. Its reports are a distillation of several years of study of a topic. The reports are widely read and quoted.

34. American Medical Association Digest of Official Actions: 1846–1958. Chicago, American Medical Association, 1959

35. DeJong RN: A History of American Neurology. New York, Raven Press, 1982

36. Kolb LC: Modern Clinical Psychiatry, 10th edition. Philadelphia, W.B. Saunders, 1982

37. Newman J (Ed): 200 Years: A Bicentennial Illustrated History of the United States. Washington, DC, US News and World Report, 1973

38. Collins AC: The Story of America in Pictures. New York, Literary Guild, 1935

39. Strecker EA: Military psychiatry WWI, in the President's Message: the leaven in war and in peace. Am J Psychiatry 100:1-2, 1944

40. Strecker EA: Presidential address delivered at the Centenary Meeting of the American Psychiatric Association in Philadelphia, May 15, 1944. New Directions in American Psychiatry, 1944–1958. Washington, DC, American Psychiatric Association, 1969

41. Glass AJ: Introduction, in Neuropsychiatry in WWII, vol. 1.

Edited by Anderson RS. Washington, DC, Office of the Surgeon General, Department of the Army, 1966

42. Group for the Advancement of Psychiatry: The VIP with Psychiatric Impairment: Report 82. New York, Group for the Advancement of Psychiatry, 1973

43. Beard CA, Beard MR: A Basic History of the United States. New York, Doubleday Doran, 1944

44. Morris RB, Irwin GW (Eds): Harper Encyclopedia of the Modern World. New York, Harper and Row, 1970

45. Menninger WC: A Psychiatrist for a Troubled World: The Selected Papers, vol. 2. New York, The Viking Press, 1967

46. History of the Medical Department in the World War, vol. 10. Washington, DC, U.S. Government Printing Office, 1929

47. Deutsch A: Military psychiatry: World War II (1941–1943), in One Hundred Years of American Psychiatry. Edited by Hall JK, Zilboorg G, Bunker HA. New York, Columbia University Press, 1944

48. Anderson RS (Ed): Neuropsychiatry in WW II, in The VIP with Psychiatric Impairment: Report 82. New York, Group for the Advancement of Psychiatry, 1973

49. Grinker RR, Spiegel JP: Men Under Stress. Philadelphia, Blakiston, 1945

50. Brill NQ, Beebe GW: A Follow-Up of War Neuroses. Washington, DC, Veterans Administration, 1955

51. Straus R: Mental Health in the Context of a Changing American Society. Unpublished report of special consultants to the Director of NIMH, December 1963

52. Barton WE: Historical perspectives in the delivery of psychiatric services, in Psychiatry in Transition, 1966–1967. Edited by Stokes AB. Toronto, Clarke Institute of Psychiatry, University of Toronto Press, 1967

53. Rennie TAC, Woodward LE: Mental Health in Modern Society. New York, Commonwealth Fund, 1948

54. Lidz T: Adolf Meyer and the development of American psychiatry. Am J Psychiatry 123:320-332, 1966

55. Bogardus EM: Measuring social distance. Journal of Applied Sociology 9:299-308, 1925

56. Allen LA: A study of community attitudes toward mental hygiene. Mental Hygiene 27:248-255, 1943

57. Ramsey GV, Siep M: Attitudes and opinions concerning mental illness. Psychiatr Q 22:428-441, 1948

58. Crocetti G, Spiro HR, Siassi I: Are the ranks closed? attitudinal, social distance and mental illness. Am J Psychiatry 127:1121-1127, 1971

Chapter 5

1. Meyer A: The "complaint" as the center of genetic–dynamic and nosological thinking in psychiatry. N Engl J Med 199:360-370, 1928. Represented in Collected Papers of Adolf Meyer, vol 3. Baltimore, Johns Hopkins University Press, 1952. Quoted in Lidz T: Adolf Meyer and the Development of American Psychiatry. J Psychiatry 123:320-336, 1966 (special section on Adolf Meyer, 1866–1950)
2. Spies T, Cooper C, Blankenhor MA: The use of nicotinic acid in the treatment of pellagra. JAMA 110:622-627, 1928; JAMA 111:584-592, 1938
3. Wise PM: Presidential address. American Journal of Insanity 58:79, 1901–1902
4. Alexander FG, Selesnick ST: The History of Psychiatry. New York, Harper and Row, 1966
5. Hart B: The Psychology of Insanity, fourth edition. New York, Macmillan, 1931
6. Hendrick I: Facts and Theories of Psychoanalysis. New York, A.A. Knopf, 1934
7. Zilboorg G, Henry GW: A History of Medical Psychology. New York, W.W. Norton, 1941
8. Bordley JB, Harvey AM: Two Centuries of American Medicine, 1776–1976. Philadelphia, W.B. Saunders, 1976
9. Meyer A: The rise to person and the concept of wholes or integrates. Am J Psychiatry 100:100-106, 1944
10. Grinker RR: Fifty Years in Psychiatry: A Living History. Springfield, Illinois, Charles C Thomas, 1979
11. Rice DP: Health statistics: past and present. N Engl J Med 305:219-220, 1981
12. Plunkett RJ, Gordon JE: Epidemiology and Mental Illness. New York, Basic Books, 1960
13. Pugh TF, MacMahon B: Epidemiological Findings in United States Mental Hospital Data. Boston, Little Brown, 1962
14. Kolb LC: The Institute of Psychiatry: growth, development, and future. Psychol Med 1:86-95, 1970

15. Barton WE: Community Psychiatry in Boston: Historical Perspectives. Paper presented to the Scientific Assembly on the occasion of the dedication of the Barton Building of the Boston State Hospital, Boston, September 29, 1966
16. Frost HP: State care of Boston's insane. American Journal of Insanity 49:301-311, 1912
17. Forbush B: The Sheppard and Enoch Pratt Hospital (1853–1970): A History. Philadelphia, J.B. Lippincott, 1971
18. Mosher JM: The insane in general hospitals. American Journal of Insanity 57:325-329, 1900
19. Lipowski ZJ: Holistic medical foundations of American psychiatry: a bicentennial. Am J Psychiatry 138:888-895, 1981
20. Hurd HM (Ed): The Institutional Care of the Insane in the United States and Canada, 2 vols. Baltimore, Johns Hopkins Press, 1916
21. Barton WE, Barton GM: Mental Health Administration Principles and Practices. New York, Human Sciences Press, 1983
22. Stevenson GS: The development of extra mural psychiatry in the United States. Am J Psychiatry 100:147-150, 1944
23. Barton WE, St. John WT: Family care and outpatient psychiatry. Am J Psychiatry 117:644-647, 1961
24. Barton WE: Administrative Psychiatry. Springfield, Illinois, Charles C Thomas, 1962
25. Cameron DE: The Day Hospital Report of 1958. Washington, DC, Day Hospital Conference, American Psychiatric Association, 1958
26. Deutsch A: The history of mental hygiene, in One Hundred Years of American Psychiatry. Edited by Hall JK, Zilboorg G, Bunker HA. New York, Columbia University Press, 1944
27. Huseth B: Halfway houses, a new rehabilitative measure. Mental Hospitals 9:5-9, 1958; quoted in Landy D, Greenblatt M: Halfway Houses. Washington, DC, HEW Vocational Rehabilitation Administration, 1965
28. Barton WE: Historical perspectives in the delivery of psychiatric service, in Psychiatry in Transition. Edited by Stokes A. Toronto, University of Toronto Press, 1967
29. Hamilton SW: The history of American mental hospitals, in One Hundred Years of American Psychiatry. Edited by Hall JK, Zilboorg G, Bunker HA. New York, Columbia University Press, 1944

30. Bryan WA: Administrative Psychiatry. New York, W.W. Norton, 1936

31. Overholser W: An historical sketch, in Centennial Papers of St. Elizabeths Hospital. Washington, DC, Centennial Commission, St. Elizabeths Hospital, 1956

32. Grob GN: The State and the Mentally Ill: A History of the Worcester State Hospital in Massachusetts, 1830–1920. Chapel Hill, University of North Carolina Press, 1966

33. Morrisey JP, Goldman HH, Klernian LV: The Enduring Asylum: Cycles of Institutional Reform at Worcester State Hospital. New York, Grune and Stratton, 1980

34. Deutsch A: The Shame of the States. New York, Harcourt Brace, 1948

35. Bulletin of Massachusetts Department of Mental Diseases, Fernald Memorial Issue. vol. 14, nos. 1 and 2, April 1930

36. Kline GM, Thom DA, Wallace GL (Eds): Bulletin of Massachusetts Department of Mental Diseases, Fernald Memorial Issue. vol. 14, nos. 1 and 2, April 1930

37. Malamud W: Psychiatric Therapies, in One Hundred Years of American Psychiatry. Edited by Hall JK, Zilboorg G, Bunker HA. New York, Columbia University Press, 1944

38. Cotton HA: Focal infections and mental disease. Am J Psychiatry 80:149, 1923

39. Neyman C, Osborn R: Artificial fever produced by high frequency current. Illinois Medical Journal 56:199, 1929

40. Bockhoven JS: Moral Treatment in American Psychiatry. New York, Springer, 1963

41. Myerson A: Theory and principles of the total push method in the treatment of chronic schizophrenia. Am J Psychiatry 95:1197-1204, 1939

42. Main TF: The hospital as a therapeutic institution. Bull Menninger Clin 10:66-70, 1946

43. Stanton AH, Schwartz MS:
    a. Management of a type of institutional participation in mental illness. Psychiatry 12:13-25, 1949
    b. Medical opinion and the social context. Psychiatry 12:243-249, 1949
    c. Observations on disassociation as social participation. Psychiatry 12:339-354, 1949

44. Wood P: Effort syndrome. Br Med J 1:767, 805, 845, 1941

45. Wilson ATM, Doyle M, Kelnar J: Hospital community as rehabilitation: the Dartford experience with ex-prisoners of war, in The Shaping of Psychiatry By War. Edited by Rees JR. New York, W.W. Norton, 1945

46. Barton WE: The psychiatric hospital as a therapeutic community, in Better Social Services for Mentally Ill Patients. Edited by Knee RI. New York, American Association of Psychiatric Social Workers, 1955

47. Jones M: Social Psychiatry: A Study of Therapeutic Communities. London, Tavistock Publications, 1952

48. Kubie L: Practical Aspects of Psychoanalysis. New York, W.W. Norton, 1942

49. Levine M: Psychotherapy in Medical Practice. New York, Macmillan, 1942

50. Meyerson A: Some trends in psychiatry. Am J Psychiatry 100:163-173, 1944

51. Weiss E (Ed): Paul Federn: Ego Psychology and the Psychoses. New York, Basic Books, 1949

52. Kolb LC: Modern Clinical Psychiatry, 10th edition. Philadelphia, W.B. Saunders, 1982

53. Saddock BJ: Group psychotherapy, in Comprehensive Textbook of Psychiatry II. Edited by Freedman AM, Kaplan HE, Saddock BJ. Baltimore, Williams & Wilkins, 1975

54. Sakel M: Zur entstehung der medikamentosen schocktherapie der schizophrenie. Wien Med Wschr 87:1108, 1937

55. Kalinowsky L: Insulin coma treatment, in Comprehensive Textbook of Psychiatry II. Edited by Freedman AM, Kaplan HE, Saddock BJ. Baltimore, Williams & Wilkins, 1975

56. Meduna JV: Die Konvulsionstherapie der schizoprenie. Psychiat Neuro Wschr 37:315, 1935

57. Cerletti U, Bini L: L'ettroschock. Arch Gen di Neurol Psichiat e Psicoanal 19:266, 1938

58. Franklin F. Offner, personal communication, Feb. 5, 1969

59. Meyerson A, Feldman L, Green I: Experience with electric shock therapy in mental disease. N Engl J Med 244:1081-1085, 1941

60. Pulver SE: The first electro-convulsive treatment given in the United States. Am J Psychiatry 117:845-846, 1961

61. Joseph Hughes, personal correspondence, May 12, 1970

62. Monez E: Tentatives Operatoires dans le Traitement de Certains Psychoses. Paris, Masson, 1936

63. Freeman W, Watts JW: Psychosurgery. Springfield, Ill., Charles C Thomas, 1942, 1950

64. Kalinowsky L: Psychosurgery, in Comprehensive Textbook of Psychiatry II. Edited by Freedman AM, Kaplan HE, Saddock BJ. Baltimore, Williams & Wilkins, 1975

65. Sweet WH: Current status of psychiatric surgery, in Controversy in Psychiatry. Edited by Brady JP, Brodie HKH. Philadelphia, W.B. Saunders, 1978

66. Clark DH: Administrative psychiatry, 1942–1962. Am J Psychiatry 109:178-201, 1963

67. Flexner A: Medical Education in the United States and Canada. Pittsburgh, Carnegie Foundation, 1910

68. Ebaugh FG: The history of psychiatric education in the United States from 1844 to 1944. Am J Psychiatry 100:151-160, 1944

69. Ebaugh FG, Rymer CA: Psychiatry in Medical Education. New York, The Commonwealth Fund, 1942

70. Russell WL: Presidential address. Am J Psychiatry 89:561, 1932

71. Austin Davies appointed. Am J Psychiatry 90:411, 1933

72. Association and Hospital Notes: sites of New York Offices. Am J Psychiatry 89:1061; 90:111; 91:407; 92:328; 96:488; 97:492

73. Sites of New York offices. APA Newsletter 3:1, June 15, 1951; 10:1, 1958; 16:1, Mar 1964; 17:1, Mar 1965

74. New York office closed. APA Operations Manual, revised edition, 1962

75. Personal letters from Drs. Bartemier, Braceland, Felix, and Gerty, 1981

76. Strecker EA: Presidential address: New directions in American psychiatry, 1944–1968. Washington, DC, American Psychiatric Association, 1969

77. Mora G: Introduction, in New Directions in American Psychiatry, 1944–1968. Washington, DC, American Psychiatric Association, 1969

78. Bowman KM: Presidential address, in New Directions in American Psychiatry, 1944–1968. Washington, DC, American Psychiatric Association, 1969

80. Appel KE: Daniel Blain, 93rd President: 1964–65, in New Directions in American Psychiatry, 1944–1968. Washington, DC, American Psychiatric Association, 1969

81. Braceland FJ: In Memorium: Daniel Blain, 1898–1981. Am J Psychiatry 139:525-526, 1982
82. Overholser W: Presidential address, in New Directions in American Psychiatry, 1944–1968. Washington, DC, American Psychiatric Association, 1969
83. Observations and recollections of Henry W. Brosin and Walter E. Barton, 1983
84. Barton WE: In Memorium: Robert Lewis Robinson, 1915–1980. Am J Psychiatry 138:696-697, 1981
85. Menninger WC: Presidential Address, in New Directions in American Psychiatry, 1944–1968. Washington, DC, American Psychiatric Association, 1969
86. Deutsch A: The Story of GAP. New York, Group for the Advancement of Psychiatry, 1959

Chapter 6

1. 200 years: A Bicentennial History of the United States. Washington, DC, U.S. News and World Report, 1973
2. Grun B: The Timetables of History. New York, Simon and Schuster, 1979
3. Wirth CL: The National Parks in America's Wonderlands. Washington, DC, The National Geographic Society, 1959
4. Danoff AP: Ten Forces Reshaping America. U.S. News and World Report 96:40-41, 1984
5. Solorzano L: Medical miracles, in Ten Forces Shaping America. U.S. News and World Report 96:51-52, 1984
6. Schwartz MD (Ed): Using Computers in Clinical Practice: Psychotherapy and Mental Health Applications. New York, The Haworth Press, 1984
7. Barton WE, Barton GM: Management information system, in Mental Health Administration: Principles and Practice, vol. 1. New York, Human Sciences Press, 1983
8. Boraiko AA, O'Rear C: A splendid light: lasers. National Geographic 165:335-337, 1984
9. Hattwick MA: Rabies, in Cecil Textbook of Medicine. Edited by Wyng Garden JB, Smith LH. Philadelphia, W.B. Saunders, 1982
10. Boardly J III, Harvey AM: Two Centuries of American Medicine. Philadelphia, W.B. Saunders, 1976

11. Goodman LS, Winetrobe MM, Damesheck W, et al: Nitrogen mustard therapy. JAMA 132:126-132, 1946; reprinted in JAMA 251:2255-2261, 1984

12. Barton WE, Barton GM: Ethics and Law in Mental Health Administration. New York, International Universities Press, 1984

13. Dublin TD: Foreign physicians: impact on U.S. health care. Science 185-407, 1974

14. Cade JFJ: Lithium Salts in the Treatment of Psychotic Excitement. Med J Aust 36:349-352, 1949

15. Malamud W, Barton WE, Fleming R: The evaluation of the effect of derivatives of rauwolfia in the treatment of schizophrenia. Am J Psychiatry 114:193-200, 1957

16. Baldessarini RJ: Chemotherapy in Psychiatry. Cambridge, Harvard University Press, 1977

17. Delay J, Denniker P, Harl J: Utilization therapeutique psychiatrique d'une phenothiazine d'action centrale elective. Ann Med Psychol 110:112-117, 1952

18. Carlson A, Lindquist M: Effect of chlorpromazine or haloperidol on formation of 3−methoxytyramine and normetanephrine in mouse brain. Acta Pharmacologis et Toxisologica 20:140-144, 1963

19. Kety SS: Biological approaches to treatment and understanding of the major psychoses, in American Psychiatry: Past, Present and Future. Edited by Kriegman G, Gardner RD, Abse DW. Charlottesville, University Press of Virginia, 1975

20. MacLean PD: A triune concept of the brain and behavior, in The Clarence Hinks Memorial Lecture. Edited by Boag TJ, Campbell D. Toronto, University of Toronto Press, 1973

21. Kolb LD: Modern Clinical Psychiatry, ninth edition. Philadelphia, W.B. Saunders, 1977

22. Arnold MD: Brain function in emotions, in Physiological Correlates of Emotion. Edited by Black P. New York, Academic Press, 1970

23. Freedman AM, Kaplan HI, Saddock BJ: The brain and psychiatry, in Comprehensive Textbook of Psychiatry II. Baltimore, Williams & Wilkins, 1975

24. Lifton MA: The evolution of biological understanding of affective and schizophrenic disorders, in Affective and Schizophrenic Disorders. Edited by Zales MR. New York,

Brunner/Mazel, 1983

25. Axelrod J: Neurotransmitters. Scientific American 230:53, 1974

26. Brodie HKH, Sabshin M: An overview of trends in psychiatric research: 1963–1972. Am J Psychiatry 130: 1309-1318, 1973

27. Kety SS, Rosenthal D, Wender PH, et al: Mental Illness in the Biological and Adoptive Families of Adopted Schizophrenics. Am J Psychiatry 128:302-306, 1971

28. Rosenthal D, Wender PH, Kety SS, et al: The adopted-away offspring of schizophrenics. Am J Psychiatry 128:307-311, 1971

29. Ham GC: Genes and the Psyche: Perspective in Human Development and Behavior. Paper presented at the annual meeting of the American Psychiatric Association, Toronto, May 9, 1962.

30. Reichman FF: Principles of Intensive Psychotherapy. Chicago, University of Chicago Press, 1950

31. Spiegelberg H: The Phenomenological Movement. The Hague, Martinus Nijhoff, 1965

32. Foy JL: The existential school, in The American Handbook of Psychiatry, vol. 1, second edition. Edited by Arieti S. New York, Basic Books, 1974

33. Havens LJ: The existential use of self. Am J Psychiatry 131:1-10, 1974

34. Bailey P: The great psychiatric revolution. Am J Psychiatry 113:387, 1957

35. Sheppard M: A critical appraisal of American psychiatry. Compr Psychiatry 12:302, 1971

36. Malamud W: The Chicago meeting. Am J Psychiatry 113:83, 1957

37. Hoch PH, Zubin J (Eds): The Future of Psychiatry. New York, Grune and Stratton, 1952

38. Barton WE: Administration in Psychiatry. Springfield, Illinois, Charles C Thomas, 1962

39. Castelnuovo-Tedesco P: The Twenty Minute Hour. Boston, Little Brown, 1965

40. Mann J: Time-Limited Psychotherapy. Cambridge, Harvard University Press, 1973

41. Strupp HH, Blackwood G: Recent Methods of Psycho-

therapy, in Comprehensive Textbook of Psychiatry II. Edited by Freedman AM, Kaplan HI, Saddock BJ. Baltimore, Williams & Wilkins, 1975

42. Berne E: Games People Play. New York, Grove Press, 1964
43. Harris TA: I'm OK–You're OK. New York, Avon Books, 1967
44. Romano J: Keynote Address in American Psychiatry, Past, Present, and Future. Edited by Kriegman G, Gardner ED, Abse DW. Charlottesville, University of Virginia Press, 1975
45. Lipowski ZJ, Lipsitt DR, Whybrow PC: Psychosomatic Medicine: Current Trends and Clinical Applications. New York, Oxford University Press, 1977
46. Beckhterev VM: Die anwendug der methode der motorischen, assoziations—reflexe zur aufdeckung der simulation. Z gesamte, Neurol Psychiatr 13:183, 1917
47. Pavlov IP: Conditioned Reflexes. London, Oxford University Press, 1927
48. Thorndike EL: Animal intelligence: an experimental study of the associative processes in animals. Psychological Monograph 2 (8), 1898
49. Skinner BF: The Behavior of Organisms. New York, Appleton-Century-Crofts, 1938
50. Miller NE: Learning of visceral and glandular responses. Science 163:434, 1969
51. Brady JP: Behavior therapy, in Modern Clinical Psychiatry, ninth edition. Edited by Kolb LD. Philadelphia, W.B. Saunders, 1977
52. Bachrach AJ: Learning theory, in Modern Clinical Psychiatry, ninth edition. Edited by Kolb LD. Philadelphia, W.B. Saunders, 1977
53. Brady JP, Brodie HKH: Controversy in Psychiatry. Philadelphia, W.B. Saunders, 1978
54. Hollingshead AB, Redlich FC: Social Class and Mental Illness. New York, Wiley, 1958
55. Srole L, Langner TS, Michael ST, et al: Mental Health in the Metropolis: The Mid-Town Manhattan Study, vol. 1. New York, McGraw-Hill, 1967
56. Leighton AH: My Name is Legion: The Sterling County Study, vol. 1. New York, Basic Books, 1959
57. Leighton AH: Psychiatric disorders in urban settings, Amer-

ican Handbook of Psychiatry, vol. 2. Edited by Arieti S. New York, Basic Books, 1974

58. Brownmiller S: Against Our Will: Men, Women and Rape. New York, Simon and Schuster, 1975

59. Kinsey AC, Pomeroy WB, Martin CE: Sexual Behavior in the Human Male, 1948. Sexual Behavior in the Human Female, 1953. Philadelphia, W.B. Saunders

60. Masters WH, Johnson VE: Human Sexual Response. Boston, Little, Brown, 1966

61. Stoller RJ: Sex and Gender: On the Development of Masculinity and Femininity. New York, Science House, 1968

62. Grinker RR Sr: Toward a Unified Theory of Human Behavior. New York, Basic Books, 1956

63. Bertalanffy L von: General Systems Theory. New York, Braziller, 1968

64. Miller JG: General systems theory, in Modern Clinical Psychiatry, ninth edition. Edited by Kolb LD. Philadelphia, W.B. Saunders, 1977

65. Much of the historical material on the evolution of the federal role in the advancement of psychiatry was taken from a pamphlet prepared for the celebration of the "Twenty-fifth Anniversary of the Mental Health Act: June 28, 29, 1971." The private foundations (Commonwealth, Falk, Grant, Ittleson, Milbank, and Van Amerigen) gave financial support for the event.

66. Joint Commission on Mental Illness and Health: Action for Mental Health: The Final Report of the Joint Commission on Mental Illness and Health. New York, Basic Books, 1961

67. Barton WE, Barton GM: Mental Health Administration: Principles and Practice. New York, Human Sciences Press, 1983

68. Sharfstein SS, Fine T, Wristel LS: Economic Fact Book for Psychiatry. Washington, DC, American Psychiatric Press, 1983

69. The Vermont Asylum for the Insane: Its Annals For Fifty Years. Brattleboro, Vermont, Hildreth and Fails, 1887

70. Musto DF: The community mental health center movement in historical perspective, in An Assessment of the Community Mental Health Movement. Edited by Barton WE, Sanborn CJ. Lexington, Massachusetts, Lexington Books, 1975

71. Ewalt JR: The birth of the community mental health movement, in Economic Fact Book for Psychiatry. Edited by Sharfstein SS, Fine T, Writsel LS. Washington, DC, American Psychiatric Press, 1983

72. Manderscheid RW, Witkin MJ, Rosenstein M, et al: NIMH report: a review of trends in mental health services. Hosp Community Psychiatry 35:673-674, 1984

73. Barton WE, Farrell JJ, Lenehan FT, et al: Impressions of European Psychiatry. Washington, DC, American Psychiatric Association, 1961

74. Peffer PA: Money: a rehabilitation incentive for mental patients. Am J Psychiatry 110:84, 1953

75. Meislin J (Ed): Rehabilitation Medicine and Psychiatry. Springfield, Ill., Charles C Thomas, 1976

76. Barton WE: Administration in Psychiatry. Springfield, Ill., Charles C Thomas, 1962

77. Greenblatt M, York RH, Brown EL: From Custodial to Therapeutic Care. New York, Russell Sage Foundation, 1955

78. Glasscote RM, Kraft AM, Glassman SM, et al: Partial Hospitalizations for the Mentally Ill. Washington, DC, Joint Information Service (APA–NAMH), 1969

79. Stanton AH, Schwartz MS: The Mental Hospital: A Study of Institutional Participation in Psychiatric Illness and Treatment. New York, Basic Books, 1954

80. Baldessarini RJ: Chemotherapy in Psychiatry. Cambridge, Harvard University Press, 1977

81. Karasu TB (Ed): The Psychiatric Therapies. Washington, DC, American Psychiatric Association, 1984

82. May PRA: Treatment of Schizophrenia: A Comparative Study of Five Treatment Methods. New York, Science House, 1968

83. Bockhoven JS: Moral Treatment in American Psychiatry. New York, Springer Publishing Co., 1963

84. Smith CG, King JA: Mental Hospitals. Lexington, Massachusetts, Lexington Books, 1975

85. Cumming J, Cumming E: Ego and Milieu, Theory and Practice of Environmental Therapy. New York, Atherton Press, 1962

86. Noshpitz JD: Milieu therapy, in The Mental Hospital: A Study of Institutional Participation in Psychiatric Illness and

Treatment. Edited by Stanton AH, Schwartz MS. New York, Basic Books, 1954

87. Jones M: Social Psychiatry: A Study of Therapeutic Communities. London, Tavistock Publications, 1952

88. Jones M: Beyond the Therapeutic Community. New Haven, Yale University Press, 1968

89. Pavlov IP: Conditioned Reflexes: An Investigation of the Physiological Activity of the Cerebral Cortex. New York, Oxford University Press, 1927

90. Skinner BF: The Behavior of Organisms: An Experimental Analysis. New York, Appleton-Century-Crofts, 1938

91. Skinner BF: Science and Human Behavior. New York, Macmillan, 1953

92. Wolpe J: Psychotherapy by Reciprocal Inhibition. Stanford, Stanford University Press, 1958; The Practice of Behavior Therapy. New York, Pergamon Press, 1969

93. Karasu TB (Ed.): Psychotherapy Research: Methodological and Efficacy Issues. Washington, DC, American Psychiatric Association, 1982

94. Barton WE, Barton GM: Mental Health Administration: Principles and Practice. 2 vols. New York, Human Sciences Press, 1983

95. Bryan WE: Administrative Psychiatry. New York, W.W. Norton, 1936

96. Myerson A: Theory and principles of the total push method in the treatment of chronic schizophrenia. Am J Psychiatry 95:1197-1204, 1939

97. Ewalt JR: Mental Health Administration. Springfield, Ill., Charles C Thomas, 1956

98. Group for the Advancement of Psychiatry: Administration of the Public Psychiatric Hospital Report #46. New York, Group for the Advancement of Psychiatry, 1960

99. Position statement on guidelines for psychiatrists: problems in confidentiality. Am J Psychiatry 126:187-193, 1970

100. American Psychiatric Association: Confidentiality and Third Parties. Task Force Report #9. Washington, DC, American Psychiatric Association, 1975

101. Confidentiality: A Report of the 1974 Conference on Confidentiality of Health Records, Key Biscayne, Florida, Nov. 9, 1974. Washington, DC, American Psychiatric Association, 1975

102. Greene BR, MacIntyre JA, Shelton BP, et al: A Guidebook to Curricula in Mental Health Administration. San Antonio, Texas, Trinity University Graduate School of Health Care Administration, 1975

103. Shortell SM: Continuing Education For the Health Professions: Application to Mental Health, Mental Retardation and Developmental Disabilities Administration. Ann Arbor, University of Michigan Health Administration Press, 1978

104. Feldman S (Ed): Report of the National Task Force on Mental Health/Mental Retardation Administration. Administration in Mental Health (Special Issue) 6:269-363, 1979

105. Talbott JA, Kaplan SR (Eds): Psychiatric Administration: A Comprehensive Text for the Clinician-Executive. New York, Grune and Stratton, 1983

106. Barton WE: What's new in administration? Hosp Community Psychiatry 34:441-443, 1983

107. Menninger WC: Psychiatry in a Troubled World: Yesterday's War and Today's Challenge. New York, Macmillan, 1948

108. American Psychiatric Association: Psychiatry and Medical Education: Report of the 1951 Ithaca Conference. Washington, DC, American Psychiatric Association, 1952

109. American Psychiatric Association: The Psychiatrist, His Training and Development: Report of the 1952 Ithaca Conference. Washington, DC, American Psychiatric Association, 1953

110. Lidz T: An outline for a curriculum for teaching in medical schools. J Med Educ 31:115-122, 1956

111. Dryer BV: Lifetime Learning for Physicians: Principles, Practices, Proposals. Chicago, AMA, 1962

112. Carmichael HT, Small SM, Regan PF: Prospects and Proposals: Lifetime Learning for Psychiatrists. Washington, DC, American Psychiatric Association, 1972

113. Bleuler M: Teaching of Psychiatry and Mental Health. Geneva, World Health Organization, 1961

114. The Pre-clinical Teaching of Psychiatry: Report #54. New York, Group for the Advancement of Psychiatry, 1962

115. Millis JS (Ed): The Graduate Education of Physicians. Chicago, AMA, 1966.

116. Coggleshall LT: Planning For Medical Progress Through Education. Evanston, Illinois, AAMC, 1965

117. Hammersley DW (Ed): Training The Psychiatrist to Meet Changing Needs. Washington, DC, American Psychiatric Association, 1963

118. American Psychiatric Association: Psychiatry and Medical Education II: Report of the 1967 Conference held in Atlanta (APA–AAMC). Washington, DC, American Psychiatric Association, 1969

119. Usdin G (Ed): Psychiatry: Education and Image. New York, Brunner/Mazel, 1973

120. Langsley DG, McDermott JF, Enelow AJ (Eds): Mental Health Education in the New Medical Schools. San Francisco, Jossey-Bass, 1973

121. Muslin HL, Thurnblad RJ, Templeton B, et al (Eds): Evaluative Methods in Psychiatric Education. Washington, DC, American Psychiatric Association, 1974

122. Rosenfeld AH (Ed): Psychiatric Education: Prologue to the 1980s. Washington, DC, American Psychiatric Association, 1976

123. Busse EW (Ed): The Working Papers of the 1975 Conference on Education of Psychiatrists. Washington, DC, American Psychiatric Association, 1976

124. Grinker RR: Fifty Years in Psychiatry: A Living History. Springfield, Ill., Charles C Thomas, 1979

125. Pardes H, Pincus HA: Challenge to academic psychiatry. Am J Psychiatry 140:1117-1126, 1983

Chapter 7

1. Carroll L: Alice's Adventures in Wonderland. Lewis Carrol was the pen name of Charles L. Dodgson (1832–1889).

2. Brosin H: Am J Psychiatry 115:369-370, 1958

3. Appel KE: Am J Psychiatry 122:16, 1965

4. Braceland FJ: Am J Psychiatry 139:525, 1982

5. Am J Psychiatry 115:561, 1958

6. Am J Psychiatry 119:380-381, 1962

7. Alexander L: Am J Psychiatry 119:16, 1962

8. Sabshin M: see Psychiatric News 9:1-34, Sept. 18, 1974

9. Braceland FJ: Am J Psychiatry 140:1241, 1983

10. Barton W: Am J Psychiatry 138:696, 1981

11. Deutsch A: The Shame of the States. New York, Harcourt Brace, 1948
12. Ewalt JR, Williams G: Action for Mental Health. New York, Basic Books, 1961
13. Barton WE: Psychiatry's Commitment to Public Service and to Improving Patient Care. Special Lecture on Administrative Psychiatry. Presented at the 136th Annual Meeting of the American Psychiatric Association. New York, May 6, 1983
14. Albee GW: Mental Health Manpower Trends. New York, Basic Books, 1959
15. The Nation's Psychiatrists. Rockville, Maryland, NIMH USPHS Publication, 1985
16. Psychiatric Services, Analysis and Manpower Utilization. NIMH, Rockville, Maryland, 1970
17. Arnhoff FN, Kumbar AH: The Nation's Psychiatrists, 1970 Survey. Washington, DC, American Psychiatric Association, 1973
18. Arnhoff, FN, Rubenstein EA, Spiesman JC: Manpower For Mental Health. Chicago, Aldine, 1969
19. Lopate C: Women in Medicine. Baltimore, Johns Hopkins University Press, 1968
20. Careers in Psychiatry. New York, Macmillan, 1968
21. Glasscote RM, et al: The Community Mental Health Center: An Analysis of Existing Models. Washington, DC, American Psychiatric Association
22. Glasscote RM: The Community Mental Health Center: An Interim Appraisal. Washington, DC, American Psychiatric Association, 1964
23. Glasscote RM: additional titles of Joint Information Service publications on CMHC:
    a. Partial Hospitalization for the Mentally Ill
    b. The Psychiatric Emergency
    c. General Hospital Psychiatric Units
    d. Legal Service and Community Mental Health
    e. The Staff of the Mental Health Center
    f. Psychiatric Treatment in the Community
24. Caplan G: An Approach to Community Mental Health. New York, Grune and Stratton, 1961
25. Williams RH, Ozarin L (Eds): Community Mental Health. San Francisco, Jossey-Bass, 1968

26. Lamb HR, Heath D, Downing JF (Eds): Handbook of Community Mental Health Practice. San Francisco, Jossey-Bass, 1969

27. Beigel A, Levenson A: The Community Mental Health Center. New York, Basic Books, 1972

28. Galt JM: The Farm at St. Anne. American Journal of Insanity 11:352-357, 1855

29. Barton WE: Administration in Psychiatry. Springfield, Ill., Charles C Thomas, 1962

30. Barton WE, Farrell JJ, Lenehan FT, et al: Impressions of European Psychiatry. Washington, DC, American Psychiatric Association, 1961

31. Copp O: Further experience in family care of the insane in Massachusetts. American Journal of Insanity 63:361-365, 1907

32. Group for the Advancement of Psychiatry: Community Psychiatry: A Reappraisal. New York, Group for the Advancement of Psychiatry, Mental Health Materials Center, 1983

33. Musto DF: The community mental health movement in historical perspective, in An Assessment of the Community Mental Health Movement. Edited by Barton WE, Sanborn CJ. Lexington, MA, Lexington Books, 1975

34. Zusman J: The philosophic basis for a community and social psychiatry, in An Assessment of the Community Mental Health Movement. Edited by Barton WE, Sanborn CJ. Lexington, MA, Lexington Books, 1975

35. Action for Mental Health: The Final Report of the Joint Commission on Mental Illness and Health. New York, Basic Books, 1961

36. Nash MD, Argyle NJ: Services for the mentally ill, a reverse of federal policy. Administration in Mental Health 11:263-276, 1984

37. American Psychiatric Association: Delivery of Mental Health Service: Needs Priorities, Strategies. Washington, DC, American Psychiatric Association, 1975

38. Barton WE, Barton GM: Mental Health Administration: Principles and Practice, 2 vols. New York, Human Sciences Press, 1983

39. Bennett AE, Hargrove EA, Engle B: Voluntary health insurance and nervous and mental diseases. JAMA 151:202-206, 1953

40. Davidson HA: Health insurance and psychiatric coverage. Am J Psychiatry 114:498-504, 1957

41. Avnet HH: Psychiatric Insurance: Financing, Short Term Ambulatory Treatment, Group Health Insurance. New York, 1962

42. American Psychiatric Association: Guidelines for Psychiatric Services Covered Under Health Insurance. Washington, DC, American Psychiatric Association, 1965 (revised second edition, 1968)

43. Reed LS, Myers ES, Scheidemandel PL: Health Insurance and Psychiatric Care. Washington, DC, American Psychiatric Association, 1972

44. Reed LS: Utilization of care under Blue Cross and Blue Shield plans. Am J Psychiatry 131:964-975, 1974

45. Reed LS: Coverage and Utilization of Care for Mental Conditions Under Health Insurance—Various Studies, 1973–1974. Washington, DC, American Psychiatric Association, 1975

46. Muszinski S, Brady J, Sharfstein SS: Coverage for Mental and Nervous Disorders: Summaries of 300 Private Sector Health Insurance Plans. Washington, DC, American Psychiatric Press, 1983

47. Sharfstein SS, Muszinski S, Myers ES: Health Insurance in Psychiatric Care: Update and Appraisal. Washington, DC, American Psychiatric Press, 1984

48. Group for the Advancement of Psychiatry: Shock Therapy. Topeka, Kansas, Group for the Advancement of Psychiatry, 1947

49. Group for the Advancement of Psychiatry: Revised Electroshock Report. Topeka, Kansas, Group for the Advancement of Psychiatry, 1950

50. American Psychiatric Association: Electroconvulsive Therapy: Task Force Report 14. Washington, DC, American Psychiatric Association, 1978

51. American Psychiatric Association Commission on Psychotherapies: Psychotherapy Research: Methodological and Efficacy Issues. Washington, DC, American Psychiatric Association, 1982

52. American Psychiatric Association: Biofeedback: APA Task Force Report 19. Washington, DC, American Psychiatric As-

sociation, 1981

53. Lewis JM, Usdin G (Eds): Treatment Planning in Psychiatry. Washington, DC, American Psychiatric Association, 1982

54. Tardiff K (Ed): The Psychiatric Uses of Seclusion and Restraint. Washington, DC, American Psychiatric Press, Inc., 1984

55. Grinspoon L (Ed): Psychiatry Update: The American Psychiatric Association Annual Review, vol. 1 (1982); vol. 2 (1983); vol. 3 (1984). Washington, DC, American Psychiatric Press, Inc., 1982–1984

56. Karasu TB (Ed): The Psychiatric Therapies. Washington, DC, American Psychiatric Press, Inc., 1984

57. Position statement on guidelines for psychiatrists: problems in confidentiality. Am J Psychiatry 126:187-193, 1970

58. American Psychiatric Association: Confidentiality and Third Parties: Task Force Report #9. Washington, DC, American Psychiatric Association, 1975

59. American Psychiatric Association: Confidentiality: A Report of the 1974 Conference on Confidentiality of Health Records, Key Biscayne, Florida, Nov. 9, 1974. Washington, DC, American Psychiatric Association, 1975

60. Barton WE: Should a national commission for the preservation of confidentiality of health records be formed? Psychiatric Opinion 12:15-17, 1975

61. Barton WE, Barton GM: Mental Health Administration: Principles and Practice. New York, Human Sciences Press, 1983

62. Hammersley DW: Psychiatric Utilization Review: Principles and Objectives. Washington, DC, American Psychiatric Association, 1968

63. American Hospital Association: American Hospital Association Quality Assurance Program. Chicago, American Hospital Association, 1972

64. Position statement on peer review in psychiatry. Am J Psychiatry 130:381-385, 1973

65. Position Statement on P.L. 92–603 (PSRO), 1974

66. American Psychiatric Association: Ad hoc Committee on PSRO's Model Criteria sets. Washington, DC, American Psychiatric Association, 1974

67. Special section on peer review. Am J Psychiatry 131:1354-1386, 1974

68. American Psychiatric Association: Manual on Psychiatric Peer Review. Washington, DC, American Psychiatric Association, 1975

69. Gibson RW (Ed): Professional Responsibilities and Peer Review in Psychiatry: Report of an APA Conference, March 11-12, 1977. Washington, DC, American Psychiatric Association, 1977

70. Talbott JA (Ed): The Chronic Mental Patient: Problems, Solutions and Recommendations for Public Policy. Washington, DC, American Psychiatric Association, 1979

71. Group for the Advancement of Psychiatry: The Chronic Mental Patient in the Community, vol. 10, no. 102. New York, Group for the Advancement of Psychiatry, 1978

72. Report of the President's Commission on Mental Health, vols. 1 and 2. Washington, DC, U.S. Government Printing Office, 1978

73. Talbott JA: The Chronic Mentally Ill: Treatment, Programs, Systems. New York, Human Sciences Press, 1981

74. Lamb HR (Ed): The Homeless Mentally Ill. American Psychiatric Association Task Force Report. Washington, DC, American Psychiatric Association, 1984

75. Finn R: A History of the Assembly of District Branches of the American Psychiatric Association, 1953–1978; a speech delivered to the Assembly on the occasion of its 25th Anniversary, May 6, 1978.
    There are two other histories of the Assembly. The first was written by Speaker Walter Obenouf (1959) and the other "the official history" written by Speaker G. Wilse Robinson in 1966. All three histories are in the archives of the American Psychiatric Association in Washington, DC.

76. The Airlie House Propositions published as a document for APA member review. Washington, DC, American Psychiatric Association, January 1966

77. 1968 council planning conference in official actions. Am J Psychiatry 126:737-775, 1969

78. Report of the trustees' policy meeting, March 1971, in official actions. Am J Psychiatry 128:385-399, 1971

79. Summary report of the special policy meeting of the Board of Trustees, Atlanta, Georgia, Feb 1–3, 1973, in official actions. Am J Psychiatry 130:731-738, 1973

80. Raw data and tape transcriptions from the Key Conference, Key Biscayne, Florida, March 20–23, 1975. Also, Report of the Joint Conference Committee to the Board of Trustees, Dec 1977, in archives of the American Psychiatric Association, Washington, DC

A brief statement about the Key Conference appears in Dr. Sabshin's Medical Director Report, Am J Psychiatry 136:1373, 1979

Index

This index was prepared and provided by the author.